OVERCOMING BLADDER DISORDERS

OVERCOMING
BLADDER
DISORDERS

COMPASSIONATE, AUTHORITATIVE MEDICAL
AND SELF-HELP SOLUTIONS FOR

Incontinence,
Cystitis,
Interstitial Cystitis,
Prostate Problems, and
Bladder Cancer

REBECCA CHALKER
AND
KRISTENE E. WHITMORE, M.D.

1817

HARPER & ROW, PUBLISHERS, NEW YORK

GRAND RAPIDS, PHILADELPHIA, ST. LOUIS, SAN FRANCISCO
LONDON, SINGAPORE, SYDNEY, TOKYO, TORONTO

FIRST EDITION

Designer: Joan Greenfield

Library of Congress Cataloging-in-Publication Data

Chalker, Rebecca.
  Overcoming bladder disorders: compassionate, authoritative medi-
cal and self-help solutions for incontinence, cystitis, interstitial cystitis,
prostate problems and bladder cancer/by Rebecca Chalker and Kris-
tene E. Whitmore, M.D.
      p. cm.
  Includes bibliographical references and index.
  ISBN 0-06-016277-5
  1. Bladder—Diseases—Popular works. 2. Urinary incontinence
—Popular works. 3. Prostate—Diseases—Popular works.
I. Whitmore, Kristene E., 1952– . II. Title.
RC919.C49 1990
616.6'2—dc20   89-45789

---

90 91 92 93 94 DT/HC 10 9 8 7 6 5 4 3 2 1

To my grandmother,
Lucille M. Stringer,
who at 93
has been a continuing source of
inspiration

R.C.

To my husband, Alan,
with deepest appreciation
for his endearing love, patience,
and generous support

K.E.W.

CONTENTS

LIST OF ILLUSTRATIONS

ACKNOWLEDGMENTS

The idea for this very large book came from a small but significant suggestion by Carol Downer, founder of the Federation of Feminist Women's Health Centers, that Rebecca write an article on stress incontinence. Later Carol developed a proposal for such a book on the subject but, alas, was sidetracked by the stepped-up attacks on abortion rights that she felt compelled to confront and, ultimately, enrollment in law school. We hope that the end result, *Overcoming Bladder Disorders,* lives up to her initial expectations.

As the concept for the project grew and began to take shape, Dr. Katherine F. Jeter, founder of Help for Incontinent People (HIP), Inc., introduced Rebecca to Kristene, and our partnership was born.

We jointly want to thank the many people who made significant contributions to the book:

Our literary agent, Sandra Elkin, a rock of Gibraltar in the sometimes uncharted waters of book publishing;

Janet Goldstein, our editor at Harper & Row, whose keen instincts helped us hone our concept and shape our material, making it far more accessible than it might have been. Special thanks are due to other staff at Harper & Row: Janet's assistant, Peternelle van Arsdale, who patiently helped us keep track of many loose ends; Ann Adelman, our excellent copyeditor; and Debra Elfenbein, our production editor, who brought order to the chaos;

Dr. Alan J. Wein, professor and chairman of the Division of Urology at the University of Pennsylvania and Kristene's husband, whose close reading of our manuscript and incisive comments improved it significantly;

Dr. Suzanne Frye, whose careful reading helped sharpen many points and encouraged us to look at some issues with fresh eyes;

Dr. David M. Banett, professor of urology, Mayo Clinic, Rochester, Minnesota, whose reading added depth in many areas;

Dr. Katherine F. Jeter of Help for Incontinent People (HIP), Inc.; Cheryle B. Gartley of the Simon Foundation for Continence; and Anne Smith-Young of Continence Restored, Inc., for reading our material on incontinence. The work of these women is of the highest order and their contributions to the field are immeasurable.

Dr. Vicki Ratner, president of the Interstitial Cystitis Association (ICA); Debra Slade, the organization's executive director; Judith Heller, treasurer; Ruth Bergman, leader of the Manhattan ICA support group; Alan Weiss and Elisabeth Suchard, co-chairs of the Canadian ICA; and many other members of the organization, for reading the material on IC and/or sharing information and encouragement. Their dedicated patient advocacy and sagacious political action on behalf of this orphan disease interstitial cystitis have dramatically changed the way we look at this disorder.

Each and every person with one of the disorders covered in this book who talked to us in person, on the phone, or in Kristene's office, and especially those with incontinence or interstitial cystitis who patiently and frankly answered Rebecca's long and sometimes nosy questionnaires;

The doctors and health-care professionals who took time to share their viewpoints on a variety of topics, especially Dr. Susan Blaivas; John Bouda of MB Products, Ltd., Asheville, North Carolina; James Mitchell Brown, Brown and Margolius, Cleveland, Ohio; Dr. Dennis Drobbit, Farmbrook Pain Control Center, Southfield, Michigan; Cara Frank, certified acupuncturist, Philadelphia, Pennsylvania; Christy A. Fleurat of Merck Sharp & Dohme International; Dr. Jean Fourcroy, president of the National Council on Women in Medicine, Inc.; Dr. Philip M. Hanno, chairman, Division of Urology, Temple University; Dr. Geraldine Hirsch, N.Y. H.E.L.P.; Paul Koprowsky; Dr. Naomi B. McCormick, professor of psychology, State University of New York at Plattsburgh; Hilda Meltzer, associate at the Center for Cognitive Therapy and faculty member of the 92nd Street Y in New York City; Dr. Edward Messing, associate professor of urology, University of Wisconsin

Hospital and Clinics; Dr. Linda Mitteness, associate professor of medical anthropology, University of California, San Francisco; Dr. Peggy Norton, assistant professor of gynecology, University of Utah School of Medicine; Dr. Neil M. Resnick, director of the Harvard Continence Center, Brigham and Women's Hospital, Boston, Massachusetts, assistant professor of medicine and director of the Geriatrics Service; Carol Nostrand, nutrition educator, New York, New York; Dr. Joseph D. Parkhurst, Bethany, Oklahoma; Charon Pierson, R.N., M.S.N., N.P., editor of *Nurse Practitioner Forum;* Dr. David R. Staskin, assistant professor, Harvard Medical School/Beth Israel Medical Center; Dr. Denise Webster, R.N., Ph.D., associate professor and coordinator of psychiatric mental health nursing at the University of Colorado Health Sciences Center; Dr. George D. Webster, associate professor of urology, Duke University Medical Center; Dr. Michael Weinstein, certified acupuncturist, Santa Monica, California; and Fran Wright, R.N., M.S.W., F.N.P.

Special thanks to Gerry Denza, who looked up *many* references; Sarah Jones, who fed us; and Ron Thompson, who nursed us through hard times.

CHAPTER 1

A New Day for Bladder Disorders

BLADDER DISORDERS PRESENT AN ENORMOUS CHAL-
lenge to both the people who have them and the doctors and other
health-care professionals who treat them. Unlike heart problems,
arthritis, or a number of other widespread disorders, bladder
problems are enmeshed in a complex web of negative social attitudes that make talking about them painful, even to our closest
relatives or friends, and make asking for help difficult if not impossible for many. Because of the stigma associated with bladder
function—and dysfunction—people who have such problems
often suffer intensely from guilt and shame, which may prevent
them from seeking the help they so desperately need. Even some
doctors are not comfortable in talking about bladder disorders,
especially urinary incontinence.

Perhaps because these problems are rarely life-threatening, their
symptoms are not taken seriously by some doctors, who believe
that they have more important things to do than deal with "a little
urinary leakage" or yet another recurrence of cystitis. To make
matters worse, many doctors do not understand how to correctly
diagnose bladder disorders and misdiagnosis is common. In most
cases, a misdiagnosis rarely leads to grave illness or death. It may,
however, condemn the sufferer, who may have waited years before
venturing to get help, to many more years of painful isolation.

If you are suffering from a bladder disorder, or someone you
care about is, you have probably discovered that this problem is

different from most other medical conditions. We hope that this book will not only serve as a guide to the diagnosis and treatment of bladder dysfunction but will also provide some much-needed perspective to help you confront a bladder problem as you would a stroke or a heart condition. With the exception of cancer, bladder disorders are not normally life-threatening. But they can dramatically diminish the quality of your life. More than anything, knowledge about treatment and coping strategies can help to minimize the impact of a bladder disorder on your life.

MYTHS AND REALITIES

In the atmosphere of shame and secrecy that surrounds bladder disorders, a number of deeply rooted myths abound. The most prominent myth is that bladder disorders are relatively rare. If you have a leaky, painful, or dysfunctional bladder, you may, like many other people, believe that you are the only person with such a condition. In fact, *millions* of people have bladder disorders. If you take a look at the box opposite, you will see that *you are not alone!*

Another widespread myth that is believed not only by bladder sufferers but by many doctors and health professionals as well, is that bladder disorders are often caused by psychological factors or stress. So, even if you manage to overcome your fears and ask for help, your doctor may fail to take your symptoms seriously. In addition, many people *and* many doctors believe that few treatments for bladder disorders exist. Neither of these assumptions is true. While some bladder disorders, like numerous other medical conditions, may be exacerbated by stress, they are *not* caused by it. Furthermore, there are quite a variety of treatments, self-help remedies, and coping techniques that can help almost everyone who suffers from bladder dysfunction.

In addition to the myths noted above, there are myths about the specific bladder disorders that discourage people from getting help:

- *That incontinence is an inevitable consequence of aging.* Incontinence is, in fact, a symptom of many health conditions to which the elderly are particularly vulnerable, but it is not caused by aging.
- *That no effective treatment for incontinence exists.* In fact, there are quite a number of treatments with which the majority of suffer-

ers can be cured or made significantly better. Almost everyone can be helped in some way.

- *That there is no effective treatment for bedwetting in school-age children or adolescents.* Waiting for bedwetting to resolve is agonizing for children and parents alike. As with adults, effective strategies for curing this problem do exist.
- *That recurrent cystitis can only be treated on an episode-by-episode basis.*

(continued)

WHO HAS BLADDER DISORDERS

Contrary to popular belief, bladder disorders are not limited to the elderly and infirm. They are pervasive.

- By a conservative estimate, at least 15 million people suffer from some form of urinary incontinence, but because of reluctance to admit urine loss, this figure could be twice as high.
- Each year, 2 million people—mostly women—are stricken with cystitis (bacterial infections in the bladder) and about 15 percent will have painful, unpredictable recurrences that will continue throughout their lives.
- Up to one-half million people—again, mostly women—have a little-understood condition called *interstitial cystitis*. This inflammation of the bladder lining causes unremitting urinary frequency and pain in many of its sufferers and has no known cause or reliable cure.
- Most men are unaware that they have a prostate until they develop an infection or have significant prostate enlargement. Although the prostate gland properly belongs to the reproductive system, as opposed to the urinary tract, disease or dysfunction in the gland directly impinges upon the urinary tract, and its symptoms are inseparable from those of bladder dysfunction. Altogether, about 5 million men each year require treatment for prostate disorders.
- Each year, about 40,000 new cases of bladder cancer—three times as many men as women—are diagnosed. Fortunately, about 90 percent of these cancers are only in the lining of the bladder and can be treated effectively.

So much, then, for the notion that bladder disorders are rare.

Although it is not known what makes some people so susceptible to recurrent cystitis, it is often possible to figure out what is triggering recurrences, and a rational program to control them can be undertaken.

- *That interstitial cystitis is a rare condition of post-menopausal women and that nothing can be done to help them.* Perhaps as many as 500,000 people have some form of this mysterious condition; far from being a post-menopausal condition, the average age when symptoms arise is forty, and 25 percent of people with the disease are under thirty years old. And although no definitive cure exists, there are numerous treatments to help mollify symptoms and control flare-ups.

- *That the cystitis-like symptoms of "urethral syndrome" are essentially stress-related or "all in your head."* This controversial condition is not well understood, but it is not a phantom condition—and there are treatments that can be used to control symptoms.

- *That male sexual activity—either too much or too little—influences prostate enlargement and that sexual dysfunction is the probable outcome of treatment.* Prostate enlargement is probably hormonally stimulated. Today, advances in equipment, surgical techniques, and patient education help preserve sexual function in most men.

- *That bladder cancer is always fatal.* Bladder cancer is not nearly as lethal as many other forms of cancer. Most bladder cancers are superficial tumors that are treatable if caught in time.

Understanding bladder disorders can help dispel these myths and help you overcome obstacles that they impose when you are seeking medical treatment.

NEGATIVE ATTITUDES

The powerful social stigma associated with bladder function presents another significant stumbling block to getting help when dysfunction occurs. We all grow up with negative attitudes toward bladder and bowel function. Before we are old enough to reason, we are taught that these normal, life-preserving functions are shameful and dirty, and that the loss of control—under any circumstances—is a grave social transgression. A highly respected cross-cultural study evaluating the toilet-training practices of twenty widely different cultures found American toilet training to be among the most coercive, both in terms of early initiation and in terms of severity of the requirements and expectations for achievement of continence.[1] The shame and guilt that we acquire from this early socialization stay with us for life, and when bladder dysfunction occurs, we may suffer the loss of self-esteem and self-image, blame ourselves for our problem, and fail to ask for help.

These decidedly unhealthy social attitudes can be overcome, but it will not happen overnight. In the meantime, as individuals, understanding the roots of our fears and guilt can help us to put them in perspective and gain liberation from them.

UROLOGY COMES OF AGE

A brief glance at medical history reveals that people have always had bladder problems and urologists have always been trying to fix them. The first urologists were Hindus of the Vedic era (about 1500 B.C.), who specialized in extracting bladder stones and in relieving urinary obstruction.[2] The Ebers medical papyrus, inscribed in Egypt at roughly the same time, provides an impressive catalog of bladder disorders, including incontinence, cystitis, frequency of urination, urethritis, prostate enlargement, and urinary retention. This priceless document also provides recipes to "regulate urine" and to "force urine out," suggesting a lively interest in the cure of such ills.[3]

Today, although 85 percent of those who suffer from bladder disorders are women, no medical specialty exists specifically for them. From the time of the ancient Hindus, urologists have been trained in men's problems and have seen themselves primarily as men's doctors. Gynecology has traditionally been the female specialty, but its focus is primarily on problems of the reproductive tract, leaving women's bladder disorders in a sort of medical limbo. Most gynecologists, internists, and family practice physicians are not trained to do *urodynamic studies*, the most basic and essential urological tests which are used in the diagnosis of incontinence, or *cystoscopic examinations*, exploratory examinations of the urethra and bladder which can identify—or rule out—many urological problems. Consequently, many bladder disorders in women go unacknowledged and untreated.

It's hard to say when things began to change, but in the last few years urologists and health professionals have begun focusing more attention upon such neglected conditions as incontinence, cystitis, and interstitial cystitis.

A momentous increase in the professional awareness of incontinence occurred when Dr. Katherine F. Jeter, the founder of Help for Incontinent People (HIP), Inc., spearheaded the National Agenda to Promote Urinary Continence in Chicago in 1984. The meeting was attended by doctors and other health-care specialists, who left the conference with a strong commitment to work toward a heightened public awareness of incontinence, and to encourage increased interest and funding of research on the subject. And in 1988—a sure sign that a disease has "arrived"—the National Institutes of Health sponsored a Consensus Development Conference on Incontinence, at which experts on all aspects of the disease testified.

Since the interstitial cystitis syndrome was first recognized in the 1920s, lack of understanding about its cause and cure condemned it to the status of an orphan disease. In 1986, a medical conference on the disease was organized by Dr. David Staskin of Boston University and Dr. Philip Hanno of Temple University in Philadelphia. The meeting, which took place in Boston, opened the way for serious dialogue about this mysterious disorder. In 1987, the National Institutes of Health sponsored a two-day workshop on interstitial cystitis—the first official recognition of this disorder, which paved the way for standardization of diagnostic criteria and government funding of desperately needed research.

At the same time that these events were occurring, changes were beginning to take place in medical schools as well. There are now about 100 female urologists in the United States, and since Dr. Elizabeth Pickett became the first board-certified female urologist in 1962, approximately fifty women have passed the rigorous urological board examination.* Dr. Suzanne Frye, who completed her residency in 1985 and now practices in New York City, is one of the women who saw intriguing possibilities in urology: "When I was trying to decide what to specialize in, I looked at urology and saw that it was, in large part, a woman's problem, and that in large part, these needs were not being met. I knew that I could help."

Another positive development in the last decade or so has been the development of the new medical specialties of female urol-

---

* Board certification requires that a doctor complete a urology residency, show proficiency in various procedures, and pass a series of difficult examinations.

ogy and *urogynecology*. Doctors who belong to the American Uro-Gynecological Society are urologists or gynecologists who have a special interest in and, hopefully, a special sensitivity to women's urological problems.

In England, things have been somewhat better in certain respects. Gynecologists are specially trained to treat women's urological problems, and there is also a well-established nursing specialty focusing on urinary disorders. Each medical district has an "incontinence adviser," a urological nurse who is available by appointment to help ensure that people have access to appropriate care.

In the United States, the job of counseling and supporting patients with urological problems on a day-to-day basis usually falls to nurses. Yet most nurses and auxiliary personnel receive only the most superficial training in this area. The training that they do receive is usually focused on rehabilitative therapy for those with spinal cord injuries, accidents, or other pelvic trauma, with little attention to less severe conditions. But things are beginning to change in this area as well. Urologic nursing has become an important new specialty and the American Board of Urological and Allied Health Professionals has approved about 300 Certified Urology Technicians.

In the future, perhaps every hospital and health maintenance organization (HMO) will have a "urological adviser" who can provide information, referral, and access to appropriate treatment. Ideally, every urologist will be sensitive to both the medical and the social ramifications of incontinence, will treat cystitis as if it is a serious illness, and will be able to quickly diagnose interstitial cystitis. And we can hope that men will have easier access to information on prostate disorders and that research will soon make the treatment of such disorders more reliable than it is at present. Finally, increased public awareness and more sophisticated screening and diagnostic techniques will help identify people who are at risk of developing bladder cancer. Then urology will truly have come of age.

WHAT THIS BOOK CAN DO FOR YOU

This book is designed to help you see the invisible but none-theless significant barriers that stand in the way of appropriate diagnosis and treatment and to help you overcome both the psychological and the social disabilities that bladder problems impose. The Self-Evaluation Checklist at the beginning of the chapters on each bladder disorder is designed to help you determine if the information in that chapter might be useful to you.

One of the most confounding aspects of bladder disorders for you and sometimes for your physician as well is that the symptoms of most bladder conditions in men and women are strikingly similar. With the exception of incontinence, bladder disorders share a constellation of similar symptoms: urinary urgency and frequency, difficulties in emptying the bladder, waking at night to urinate, blood in the urine, and bladder discomfort or pain. Because of these similarities, misdiagnosis is frequent and treatment often fails, leaving you worse off than before. The Symptom Chart for Bladder Disorders on pages 28–29 graphically illustrates these similarities, emphasizing the necessity of a careful review of your medical history, a thorough examination, and a judicious interpretation of test results.

Many people who have bladder dysfunction feel as if they have lost control over their lives. Chapter 2, Taking Control of Bladder Problems, offers concrete guidelines to help you become more assertive about your special needs and your right to treatment. This chapter also offers suggestions for locating a doctor who can help you and includes information on how to prepare for your doctor's visit so that you can get the help you need.

Chapter 3, Anatomy 101, provides a guided tour through the urinary tract and prostate, so that as you read about each disorder you can see how these organs function and what can go wrong.

Chapters 4 through 8 are about the various bladder disorders. The goal of these chapters is to give you a complete picture of each condition. You will find information on symptoms, signs that you or your doctor can observe (referred to in medical shorthand as "signs and symptoms"), and the causes, if they are known. The information on medical tests will guide you through diagnosis and give you a thorough review of the available medical treatments. You will also find information on alternative treatments and self-help remedies which can often be used alone, or as adjuncts to medical therapy.

We feel very strongly, as do many experts in the field, that treatment of bladder disorders should begin with the most conservative remedy that is likely to provide relief and work systematically through to more invasive options. To help you in your decision about having a particular treatment, we have noted potential risks and benefits, as well as the advantages and disadvantages of each procedure. At certain junctures, we have also provided key questions that you can ask to make sure you are getting the appropriate tests and proper treatment.

Of all of the difficulties that people with bladder disorders face, sexuality perhaps looms the largest and lends itself the least to quick-fix solutions. Chapter 9, Staying Sexual: Strategies for Enhancing Sexuality, looks at the questions people with bladder disorders ask most frequently about sex and offers some suggestions for working through them. In researching this book, Rebecca interviewed many people about the impact of bladder dysfunction on sexuality and designed a special questionnaire on the subject to people with interstitial cystitis. Many openly shared their fears and frustrations on this sensitive subject. She also talked with a number of sex therapists who have worked with people who have bladder disorders about the coping strategies they most frequently recommend.

If you already have a bladder disorder, you may view your condition as inevitable. However, with appropriate diagnosis and treatment bladder problems can often be cured, or if not, they can be improved significantly. But sometimes things simply can't be fixed, and coping techniques become all-important. Chapter 10, Coping Strategies for Everyday Survival, is a compilation of inventive coping mechanisms that have been developed by people like yourself who have had long and often bitter experience with bladder disorders. There are some ingenious, even brash, ideas for gaining access to restrooms and tips on planning family or business trips with a demanding bladder in mind. Absorbent products, once sold only by medical supply houses, have proliferated and have helped numerous people cope with the involuntary loss of urine, but you may still be unaware of their existence. This chapter provides a brief survey of the range of products and devices that are available.

Humor can be one of the most powerful implements in the tool kit of anyone with bladder dysfunction. Chapter 10 closes with a collection of anecdotes—and even a tidbit of fantasy—about living with leaky, sluggish, or painful bladders. These wry, often piquant stories, told by veterans of the bladder wars, convincingly affirm that you can survive a debilitating bladder disorder and, sometimes, even laugh in its face.

The Index of Diagnostic Tests on page 278 provides detailed information about how these tests are done, including risks and side effects.

The Drug Glossary on page 295 lists the drugs that are typically used for urological problems. We have noted how each drug works, which conditions it is commonly prescribed for, what its side effects are, more serious effects, and who should not take it.

Since bladder disorders have been such a dark secret for so long, we don't have even the most rudimentary vocabulary for expressing our needs and problems. Normally, technical terms are described in the text the first time that they occur, but because the terms are used over and over and you may not read the chapters in order, we have included a Glossary of Urological Terms (page 311) to provide you with a working understanding of the basic vocabulary of urology.

A NEW DAY FOR BLADDER DISORDERS

At last, bladder disorders have begun to emerge from the shadows and have become the subject of a flood of newspaper and magazine articles and a frequent talk show topic. Now, absorbent products, once advertised only in specialty catalogs, have taken their place on the TV screen beside commercials for breakfast cereals, light beer, and Japanese-made cars. In 1986, President Reagan's very public prostatectomy brought prostate problems out of the doctor-advice columns and into the arena of hard news, proving once and for all that bladder disorders are just as important and as worthy of public discussion as osteoporosis or heart bypass operations.

ABOUT THE AUTHORS

Rebecca Chalker: I am a writer and journalist whose work has focused primarily on the areas of women's sexual and reproductive health. My goal in writing about medical subjects is to translate difficult and often inaccessible information so that anybody—including myself—can understand it. When I developed the condition called "urethral syndrome" in 1982, I could not find a single book on the subject or even a *paragraph* in a book that described the condition. And I experienced many of the frustrations and encountered some of the obstacles that people with bladder disorders often face in seeking treatment. Later, while I was working on a proposal for a book on stress incontinence, I learned about interstitial cystitis and found out more about "urethral syndrome." Becoming knowledgeable about these disorders and the difficulties many people, like myself, have in getting proper diagnosis and treatment helped me to see how information on these and other bladder conditions is badly needed. Urological disorders have not been studied as extensively as many other conditions have, and even the medical profession doesn't understand them very well. For this reason, I found writing about them to be particularly challenging.

Dr. Kristene Whitmore: I am one of about fifty board-certified female urologists in the United States. As assistant professor of urology and director of the Incontinence Center at the Graduate Hospital in Philadelphia, I have become very aware of the ramifications of bladder dysfunction. When I finished medical school and was trying to decide on a specialty, I was attracted to urology because of the diversity of the conditions, which makes it interesting, and because there is ample opportunity to have, on the one hand, a lot of direct patient contact and, on the other, room for extensive research and development of new techniques and treatments. I also realized that women constitute 50 percent of urological patients, but that there were very few female urologists. After I began practicing, I became especially interested in incontinence and interstitial cystitis because the current available treatments could not provide all of the answers for my patients. Because of this deficiency, I began doing research in these two areas, hoping to discover new and more effective treatments of my own. I also do a lot of speaking about bladder problems, both to my colleagues in the medical community and to the public. Although sometimes

11

this is hard because my practice is so demanding, I do it because I think it is important to raise the visibility of bladder disorders, which have been invisible for far too long.

Throughout the book we refer to ourselves by our first names. Because of the complicated nature of many of my patients' problems, I deal with them for prolonged periods of time, and we build up trusting relationships. In these cases, we both find it more comfortable to be less formal; however, this may not be either desired or preferred by some doctors and patients. For the purposes of this book, it seems unnecessary to maintain such a formal distance, as we speak directly and intimately to the reader.

Although we have very different backgrounds and training, we have common goals in writing this book. We want to simplify the complexities of bladder disorders for you so that you can understand what has gone wrong and why. We want to help you overcome the difficulties many people have in getting proper diagnosis and treatment. But we want to do more than just provide information. We want to help change the way that people—and their doctors—look at bladder disorders.

CHAPTER 2

Taking Control of Bladder Disorders

IN SEEKING TREATMENT FOR A BLADDER DISORDER, you may encounter stumbling blocks along the way. You may need to overcome your own fear of admitting your problem to family members, friends, or doctors. Or you may have to overcome your own conviction that nothing can be done for you. You may also experience feelings of isolation—even in your own home—because of a bladder problem. If you do get up the nerve to speak to a doctor, you may find indifference or an unfamiliarity with proper diagnostic procedures and treatment. If the latter is the case, you may be faced with misdiagnosis, which in turn can lead to mistreatment. If you have not yet seen a doctor or other qualified health professional, your decision to get help is the first step toward gaining control of a leaky, painful, or dysfunctional bladder. If you have received treatment but it did not help you enough or failed altogether, it is certainly worthwhile to consult a new practitioner and perhaps try a different approach.

This chapter is designed to help you overcome the barriers to getting help for bladder disorders. It provides information on how to be more assertive about the special needs that bladder problems impose and suggests how a patient advocate can help you get competent, respectful care; and it introduces you to several educational organizations and support groups that provide up-to-the-minute information on the latest diagnostic techniques, treatments, products, and publications on bladder disorders. There are also a number of suggestions on how to find a doctor or surgeon who has an interest in your problem and is qualified to help you.

GETTING ASSERTIVE

To assert, according to the *Random House Dictionary of the English Language,* means "to state with assurance, confidence or force; to state strongly or positively." Being assertive *doesn't* mean being aggressive, which is characterized by "unprovoked offensiveness, attacks, invasions or the like." These definitions seem straightforward enough, but they do not convey the social overlay that makes "assertive" an extremely loaded term which, in fact, has separate connotations for women and men.

Men are brought up to be assertive, to confidently claim the rights that they know are theirs. Women are brought up to be meek, compliant, and non-assertive. When women are assertive, they are often accused of being *aggressive* and are criticized as "being demanding." For many women, non-assertive behavior includes not making eye contact, keeping eyes downcast, maintaining demure (modest or reserved) behavior; using indirect forms of speech; practicing self-censorship by avoiding situations in which they must take a stand or assert preferences; being reluctant to disagree; or being reluctant to express personal needs or preferences. Women often compensate for non-assertiveness by being coy, seductive, or manipulative. Assertive behavior, on the other hand, is characterized by direct eye contact, direct communication, and honest, confident expression of needs and preferences. Some men have problems being assertive, but they often cover these up by brash or aggressive behavior.

In a doctor's office, the lack of assertiveness, coupled with shame about admitting a bladder problem, often leads to being afraid to ask questions, failing to volunteer potentially helpful information, and agreeing to diagnostic procedures or treatments you don't understand or don't want. Learning to be assertive through supportive counseling, books on the subject, or assertiveness training can help you overcome the fear of talking about your problem and help you get appropriate diagnosis and treatment.

Assertiveness Training

Assertiveness training, which is rooted in the behavioral approach to psychotherapy, helps to identify non-assertive ways of thinking, behaving, or relating and attempts to replace these negative, counterproductive patterns with positive, assertive responses. The techniques used include consciousness raising about sex roles, role playing, practicing communication skills, and positive reinforcement. Most therapists with a behavioral, cognitive, or feminist perspective utilize some form of assertiveness training in their practices, and classes are often taught at YW (or M) CAs or YW (or M) HAs, alternative learning centers, and in university or community college continuing education courses. Many corporations also hire assertiveness trainers to help their employees become more effective communicators. Assertive techniques can be learned in a few weeks and most of these courses are affordable for the average person. Several excellent books on assertiveness are listed in the Resources section at the end of this chapter.

Having a Health Advocate

In addition to assertiveness training, another key to overcoming barriers to effective care is having the support of a health advocate. Rebecca worked in a clinic for several years and frequently served as an advocate for clients who needed hospitalization. She found that people often didn't have enough information about their condition to ask appropriate questions, and when they did, they were often too ill or disoriented by unfamiliar office or hospital routine to ask critical questions in the limited time they had with the doctor.

A health advocate can be a friend or family member who accompanies you to the doctor's office, hospital, or nursing home to ensure that your needs are taken care of and your rights respected. He or she can help you remember all of the questions you want to ask, mediate situations where substandard care occurs, and take notes if your situation is complicated. An advocate can also provide support for you at home if there are many restrictions or instructions that you must follow. In terms of bladder disorders, patient advocates can be very useful in helping you to communicate effectively about a subject that may be embarrassing to you. They can also be particularly useful in seeing that your care in a nursing home is adequate. For people who are incontinent, having someone advocate for you can often mean the difference between self-sufficiency and becoming dependent upon absorbent products and catheters.

EDUCATIONAL ORGANIZATIONS

In the past six or seven years, several educational and patient advocacy organizations have come into being to provide much-needed information and support for people with various bladder disorders. These organizations can provide you with a wide range of information on the medical, social, and psychological aspects of bladder disorders. They have newsletters which are packed with the latest information on refinements in existing treatment, experimental treatments, absorbent products, new books on bladder disorders, important scientific articles, and self-help tips from subscribers. They also offer a variety of pamphlets and audio and video materials on various bladder disorders, and run support groups or provide information about how you can start one in your hometown.

The following educational organizations provide information and/or coordinate support groups for various disorders:

Incontinence: Help for Incontinent People (HIP), Inc.; The Simon Foundation for Continence, Inc.; and Continence Restored, Inc. (See Chapter 4, pages 94–96.)

Interstitial cystitis: The Interstitial Cystitis Association. (See Chapter 6, page 177.)

Ostomies: The United Ostomy Association. (An ostomy is a surgically constructed outlet in the abdominal wall to drain the contents of the bladder or bowel. See Chapter 10, page 266.)

SUPPORT GROUPS

Many people with bladder disorders acknowledge that getting information or finding someone else who had the same problem was the turning point in their struggle with the disorder. Sometimes these contacts occur by sheer chance, by reading an article in a magazine or newspaper or seeing a fellow sufferer on TV. But often they occur when you actively seek out a group where you can meet people like yourself who are trying to educate themselves and take control of dysfunctional bladders and disrupted lives.

Susan, who has suffered from incontinence since birth, joined a group two years ago. "My parents and older brother and sister were normal," she says. "I always felt so different. I had met people on my numerous trips to the hospital who were incontinent. But it was such a revelation to go to a support group meeting and find functioning adults who had the same problem I did."

Sherry, an interstitial cystitis sufferer, says, "I was really going down the tubes. I had just been diagnosed after having symptoms for eight years, and I was having to make some radical readjustments to the hard realities of having IC: 'We don't know the cause, we don't know the cure, you'll probably have to have it for the rest of your life.' My family was very sympathetic, but I really needed to talk to someone who understood on a gut level what it meant to have pain twenty-four hours a day, never be able to have a cup of coffee, and not be able to have sex without experiencing pain. When I found my support group, I felt like I didn't have to apologize anymore for how miserable I was."

Lloyd had surgery for prostate cancer last year. He had no incontinence prior to the surgery, but suffered constant urine loss and lost his ability to have an erection afterward. His wife was extremely helpful and caring, especially about the changes in his sexual function, but he wanted to talk to other men with the problem. "I had never heard the word 'prostate' spoken out loud until my doctor said it to me, and I didn't even know if other men had the same problem." A friend of Lloyd's wife suggested that he attend an incontinence support group. "There were *two* men there with similar problems," Lloyd remembers. "They spoke openly about their problems and gave me several ideas about how to manage my situation better."

Joining or starting a support group can be a very assertive thing to do. As Susan, Sherry, and Lloyd discovered, just one meeting can break the cycle of isolation and desperation so many people feel. Groups can also offer emotional support, information about good doctors, new treatments, and coping strategies. If you are the kind of person who doesn't like to join groups, attendance at one or two meetings might give you all the information you need to get help. If you are housebound or in a nursing home, ask the group leader to send you notes of the meeting, if they are compiled, or ask for the number of someone who would be willing to talk to you on the phone after the meeting. Perhaps a friend, family member, or a therapist or social worker could help start a group in your nursing home.

If no support group for your problem exists in your area, you can certainly start one. Contact one of the organizations listed above and ask how you can do this. Of course, to start a support group, you need bodies—people who have the same disorder that you have. You can probably get a free room at a local hospital, church, or community center and put a notice in your local newspaper for the first meeting. If enough people show up (and they probably will), you can reserve the room again and invite a guest speaker to talk about the topic people are most interested in.

FINDING THE RIGHT DOCTOR

If you are seeking help for the first time, or have not been satisfied with your treatment and are looking for a new doctor, you will want to choose your physician with great care. If your problem is your prostate, or you have bladder cancer, you have a pretty good chance of getting competent treatment. Urologists specialize in these conditions and have a lot of experience in treating them. Nevertheless, you may still have individual preferences that make finding the right doctor an important issue. If your problem is incontinence, you need to make sure that your doctor is familiar with *urodynamic tests,* the tests that can identify the type and severity of urinary loss, and *the range of treatment options*—not just drugs and surgery. The same principles apply to clinics. If a clinic advertises itself as an "incontinence clinic," make sure that it provides a wide range of support and services. If you have cystitis, you want to be sure that your doctor takes your symptoms seriously, i.e., doesn't think that repeated recurrences are "all in your head." If you have cystitis-like symptoms but no bacteria in your urine, you need to find a doctor who can determine whether you need to undergo testing for interstitial cystitis. If you have been diagnosed with IC and are having trouble controlling your symptoms, you certainly want to find a doctor who is willing to work with you in very creative ways to manage your symptoms. If you have been diagnosed with bladder cancer, the question of your care is all-important, and you may want to find a surgeon whose philosophy of treatment seems most reasonable to you. If you belong to a health maintenance organization, you may not have the wide selection of doctors to choose from that people with private insurance have, but there are still circumstances when you can be referred to an outside physician. If you are on Medicare, your selection may also be limited, but that should not stop you from asking pointed questions about your doctor's experience and expertise.

Which Specialist Should I See?

In addition to urologists, there are several other medical specialties that deal with different aspects of bladder disorders. In choosing your doctor, it is useful to be aware of what these specialties are and how they can help you.

- If you are a man who is suffering from urinary dysfunction, then a urologist is probably where you should start. Most urologists focus on men's bladder problems, and many even specialize in sexual dysfunction as well.
- If you are a woman who is suffering from interstitial cystitis, a urologist is also probably your best bet, but you need to find one who has a specific interest in treating this disorder—and the only way to find this out is to ask.
- If you are a woman who suffers from recurrent cystitis, you are probably already under the care of a gynecologist, internist, or family practice physician. Whether or not these doctors are qualified to treat cystitis depends not so much upon their training as upon whether they are willing to help you figure out why you are having repeated recurrences, and help you make a plan for controlling them. If you are having frequent recurrences, perhaps you might want to find a urologist who specializes in female urology or gynecologist who is a member of the American Uro-Gynecological Society (AUGS). By membership in this organization, these doctors have expressed a special interest in treating disorders of the female urinary tract.
- If you are elderly and suffer from incontinence and/or prostate problems, you might want to seek out a gerontologist, an internist who specializes in treating the medical problems of older people.
- Many people primarily depend on an internist or family practice physician for their care. Many doctors in these specialties are now more informed about bladder disorders, especially inconti-

nence, and may be able to evaluate your problem appropriately and determine if you need to be referred to a specialist for treatment. In any event, you need to ask specific questions, like the ones suggested below, as you would of any doctor, to assess his or her ability to treat bladder disorders.

Ask Around

If you are serious about getting proper diagnosis and treatment for a bladder disorder, you will need to pick your physician with great care—as much care as you might expend on picking a school for your child, planning a major vacation, or buying a new house. Here are some suggestions for going about this process:

- If you belong to a support group, ask several members whom they go to. If you are not in a support group, you might consider joining one, or at least going to one or two meetings, for this reason.
- Ask friends, relatives, or fellow employees for the names of doctors they regard highly.
- Ask a doctor or nurse you trust whom they would go to for a similar problem.
- If someone recommends a doctor, ask them if they know anyone else you might contact who has been treated by him or her.

Once you have several recommendations, call each doctor's office or clinic and get as much information as you can over the phone.

- Ask if the doctor treats many other people with your condition.
- Ask if he or she has had much success in treating people with your condition.
- If you are calling a clinic or incontinence center, ask if there is a brochure or other information on its services that can be sent to you.

WHERE TO FIND DOCTORS WHO SPECIALIZE IN BLADDER DYSFUNCTION

Many members of the following professional organizations have a special interest in bladder disorders. If you are unable to find a doctor or clinic that treats bladder disorders and can provide you with a range of treatment options, perhaps you can find one through these organizations. (When you write or make your phone call, be very specific about your needs.)

- **American Board of Allied Urological Health Professionals,** c/o Anne Smith-Young, 407 Strawberry Avenue, Stamford, CT 06902 (203) 323-1227.
- **American Urological Association (AUA),** 1120 North Charles Street, Baltimore, MD 21201 (301) 727-1100.
- **American Urological Association Allied,** 11512 Allecingie Parkway, Richmond, VA 23235 (804) 379-1306.
- **American Society of Clinical Oncology (ASCO),** John Yarbro, M.D., Department of Medicine, University of Missouri Medical Center, Columbia, MO 65212.
- **American Society of Genitourinary Surgeons (ASGS),** George Drach, M.D., Depts. of Surgery/Urology, Arizona Health Science Center, 1501 N. Campbell Avenue, Tuscon, AZ 85724 (606) 626-6236.
- **Canadian Urological Association,** Dr. O.H. Millard, President, 620-5991 Spring Garden Road, Halifax, Nova Scotia, B3H 1Y6, Canada.
- **Gerontological Society of America,** 1411 K Street NW, Washington, D.C., 20005 (202) 842-1275.
- **International Continence Society (ICS),** Paul Abrams, F.R.C.S., Consultant Urologist, Southmead Hospital, Bristol BS10 5NB, United Kingdom.
- **Society of Urological Oncology (SUO),** Urology Department, Brigham and Women's Hospital, 45 Francis Street, Boston, MA 02115 (617) 732-6325.
- **Urodynamics Society,** c/o Division of Urology, Hospital of the University of Pennsylvania, 5 Silverstein, 3400 Spruce Street, Philadelphia, PA 19104 (215) 662-2891.
- **Urology Nurses' Interest Group** (Canada), Humber College, 205 Humber College Blvd., Etobicoke, Ontario, Canada, M9W 5L7.

Asking the Right Questions

Finding a doctor is just the first step. Regardless of how well recommended or well qualified your doctor is, he or she does not have a crystal ball. Don't leave it up to the doctor to ask all the right questions. Either note your concerns on a written health history or, if the doctor or nurse is taking the information orally, *bring them up.* Be very specific about your symptoms. Make sure that your needs are met. Ask questions whenever anything is not clear.

Regardless of the type or severity of your bladder problem, ask direct questions such as:

- Is this test conclusive?
- Can there be other things causing my condition?
- Are there more conservative [i.e., less risky] treatments?
- Why won't this or that treatment work for me?
- What are the chances of a complete cure with this treatment?

If your doctor fails to address an issue that is important to you or answers your questions evasively, this is a good clue that he or she is not interested in your bladder problem, or even perhaps may be uninformed or uncomfortable in dealing with bladder disorders. In this case, you might ask him or her for a referral, saying, "Do you know a doctor who is interested in female urology?" Most doctors will be glad to refer you to another physician who may be better equipped to handle your problem. By being assertive and by asking pointed questions you should begin to get an idea whether your doctor has the expertise and enthusiasm to treat your bladder condition.

Choosing a Surgeon

Because the risks of surgery are so much higher than in other treatments, choosing a surgeon is a much more serious proposition. If you are considering surgery, in addition to using the tactics above you might want to do the following:

- If your doctor is volunteering to do your operation, ask how many surgeries of this type he or she has done in the past, and what the success rate has been.

- Ask your doctor if he or she would mind recommending some-one for a second opinion.
- Talk to a urological nurse or resident physician and ask for rec-ommendations.
- You may want to review the medical literature on your condition and see which doctors have written articles on the type of surgery you will be having. One way to do this is to run a Med-Line search, which will provide you with a computer printout of rele-vant articles for about $50. You can get the information free in book form from the *Index Medicus* at many medium-sized libraries.

If you have had a thorough evaluation and surgery has been suggested to you, it is essential that you ask your doctor some hard questions:

- What is my precise diagnosis?
- What other treatments are used for my condition?
- How restricted will my activities be after surgery?
- Will I have to have a catheter after surgery?
- How long will I be hospitalized?
- Is there a likelihood that I will also have to take drugs after surgery?
- What are the potential complications of this procedure?
- How long will I have to be out of work?
- How long will I have to abstain from sexual activity, especially intercourse?
- How long will my ability to lift heavy objects be restricted?
- When will I be able to participate in my usual sports or recrea-tional activities [name the activities]? *

If your doctor has suggested surgery and dismisses other op-tions as "a waste of time" or doesn't appear to be familiar with alternatives, you might do well to get a second opinion. Cheryle Gartley of the Simon Foundation also recommends making sure that you and your doctor have similar definitions of "success." She suggests asking questions like "Will I still need to wear pads?" and "Will this surgery be final, or is there a possibility that another procedure might be necessary in the future?"

* Special thanks to Charon Pierson, R.N., and Cheryle Gartley of the Simon Foundation for contributing to this list.

A successful surgery takes both a skilled surgeon and a knowledgeable, cooperative patient. In order to get the best outcome possible, it is essential that you follow all of your surgeon's instructions both before and after surgery.

Preparing for Your Doctor's Visit

We often spend days thinking about what to wear to a big party, then spend hours getting ready, but we don't spend five minutes preparing for a doctor's visit. Yet the outcome of some doctor visits can have a profound impact upon the quality of our lives. Because your health, and sometimes your life, is at stake, your doctor's visit —especially the first one—is worth at least as much forethought and preparation as a special social event. Here are some suggestions for things you might do beforehand to help make your visit more valuable:

- Make a two- or three-day voiding diary (see pages 26–27).
- Make a written summary of your medical history, including diseases you have had, current medical conditions, hospitalizations, surgeries, and allergies to medicines or foods.
- Make a list of your symptoms. (You might want to consult the Symptom Chart [see pages 28–29] to make sure you don't leave any out.)
- List all prescription and over-the-counter drugs you are currently taking, including birth control pills and any "recreational" drugs, and note any drugs you have taken and how long you took them.
- Write a brief summary of your recent sexual history, including the number of partners you have had, the types of activity you engage in, i.e., vaginal intercourse, anal intercourse, or sexual activity that does not involve vaginal penetration. If applicable, include your contraceptive history. (Your sexual history isn't applicable to every type of bladder disorder, but can be very relevant to recurrent cystitis and prostate problems.)

The tests that are usually done for the different bladder disorders are mentioned in each chapter, and discussed in detail in the Index of Diagnostic Tests beginning on page 278. You might want to check the section on Diagnosis in specific chapters, then review how these tests are carried out and what they can tell you about your condition. This will help you know what to expect when you go for your visit. Then if a certain test is omitted, you can ask why it is not useful in diagnosing your condition.

These simple pre-visit tasks will enable your doctor to better understand your case and thus to know if he or she can help you. They should also save valuable time during your visit that could be spent talking about your bladder problem.

Requesting Your Medical Records

If you are changing doctors or obtaining a second opinion, you might try calling the doctor you last saw, or the one you saw the longest, and get any information you do not currently have. You might consider requesting your medical records by getting a release form from your old doctor. It is your right by law to request your medical records and have them sent to your own address or to the physician who will be treating you. If you have had X-rays, you can go to the radiologist who made them, or to the hospital radiology department, sign a release, and have them sent to you or your doctor. Otherwise, your doctor can request these records if he or she thinks it is necessary.

If you have been hospitalized, you can obtain copies of your chart from the medical records office and of any biopsies or other surgical procedures from the pathology department of the hospital.

REACHING OUT

More than some diseases, bladder disorders have a way of taking over your life. Depending on what type of disorder you have and how serious it is, your bladder can dictate what you can and can't do, where you can go, how long you can be gone, whom you can see, whether you get any sleep at night, how you perform on your job, whether you are able to work or advance in your career, and even how you feel about yourself. Unlike some conditions, bladder disorders usually don't get better on their own, so if you don't take action, they may stay the same—or possibly get worse. By following the advice in this chapter, you can begin to overcome your bladder disorders. Reaching out can help break the cycle of embarrassment and isolation that bladder disorders can impose and help you get a proper diagnosis and the best available treatment.

VOIDING DIARY

Number of Accidents Today _____

Time of Day	Type and Amount of Fluid Intake	Amount Voided (in ounces)	Amount of Leakage*	Activity Engaged in When Leakage Occurred	Was Urge Present?
6:30 A.M.		8 oz.			Yes
7:30 A.M.	Coffee 7oz.		2	Washing dishes	No

* Estimate the AMOUNT OF LEAKAGE according to the following scale:

  1 = damp, few drops only

  2 = wet underwear or pad

  3 = soaked clothing or emptied bladder

27

SYMPTOM CHART FOR BLADDER DISORDERS

	Incontinence
Key: X = Primary symptoms O = Secondary or less frequently occurring symptoms NOTE: Not all symptoms may be present.	
Involuntary loss of urine	X
Frequency of urination	O
Urgent need to urinate	X
Painful urination	
Small amount of urine	X
Waking at night to urinate	O
Bladder pain relieved by voiding	
Difficulty in emptying bladder	X
Difficulty in starting urinary flow	O
Decreased stream	X
Bladder, urethral, or vaginal pain	
Perineal or anal pain	
Painful intercourse	
Painful ejaculation	
Visible blood in urine	
Blood in semen	
Lower-back pain	
Fatigue	
Chills/fever	

Irritative Voiding Symptom — Frequency of urination through Waking at night to urinate

Obstructive Voiding Symptom — Bladder pain relieved by voiding through Decreased stream

Cystitis	Interstitial Cystitis	Prostatitis	Benign Prostate Enlargement	Prostate Cancer	Bladder Cancer
O	O	O	O	O	O
X	X	X	O	O	O
X	X	X	O	O	O
X	O	O			O
X	X	X	X	O	O
X	X	X	X	O	O
	X	O			
	X	X	X	O	
X	X	X	X	O	O
	X	X	X		
X	X	O			
	X	X	O	O	
O	X	X			
	X	X	X	O	
	O	O	X	O	X
		X	O	O	
	O	X	O	X*	
X	X	X	O	O*	O*
O		X†			

* Occurs late in disease process
† Occurs only in acute bacterial prostatitis

RESOURCES

The Assertive Woman, Stanlee Phelps and Nancy Austin. 2nd ed. San Luis Obispo, CA: Impact, 1975.

The New Assertive Woman, Lynn Z. Bloom, Karen Coburn, and Joan Pearlman. New York: Delacorte Press, 1975.

Your Perfect Right, Robert E. Alberti and Michael L. Emmons. 5th ed. San Luis Obispo, CA: Impact, 1970.

CHAPTER 3

Anatomy 101:
The Healthy Bladder

THE BLADDER HAS TWO FUNCTIONS: THE STORAGE and the evacuation of urine. *Continence* is the storage of urine until an appropriate time and place can be found to empty it, and *micturition* (a fancy medical word for urination) is the process of emptying it. These two seemingly straightforward functions constitute an exquisitely subtle cycle of events that is controlled by both voluntary and involuntary nerves. Because of the dynamic interplay between the voluntary and involuntary nervous systems, the bladder is one of our most complex and sophisticated organs.

This brief tour through the urinary tract and its neighbor, the prostate, is designed to dispel some misconceptions about their function and to help you understand how they can malfunction and why. Much remains to be understood about the intricacies of the bladder, yet what is known can be simplified for our purposes and, with a little help from the accompanying illustrations, can be readily understood.

HOW THE BLADDER WORKS

In the healthy intact bladder, urine can be stored under enormous pressure, for example, when a runner does a sub-four-minute mile, a gymnast does a high double flip, or an astronaut exits in the atmosphere in a spaceship at Mach 7. If the bladder didn't

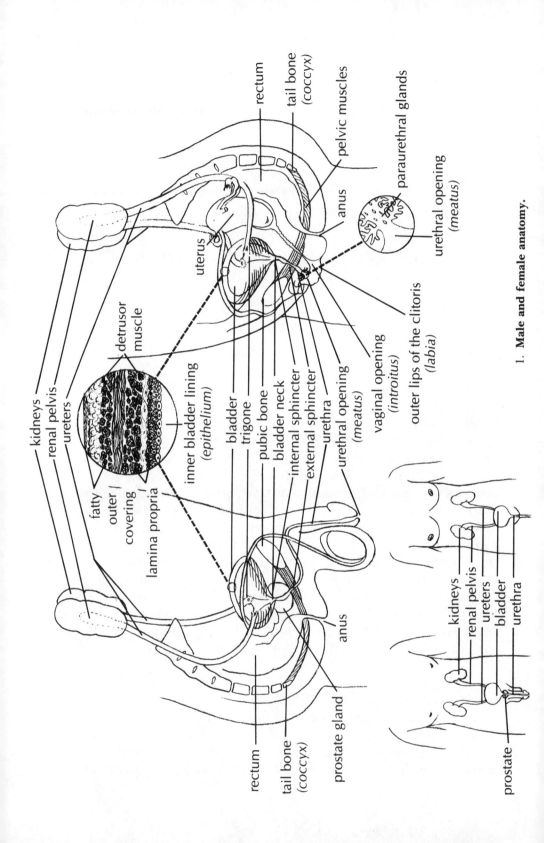

1. **Male and female anatomy.**

have a pretty efficient containment mechanism, athletes, astronauts, and just plain folks stooping to pick up a package or playing a Sunday afternoon game of volleyball would lose urine on a fairly regular basis.

The kidneys constantly filter water and waste products from the bloodstream through an intricate maze of microscopic tubes and blood vessels. This filtration process results in urine, which is 95 percent water and 5 percent waste material. The urine collects in a sort of holding tank called the *renal pelvis,* and from there travels down the *ureters,* two slender tubes about 8 to 10 inches long, which enter the back wall of the bladder roughly two thirds of the way from the top. The ureters are not merely hollow straws. They have a muscular outer coating that is constantly contracting and relaxing, similar to the muscular contractions *(peristalsis)* that move food through the bowel, forcing the urine downward and actively preventing it from moving back up into the kidneys. This function is an essential life-preserving feature of the urinary tract, since urine has a tendency to become infected when it stands still or backs up. Small amounts of urine are intermittently emptied into the bladder from the ureters about every 10 to 15 seconds.

The bladder is a hollow sac, slightly smaller than a regulation softball when full, and holds anywhere from 8 to 12 ounces of urine—about as much as a can of soda—under normal conditions. This is the bladder's *functional capacity.* Its *true capacity,* the amount it will hold if artificially distended while you are under anesthesia, is anywhere from 25 to 30 ounces (750 to 1,000 ml). When the bladder is empty, it is collapsed, like a rubber ball with the air let out. The bladder is kept in place by ligaments attached to adjacent organs and to the bones of the pelvis.

The wall of the bladder is composed of three layers: the fatty outer covering, the central muscular layer called the *detrusor,* and the inner mucous lining. This lining, called the *transitional epithelium,* is subdivided into several layers of cells. The transitional layer and the detrusor are separated by a thin membranous layer of connective tissue called the *lamina propria.* The lamina propria doesn't have much significance to the average person, but it has great significance to your doctor when he or she must diagnose bladder cancer that may invade the deeper layers of the bladder wall.

The bladder's sensory nerves, the ones that tell you it's time to urinate, are thought to be concentrated in the *trigone,* an upside-

33

down triangular area of tissue on the wall of the bladder. The ureters enter the bladder near each corner of the trigone's top (the base of the upside-down triangle). The apex of the trigone (the pointed end of the triangle) terminates near the opening of the *urethra.* This conjunction of bladder and urethra is known as the *bladder neck.* While urine is being stored, no urine backs up into the ureters because of a flap-valve mechanism created by the way the ureters enter the bladder wall. This mechanism is augmented by contraction of the muscle fibers around the ureteral opening during urination.

The urethra is a thin tube connecting the bladder to the outside of the body. The female and male urethras are similar in some respects and significantly different in others. The main similarity is that their walls consist primarily of smooth muscle and an inner lining of mucous cells. The main differences are that a man's urethra is much longer; it passes through the prostate, which women do not have; and because it transports semen, it also has a role in sexuality and reproduction.

In women, the urethra runs from the neck of the bladder along the top of the vagina to the urethral opening *(meatus),* which is located just above the entrance to the vagina—called the *introitus.* (See illustration 2.) When you are not urinating, the urethral tube is collapsed and held closed by tiny but very powerful internal and external *sphincter muscles.* In women, these two muscles are so close together that they are often thought of as a single muscle.

Since men handle their genitals many times each day from the time they are toilet-trained, they are very familiar with the location of the urethral opening. They are less familiar, however, with the urethra's more remote anatomy. Depending on the length of the penis, the male urethra is about 8 to 10 inches long. The innermost portion, similar in length to the entire female urethra, begins at the bladder neck and passes through the core of the prostate gland, and is called the *prostatic urethra.* This is the part that can be pinched or blocked as the prostate enlarges. The prostatic urethra is bounded on both ends by the *internal* and *external sphincter* muscles. The internal sphincter is an involuntary muscle and the external sphincter is largely a voluntary muscle. The remainder of the male urethra doesn't have any muscles and serves primarily as a conduit for urine and semen.

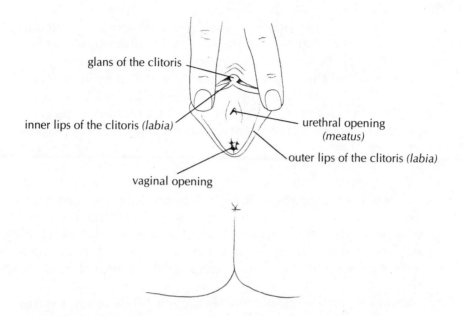

glans of the clitoris

inner lips of the clitoris *(labia)*

urethral opening
(meatus)

outer lips of the clitoris *(labia)*

vaginal opening

2. **Woman locating urethral opening.** The urethral opening is buried in the tissue just above the vaginal opening. Sometimes it is hard to see because it is buried in the mucous membrane lining beneath the clitoral lips. Using a light and mirror, you can locate your own urethral opening as the woman in the illustration is doing, by spreading the outer and inner lips (or *labia*) with your fingers. Some women mistakenly believe that urine comes from deep within the vagina, so locating the *meatus* for the first time can be quite a revelation.

The Bladder's Nervous System: Messages Traveling on Parallel Tracks

There is a center at the base of the brain, called the *pons micturition center,* that controls the storage and evacuation of urine, somewhat like a switching station for trains. Two types of tracks emerge from the *pons,* heading for different destinations. One track carries the voluntary (or *somatic*) nerves and the other carries involuntary (*sympathetic* and *parasympathetic*) nerves. The destination of the voluntary track is the external sphincter of the urethra. This muscle is the first one you relax when you urinate. The involuntary track branches, with the sympathetic track going to the trigone and the

35

internal sphincter of the urethra and the other, the parasympathetic track, going to the detrusor muscle.

If you look at illustration 3, you will see a schematic representation of the nerves that control the bladder. The storage phase of the voiding cycle is primarily controlled by the involuntary *(sympathetic)* nerves, and the emptying phase is controlled by involuntary *(parasympathetic)* and voluntary *(somatic)* nerves. Each of these nerve tracks is made up of certain types of fibers and receptors that react to specific substances called *neurotransmitters.* The sympathetic track is composed of *adrenergic* fibers and receptors that respond primarily to *norepinephrine,* a hormone produced by the adrenal glands. The parasympathetic track is made up of *cholinergic* fibers and receptors that respond to *acetylcholine,* a potent substance that helps facilitate nerve transmission. Deficiencies in these substances can cause certain types of incontinence. Some drugs are able to stimulate or block adrenergic and cholinergic nerve receptors, and thus increase or decrease the activity of the bladder muscle and the urethral sphincter.

The voiding cycle begins as the bladder fills. The bladder stores urine comfortably for 2 to 5 hours, depending upon fluid intake and normal kidney function. As the bladder fills with urine, we get the vague perception of a need to urinate. Eventually this sensation becomes stronger until—at some point that varies from person to person—the urine reaches a critical level and the nerves in the bladder wall signal the brain that the bladder is nearly full—an involuntary signal. This is perceived as a frank urge to empty the bladder. Ever since we were toilet-trained we have been conditioned to voluntarily hold the urine until it could be emptied appropriately. If no toilet or other acceptable place is available, most people can usually wait a while longer. But soon, the need to find a suitable spot to urinate becomes all-consuming. As the bladder begins to reach its functional capacity, sensory nerves send a "getting full" message up the sympathetic track to the *pons,* where it is processed. When you are ready, a return message travels down the somatic or voluntary track, allowing you to consciously relax the external sphincter muscle. At the same time, the *pons* sends a message down to the parasympathetic track, telling the detrusor muscle to contract and a signal down the sympathetic track to relax the involuntary external sphincter. If all of these messages arrive on time, and are strong enough, urination occurs.

If you do not voluntarily urinate, several things might occur.

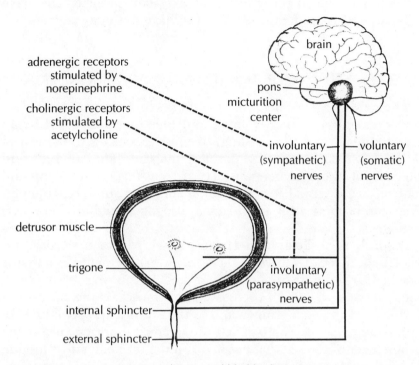

adrenergic receptors
stimulated by
norepinephrine

cholinergic receptors
stimulated by
acetylcholine

brain

pons
micturition
center

involuntary
(sympathetic)
nerves

voluntary
(somatic)
nerves

detrusor muscle

trigone

involuntary
(parasympathetic)
nerves

internal sphincter

external sphincter

3. a. Nerves that control bladder function

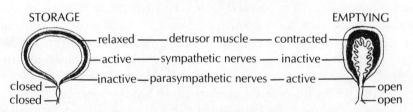

STORAGE

relaxed —— detrusor muscle —— contracted
active —— sympathetic nerves —— inactive
inactive — parasympathetic nerves — active
closed
closed

EMPTYING

open
open

b. Coordination of nerve signals for efficient urination

3. a. **Nerves that control bladder function.** This schematic illustration indicates the pathways of bladder nerves. Both voluntary and involuntary nerve signals to and from the bladder are processed in the *pons.* These nerves pass through the *pons micturition* center located near the base of the brain, where their messages are processed. For efficient storage and evacuation of urine, the activity of these nerves must be precisely coordinated.

b. **Coordination of nerve signals for efficient urination.** For storage of urine, the detrusor muscle must be relaxed and the sphincter muscles must be tightly closed. For urination to occur, the detrusor muscle must contract and the sphincter muscles must be relaxed.

37

You could lose some or all of the urine involuntarily. Or you might develop a spasm in the internal or external sphincter and have difficulty releasing the urine when you have found a place.

MUSCLES THAT HELP THE BLADDER FUNCTION

The pelvic organs, including the uterus in women and the bladder and rectum in both women and men, are supported by an overlapping hammock, or sling, of muscles variously referred to as the *pelvic muscles* or the perineal muscles. The strength and integrity of these muscles, which are entirely under voluntary control, are essential to the maintenance of urinary continence. They can become weak from lack of use, age, childbirth, surgery, or injury.

If you look at illustration 4, you will see part of the broad, flat triangular sheet of muscle, called the *urogenital diaphragm*, that is attached to the pubic bone in front and to the ischial bones (the ones that you sit on) on each side. This muscle is pierced by the urethra and vagina in women and by the urethra and penis in men. The *pelvic diaphragm* (also called the *levator ani* muscle) is a much larger sheet of muscle that lies beneath the urogenital diaphragm. This broad muscle is hung between the coccyx and the pubic bone like a hammock and is pierced by the rectum. If these muscles are in good shape, when you contract them, you can stop or prevent the flow of urine or a bowel movement. (Information on how to exercise these muscles and make them stronger can be found on page 65.) The *bulbocavernosus muscle* and the *anal sphincter muscle* lie on top of the broad pelvic muscles, encircling the urethra, vagina, and anus in women and the urethra and anus in men, forming a sort of figure-eight. These muscles, often referred to as the *pubococcygeal muscles,* also play a major part in maintaining continence.

THE NORMAL PROSTATE

Technically, the prostate is not a part of the male urinary system. It belongs, rather, to the male genital, or reproductive, system; but by virtue of its location and interdependence with the male urethra, the prostate strongly influences the normal function of the

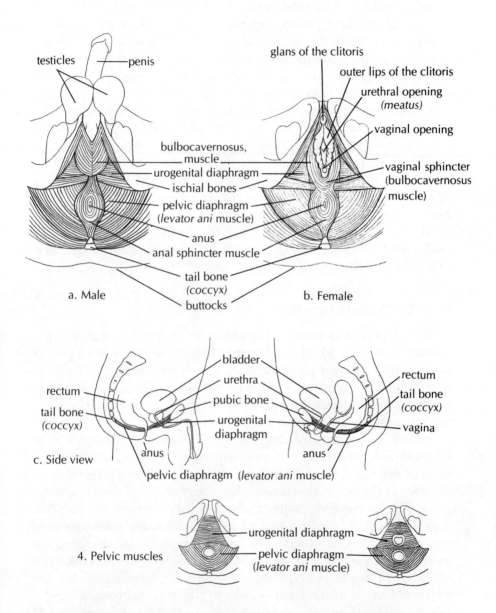

a. Male

b. Female

c. Side view

4. Pelvic muscles

4. Pelvic muscles. In terms of continence, the most important muscles are the urogenital diaphragm and pelvic diaphragm (also called the *levator ani* muscle).

These muscles form a secure hammock, or sling, that supports the bladder and other pelvic organs. These are the muscles that you want to contract when you are doing pelvic muscle exercises.

bladder and urethra. If you look at illustration 5, you will see the prostate and its relationship to the bladder and urethra.

The walnut-sized prostate gland, weighing about an ounce (20 grams), surrounds the urethra like a fat cuff just below the bladder. The urethra, about the size of a soda straw and slightly bent, passes through the heart of the gland. This segment, the *prostatic urethra,* is bounded on the bladder end by the internal sphincter and at its exit from the prostate by the external sphincter. The prostate is primarily composed of glandular and fibrous connective tissue and is divided into three distinctive zones. The *central zone* is composed primarily of glandular tissue and the *prostatic ducts* that empty into the urethra. Most benign prostatic enlargement occurs in this zone. The *peripheral zone* contains primarily fibrous tissue. Most cancers of the prostate originate in this part of the gland. A third zone, the narrow *transitional zone,* separates the two. The entire prostate is encased by a thin layer of fibrous muscular tissue called the *prostatic capsule.*

How the Prostate Functions

The glandular portion of the prostate secretes an alkaline, opalescent fluid through about fifty *prostatic glands* that open into the urethra through tiny prostatic ducts. The twin *seminal vesicles* (only one is visible in illustration 5), which lie just adjacent to the prostate, also manufacture an alkaline fluid that empties into the prostatic urethra through two small *ejaculatory ducts.* The sperm are manufactured in the testicles and stored in the *epididymis,* a sort of holding tank, where they await ejaculation. The muscular contractions of ejaculation propel the sperm through a tube, called the *vas deferens,* to the seminal vesicles, where they are mixed with seminal fluid. The sperm and seminal fluid, now called semen, are emptied into the prostatic urethra and mixed with prostatic fluid squeezed out of the prostatic ducts. The secretions made by the prostatic glands increase the bulk of the semen by about 15 percent. The alkalinity of this fluid helps the sperm survive, especially if they are deposited in the acidic environment of the vagina. Prostatic fluid is produced continuously, not only when sexual activity occurs. If ejaculation does not occur, the fluid seeps through the ducts and is carried out with regular urination, or is perhaps discharged in nocturnal emissions, commonly known as "wet dreams."

When the prostate functions normally, men are not aware of its

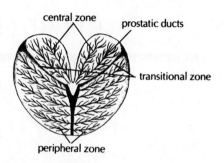

central zone

prostatic ducts

transitional zone

peripheral zone

5. **The normal prostate.** This illustration shows the prostate gland and its relationship to the bladder and urethra. You can see how the urethra passes through the core of the gland, bending slightly. You can see a number of the prostatic glands, which manufacture an alkaline fluid that becomes part of the semen. The inset in the lower left-hand corner of the illustration shows the three zones of the prostate.

existence. But when it becomes infected, enlarged (a completely normal process), or diseased, it can cause many problems. Chapter 7, Prostate Problems, can help you recognize the signs and symptoms of prostate disorders, understand what types of problems can occur, and see how they are treated.

Now that you have seen how the bladder and prostate function, you are ready to move into the chapters on the different bladder disorders. As you read through these chapters, you may want to refer back to the illustrations frequently when reading about the causes, diagnosis, and treatment of bladder dysfunction.

CHAPTER 4

Incontinence

HILLARY, WHO TEACHES FRENCH AT A SMALL COLLEGE near Philadelphia, had her third child two years ago at the age of thirty-five. "We were really looking forward to this baby," she recalls. "But I've had nothing but trouble since he came. Now I leak whenever I cough, laugh, sneeze, or pick him up." Hillary's muscles were torn during her delivery, causing urinary incontinence. "When I asked my doctor about the leakage, he said it was common with births like mine, and gave me some pills," she recalls. "I used to belong to a tennis club and had gotten good enough at the game to hold my own in tournaments, but I stopped playing because wondering if I was going to get through a game without major leakage was just too nerve-wracking." Hillary became very frustrated at the limitations incontinence imposed. "I got tired of having to arrange my life around a leaky bladder," she says. "After a while, it seemed that the only safe thing I could do was to watch TV—if I didn't laugh too much."

Hillary is typical of many people who suffer from incontinence. A friend recommended that she see Kristene for an evaluation. After a complete urologic work-up, she recommended a course of pelvic muscle exercises, monitored by a biofeedback device. She also told Hillary about several organizations that provide information on incontinence and a catalog that contains a wide range of absorbent products. "I felt so helpless all that time," Hillary says. "It was such a relief to be doing something about my problem."

Self-Evaluation Checklist

You don't have to go through the Self-Evaluation Checklist below to figure out if you are incontinent. The symptom is unmistakable: damp or wet underwear and clothing. However, you may believe that incontinence is unusual and that little can be done about it. On the contrary, most incontinence can be cured or be made significantly better with appropriate diagnosis and treatment. The checklist notes many of the ways that incontinence can be experienced and some of the ways that it can impact on your life. So, if you answer "yes" to several questions on the list, you might want to consider having your incontinence evaluated.

SELF-EVALUATION CHECKLIST

___ Do you leak urine when you sneeze, cough, laugh, or make sudden movements?

___ After feeling a strong urge to urinate, are you unable to make it to the toilet before urine begins to leak out?

___ Do you wet the bed?

___ Do you feel that your bladder does not empty entirely, causing you to urinate more frequently?

___ Have you tried incontinence exercises, but failed to get results?

___ Have you given up sex because of embarrassment about urinary leakage?

___ Have you had surgery for incontinence and still leak?

___ Have you had prostate or other pelvic surgery which resulted in incontinence?

___ Do you wear diapers or pads because of incontinence?

___ Has it been recommended that you take hormone replacement therapy?

___ Have you stopped doing many things you enjoy because of the threat of urinary leakage?

___ Does incontinence make travel difficult for you?

___ Have you curtailed dating or other social relationships because of incontinence?

___ Do you have a relative or friend in a nursing home who suffers from incontinence?

___ Does your child wet the bed or have embarrassing episodes of incontinence away from home?

WHAT THIS CHAPTER CAN DO FOR YOU

As you will soon see, incontinence is a complex, often misdiagnosed condition with multiple causes and, in many cases, no magical cure. There are, however, numerous treatments available, and the key to getting the best treatment possible is getting a correct diagnosis. This chapter covers the topic of diagnosis in detail, providing information about which tests are appropriate for each type of incontinence and what the test results can (or can't) tell you about your condition. Once you have gotten a diagnosis, you will want to know about treatment. This chapter also covers the range of treatments that are available and reviews the advantages and disadvantages of each. Some will treat only the symptom, while others will cure or improve your condition a great deal. If, for various reasons, cure or improvement is not possible, there are still numerous things that can be done to help you continue to be active.

WHO HAS INCONTINENCE?

Conservatively, 10 to 15 million people in the United States are reported to have some degree of incontinence, but because of reluctance to report the condition, this figure could easily be as high as 30 million. *Campbell's Urology,* a standard urology text, states that "50 percent of women who have never delivered a child occasionally experience stress urinary incontinence in sufficient quantity to be socially embarrassing."[1] Many women can become incontinent after childbirth, hysterectomy, or other pelvic surgery. From 0.5 to 2 percent of men develop incontinence after surgery for prostate enlargement, and between 5 and 15 percent will experience urine loss after surgery for prostate cancer. About 30 percent of older people who live at home are incontinent and 50 percent of all nursing home residents suffer from severe wetness. Among young children, 10 percent of five-year-olds—more boys than girls—and 5 percent of ten-year-olds continue to wet the bed and have daytime accidents. By the age of fifteen, about 2 percent of children are still having bedwetting episodes. In short, about one person in twenty-five in the United States and Canada suffers from incontinence, making it one of our most common medical problems.

Many People Are Reluctant to Seek Help

Many people with incontinence are not only afraid of admitting their condition, they are also reluctant to bring the subject up with a doctor or other practitioner. Surveys show that *only one person in twelve actively seeks help.* One survey done by Help for Incontinent People (HIP), Inc., revealed that those who do seek help wait an average of nine years before taking action.[2] And of those who do discuss the subject with their physicians or with another health professional, only about one third receive appropriate therapy.

Each year, more than $10 billion is spent on incontinence. This figure is greater than *the entire $8 billion annual budget of the National Institutes of Health.* Unfortunately, the bulk of this money is spent on maintenance and mop-up, rather than on research aimed at developing better diagnostic techniques and more effective forms of therapy.

The Good News About Incontinence

To counterbalance this very dismal state of affairs, there is some good news. Incontinence has been the focus of quite a bit of research in the last few years and some significant progress has been made in terms of diagnosis, management, and treatment. Today, if all of the people who suffer from incontinence sought and received appropriate help, more than one half could be cured, another third could be helped significantly, and most of the rest could be made more comfortable.

WHAT IS INCONTINENCE?

When you finally get up the courage to tell your doctor that you have urinary leakage and are interested in getting help, you may, like many people in the past, run into a brick wall. One reason doctors may seem so unconcerned is that their definition of incontinence may not be the same as yours. If you lose urine twice a month, your doctor may not think it is very serious, but if you are teaching a class, or you are in the middle of a business meeting, a tennis game, shopping, or whatever, the involuntary loss of urine may be a significant problem for you.

Even among people who have incontinence, definitions differ.

Many people, like Renee, find the leakage of even minor amounts of urine disconcerting and disruptive. "I leak occasionally—maybe about once or twice a month, not frequently enough to wear a pad all the time. I always think, I didn't leak yesterday, I probably won't today. Then I am upset when it occurs, especially if it gets on my clothes. Whenever that happens, I'll use any excuse to leave work to go home and change. I have even walked out in the middle of some very funny movies."

Lauren looks at urinary leakage quite differently. She developed moderate incontinence after the birth of her son. "I was forced to push the baby out before I was ready and my muscles were stretched during the delivery," she says. "Now I have to use absorbent pads all the time." Lauren has run several marathons and continues to train regularly. "Running is the worst," she says. "I have to carry a pad and change along the way. That isn't always easy, but I don't have any choice."

Even though Lauren's daily urine loss is much more than Renee's occasional leakage, the problem is much more traumatic to Renee. Part of what bothers Renee is the unpredictability of her leakage. It's just infrequent enough for her to pretend to herself that it's not a problem—until the next accident. Lauren has accepted the fact that she has significant leakage, but it hasn't changed her life in any appreciable way. Yet they are both *incontinent*.

When doctors and other health professionals don't respond to queries about incontinence with interest and concern, people tend to get discouraged and give up, instead of pursuing the issue further. Dr. Katherine Jeter, who has worked with incontinent people for many years, states emphatically, "Some health professionals refer to a person as being 'slightly incontinent.' That is like being 'a little pregnant.' The unexpected loss of urine in any amount, on a regular basis, in an inconvenient place is incontinence."[3] Regardless of the definition of incontinence, *any amount of urine loss that is troublesome to the person experiencing it (or to others)* ought to be taken seriously by practitioners.

In an effort to correct this problem, the International Continence Society formulated a definition of incontinence that simply states: Incontinence is "a condition in which involuntary loss of urine is a social or hygienic problem. . . ."[4] That is, you should be classified as having incontinence if urine loss is a problem for you or for those around you.

The Big Myth About Incontinence

"Incontinence, like retention, is a symptom, and not a disease," wrote Dr. Van Buren, an English physician, in a treatise on genital disorders in 1874.[5] This was a fairly sophisticated view that has in large part gotten lost in modern medicine. Today, although a number of well-known urologists and gerontologists have raised their voices in protest, the prevailing assumption among physicians and other practitioners who work with the elderly is that incontinence is a normal part of aging. Perhaps it is this prejudice that allows physicians to dismiss the condition as inevitable and serves as the rationale for not taking the symptoms or consequences of incontinence seriously. It *is* true that organs and bodily functions become more fragile and vulnerable to accident and disease as we grow older, but rather than causing incontinence, aging merely *predisposes* us to certain ailments or conditions that can result in the inappropriate loss of urine.

TYPES OF BLADDER DYSFUNCTION

One of the difficulties lay people encounter in dealing with incontinence is that there are several different types, and more often than not, they are intermixed. Another difficulty is that doctors have a number of ways of looking at incontinence. One may tell you that you have a "neurogenic bladder." If you seek a second opinion, another may say that you have "an unstable bladder." Yet another might say that you have "storage failure." And you are left feeling as though you have just heard a sentence out of a science fiction novel—in another language. It's very important, however, for you to understand why your bladder or urethra (or both) is malfunctioning, so you can ask specific questions to make sure you are getting proper treatment. (At this point, you might want to refer back to Chapter 3, which explains normal bladder function in detail. That information should be helpful in understanding what can go wrong.)

When you go to your doctor and have a complete urologic exam, you will probably be told that you have one of the following types of incontinence:

- *stress incontinence,* in which urine leaks in response to a cough, sneeze, laugh, or sudden movement;

- *urge incontinence,* in which you feel an urge to urinate but may not have time to get to the toilet; *reflex incontinence,* a variation of urge incontinence in which you urinate suddenly without any warning;
- *overflow incontinence,* in which the bladder overfills and leaks without any warning and without any feeling.

These labels are roughly descriptive of what *triggers* incontinence. They tell you little about what has gone wrong. Because incontinence is so complex, many doctors have come to look at bladder disorders from a "functional" perspective, simply looking for what can go wrong with (1) the bladder, (2) the urethra, or (3) both.[6] Looked at in this way, complexities of bladder dysfunction can be understood by anyone.

What Can Go Wrong?

The bladder slowly fills and stores urine comfortably for several hours and then, when you are ready, you begin urination voluntarily and the bladder empties completely. Incontinence occurs when the bladder either *fails to store urine properly* or *fails to empty it completely.*

The failure to store urine can be due to (1) an overactive bladder muscle, or (2) a displaced or damaged urethra. Incontinence can occur if the bladder muscle is overactive and contracts at unpredictable times. When this occurs, you will have an urge to urinate, but you may not have time to get to the toilet. This is *urge incontinence.* If such leakage occurs without warning, the term *reflex incontinence* may be used.

The failure to store urine properly also occurs when a cough, a laugh, a sneeze, or a sudden movement puts extra pressure or "stress" on the bladder. In its normal position, the urethra is able to withstand an enormous amount of pressure—that of a deep belly laugh or extreme physical exertion. But if the pelvic muscles are stretched or damaged and the urethra slips out of its normal position, it cannot maintain sufficient pressure and has a harder time remaining closed. Stress incontinence results. If the sphincter muscle is actually damaged and cannot close completely under any circumstances, it becomes like an open pipe, and severe or total incontinence occurs.

Failure to empty the bladder completely can be due to either an underactive bladder muscle or a blocked urethra. If the nerves of the bladder are not functioning properly, the bladder muscle will not contract hard enough, and just a little bit of urine will come out, leaving the remainder to collect in the bladder as water does in a reservoir. When the reservoir gets too full, a little bit may leak through the dam (the urethra) whenever the pressure increases. This is called *overflow incontinence*. If the urethra is partially blocked, for example, by an enlarged prostate, the bladder can also become too full and overflow, also causing overflow incontinence. If the urethra is totally blocked, nothing will come out and you will have total urinary retention. This can be very uncomfortable and causes many people to go to their urologist or to the emergency room in severe pain, needing to have their bladder drained.

In order for normal urination to occur, the bladder muscle and the urethra must function in a coordinated fashion. The bladder muscle must *contract* and the urethra must *relax* at precisely the same time. If the urethra does not relax because its nerves are not functioning properly, voluntary urination cannot occur. This lack of coordination is called *bladder-sphincter dyssynergia* and can result in retained urine.

Regardless of the cause or causes of urinary leakage, incontinence is nearly always a result of one or more of the above factors. The chart below will help you to see the different types of malfunction that can occur in the bladder, the conditions that underlie each type of failure, the types of incontinence that can result, and what you might experience with each type of malfunction.

Stress Incontinence

Stress incontinence is the leakage of urine that occurs when sudden pressure or "stress" from a source outside of the bladder is applied unequally to both the bladder and the urethral sphincter mechanism. (In a way the name is unfortunate because it suggests that incontinence is caused by emotional stress, which it is not.) The classic examples of such stress are coughing, sneezing, and laughing, sudden movements such as bending or lifting, and athletic activities of all sorts. When the bladder is well supported by the muscles of the pelvic floor (see page 38 for a description of these muscles), pressure is applied about equally to the sphincter muscle and to the bladder, and continence is maintained (see illustration 4). If the urethra has slipped from its normal position,

THE FUNCTIONAL CAUSES OF INCONTINENCE*

Malfunction	Underlying Conditions	Types of Incontinence	What You Experience
Failure to store			
Because of the bladder	overactive or unstable bladder muscle	urge incontinence	you feel it coming but can't stop it
Because of the urethra	displaced urethra	stress incontinence	you leak after sudden movement
		reflex incontinence	you can't feel it coming
		total incontinence	you leak all the time
Failure to empty			
Because of the bladder	underactive bladder muscle	overflow incontinence	bladder leaks unexpectedly
Because of the urethra	obstruction from enlarged prostate	overflow incontinence	bladder leaks unexpectedly
	lack of coordination between bladder and sphincter	bladder-sphincter dyssynergia	urgency, frequency, voiding small amounts of urine

* Adapted from A. J. Wein, "Classification of neurogenic voiding dysfunction," *J. Urol.*, 125:605–609, 1981.

to the pelvic muscles can also cause the uterus to drop
into the vagina. Your doctor can usually feel the degree
by inserting one finger into your vagina and pressing
our abdomen with the other hand, while you cough or
with your abdominal muscles. You should be able to
otrusion as well, by putting your finger in your vagina
ng. If the cystocele is large enough, you can even see it
a mirror between your legs and straining. A portion of
e tissue along the roof of the vagina will move closer
vaginal opening, or may actually protrude. This may
n during orgasm, and can easily be felt with your fin-
tocele and/or urethrocele does not necessarily cause in-
, but their presence is definite evidence of pelvic muscle
r damage, which does cause it.

ATION OF STRESS INCONTINENCE

g how severe incontinence is can be very useful in deciding
ment is most appropriate. Many urologists classify stress incon-
ed on the following criteria:

mild stress incontinence, the bladder and urethra are in their
normal position and you experience leakage only upon
coughing, laughing, straining, etc.;
moderate stress incontinence, the bladder and urethra protrude into the vagina;
severe stress incontinence, in which the urethra does not
work at all.[7]

illary, whose story appears at the beginning of this chap-
o see Kristene, it was clear that her bladder and urethra
uded somewhat into her vagina. Kristene found that
a cystourethrocele, which indicated Type II stress in-

tinence

point during the filling stage of the voiding cycle, we
t sensation of filling. Then, gradually, over a period of

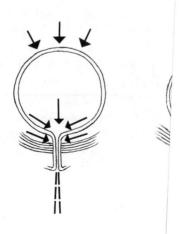

6. **How urine loss occurs from stress inc**
pressure on the bladder and urethra is tran
able to remain closed. If the bladder has sli
pressure will be higher inside the bladder,
and leakage will occur.

due most often to muscles damage
pelvic surgery, especially hysterecto
bladder, but a similar amount of pr
sphincter area, the urethra does n
curs.

Stress incontinence caused by we
be mild, but can be severe enough to
times a day. How severe the incor
weak or damaged your pelvic muscl
the bladder and urethra are. Stress
diagnosed by looking at how mu
protrude (or herniate) through the
If the urethra slips from its norma
the pressure of a cough or laugh,
the vagina, you have a *urethrocele*. I
you have a *cystocele*. If both the bla
you have a *cystourethrocele* (see illus

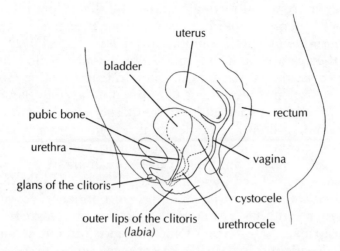

7. a. Cystocele and urethrocele

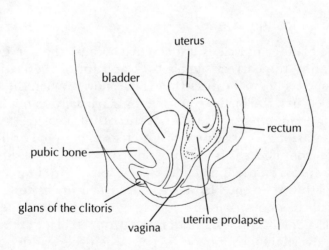

b. Prolapsed uterus

7. a. **Cystocele and urethrocele.** b. **Prolapsed uterus.** These illustrations show the normal position of the female bladder, urethra, and uterus. In *a*, the dotted line shows the altered position of the bladder and urethra. The pelvic muscles sag and the bladder protrudes through them, in many cases resting against the vagina. In severe cases, the urethra may protrude through the vaginal opening.

time, the sensation becomes stronger, until there is a frank *urge* to urinate. If no toilet is handy, most people can voluntarily prevent the bladder from contracting and tolerate the urge until one can be found. In some people, however, a strong urge to urinate comes on quite suddenly and involuntary urination occurs quickly, often before they can make it to a toilet. The amount of time between episodes of urinary leakage varies, and urine loss is often moderate to severe. Urge incontinence is most often the result of an overactive (hyperactive, hypersensitive, or spastic) bladder muscle and usually occurs when the bladder contracts involuntarily (involuntary bladder contraction). Urge incontinence can also occur if you have a bladder infection, which causes the lining of your bladder to become irritated and hypersensitive.

Reflex incontinence, a variation of urge incontinence, occurs when the bladder contracts involuntarily but you don't experience an urge to urinate. This type of incontinence without sensation is often the result of spinal cord injury or is caused by certain tumors, diseases, or surgery that interrupt the transmission of nerve impulses from the nervous system to the bladder and urethra.

Overflow Incontinence

If the bladder muscle is underactive because the nerves are not transmitting the correct signals back and forth, the bladder may fill beyond its normal capacity and "overflow." When the desire to urinate occurs, the bladder empties only partially or not at all and straining to empty it is usually not successful. Leakage may occur without warning, or may manifest itself as a continual dribble. This type of incontinence is frequently caused by diabetes, a slipped disc that may press on the spinal nerves, or a spinal cord injury in which nerve pathways to the bladder are disturbed or disrupted. It can also result from obstruction (blockage) of the urethra due to prostate enlargement, stones, tumors, or a dropped bladder (cystocele). Rarely, overflow incontinence occurs when the bladder and urethral muscles get out of sync and contract instead of relaxing when the bladder muscle contracts.

Mixed Incontinence

It is quite possible, and all too common, to have more than one type of incontinence at the same time. About one third of older women who have stress incontinence also have urge incontinence as the result of a hyperactive bladder.[8] Older men often have urge incontinence coupled with overflow incontinence that occurs because of obstruction of the urethra, usually from prostate enlargement.

CAUSES OF INCONTINENCE

Since incontinence is merely the sympton of bladder dysfunction, it is not useful to treat just the symptom. It is necessary to pinpoint, as precisely as possible, the underlying cause of incontinence and, if possible, treat that instead. There are numerous causes of incontinence. Some are temporary and relatively easy to treat. Others are long-standing, entrenched conditions that are often more difficult to deal with. Because of these differences, physicians have found it useful to separate the causes of incontinence into two categories: *transient* causes that are usually of recent origin and are often treatable and reversible; and chronic or *established* conditions. Transient conditions account for at least 50 percent of incontinence in elderly women and men, with the other half being caused by established conditions. Established causes of incontinence are more common among women twenty to sixty years of age.

Temporary or transient causes of incontinence include:

- *drugs:* It is not uncommon for an elderly person to be taking several over-the-counter (OTC) remedies in addition to prescription drugs. Both prescription and OTC drugs often contain ingredients that interfere with the function of the bladder and urethral nerves and muscles.
- *mental impairment:* Mental dysfunction ranges from depression to disorientation, and in more severe forms, a person may be unaware of the need to urinate.
- *estrogen deficiency:* The healthy function of the female bladder and urethra are dependent to some extent upon the amount of estrogen (the hormone responsible for menstruation in women) that is produced. With menopause, estrogen production is decreased, and in some women, urethral tissues become more fragile and susceptible to damage or infection.
- *restricted mobility:* Severe illnesses, accidents, strokes, and surgery

55

may result in confinement to bed or to a wheelchair, limiting your ability to get to the toilet in time.

- *urinary tract infections:* Bladder infections are common among the elderly and are often associated with a temporary or long-standing indwelling catheter.

Established long-standing causes of incontinence include:

- *abdominal or pelvic surgery:* These include hysterectomy, previous incontinence surgery, surgery for prostate enlargement, cancer of the prostate, or extensive pelvic surgery for colon, cervical, or ovarian cancer.
- *childbirth:* Pelvic muscles that surround the vagina can be stretched or torn during delivery. As a result, the bladder may sag from its normal position, resulting in stress incontinence.
- *a weak or damaged urethral sphincter muscle:* Stress incontinence can be caused by hysterectomy or complications from incontinence, prostate or bladder surgery, certain drugs, pelvic radiation, or estrogen deficiency.
- *urethral obstruction:* Obstruction can be caused by prostatic enlargement, bladder stones, a dropped bladder (cystocele), scarring from surgical procedures, or from infections such as gonorrhea.
- *diseases such as Alzheimer's, Parkinson's, diabetes, or multiple sclerosis:* These conditions can damage the nervous system and interfere with nerve function.
- *strokes, spinal cord injuries, or tumors:* These conditions can block nerve impulses.
- *damage to bladder nerves:* Any kind of pelvic surgery or injury can damage or sever nerves that control bladder function.
- *cystitis:* Infection or inflammation of the bladder can be caused by an indwelling catheter, radiation therapy, chemotherapy for bladder, prostate, or uterine cancer, stones in the bladder or prostate, or interstitial cystitis, and may result in incontinence.
- *obesity:* Large internal fat deposits may cause increased pressure on the bladder.
- *alcohol:* A central nervous system depressant, alcohol can temporarily or permanently deaden the nerves that transmit the signals for storage or release of urine. Alcohol is also a diuretic that causes the kidneys to make more urine. It may also irritate a sensitive bladder or precipitate urinary retention by deadening

the perception of the need to urinate. In the long run, alcohol can damage the bladder nerves, causing permanent inefficient bladder emptying.

- *birth defects, especially spina bifida:* In this condition, the spinal cord herniates through the membrane covering the spine, causing bladder dysfunction and other problems. Often the bladder does not function at all, and urine has to be drained with a catheter.

If you have any of these conditions or diseases, be sure to mention them to your doctor when he or she is taking your medical history. Although long-standing causes of incontinence are more difficult to treat, two thirds of the people with these conditions can be cured or improved significantly with appropriate evaluation and therapy.

DIAGNOSIS

Getting a diagnosis involves two things: finding a clinic or doctor who is experienced in treating incontinence; and communicating your needs to the practitioner you have selected. For many people, these are easier said than done. But having confidence that your condition can be diagnosed, and that it is your right to obtain treatment, will help you overcome the obstacles you might encounter—or imagine you will.

Finding a Doctor

Chapter 2 contains a number of general suggestions for finding a doctor who can help you. In addition, you need to ask some specific questions:

- Does this doctor treat other people with incontinence?
- Does he or she have an interest in treating incontinence?
- Is urodynamic testing available?
- Does this doctor or clinic offer a range of treatment options?

A qualified doctor, or a genuine incontinence clinic, should provide both *urodynamic testing* and *a range of treatment options,* including bladder training and biofeedback programs, as well as drugs and surgery. Ideally, a nurse or social worker should be on staff to answer questions and to give you additional information and support. If these specific services are not available, you need to look further.

Communicating Your Needs

Once you have found a doctor or clinic, you have to describe what is wrong. But many people find that communicating about the loss of bladder control to a complete stranger can be extremely difficult. Even people who have been with a doctor for many years often find it uncomfortable to discuss the subject of incontinence. Or, as often happens, people bring the subject up with their doctor, as Hillary did (page 42), only to have it shrugged off with a prescription, without either proper evaluation or information about potential treatments.

If you find it too difficult to discuss incontinence with a doctor, you might try talking to a nurse. *The HIP Report* (see Resources on page 97) suggests calling the nursing office of your local hospital and asking to speak to a nurse in urology, rehabilitation, or geriatrics, or to an enterostomal therapist.[9] Nurses in these specialties should know doctors or clinics in the area that treat people who have incontinence. They may be busy when you call, but if you leave your number someone will probably call you back. If you don't get a response in a couple of days, try again. When you do get someone on the phone, tell them that you are looking for a doctor or clinic that specializes in treating incontinence.

Your Medical History

Your medical history often provides vital clues to the underlying cause of incontinence and helps your doctor decide which tests are necessary. In taking your history, your doctor will be looking for information on:

- When you first experienced incontinence, even if it was many years ago.
- If you have a family history of incontinence.
- How often you experience urinary leakage.
- How much urine you lose each time.
- If you have difficulty in emptying your bladder completely.
- If you have any warning before leakage occurs.

- If you have noticed any pattern to leakage, especially regarding the time of day or night it is most likely to occur, or what kind of movement is most likely to precipitate urine loss.
- If urine loss is associated with taking certain drugs or eating or drinking certain foods.
- If you are using absorbent pads, what type you are using, how many a day you use, and how wet they usually are.
- What kinds of treatments you have tried, if any.
- What kinds of drugs, both prescription and over-the-counter, you are currently taking.
- Any surgery you have had, especially pelvic or back surgery.
- If you are female, how many vaginal births and/or Cesarean deliveries you have had, or whether you are post-menopausal.
- If you are male, if you have had any prostate problems in the past or if you are experiencing any symptoms of prostate enlargement (see page 197 for these symptoms).
- Whether you have had any radiation therapy or chemotherapy for cancer.

Voiding Chart

Your doctor may ask you to keep a voiding chart for up to a week, noting fluid intake, frequency of urination, output of urine each time you urinate, number of times you leak each day, how much you leaked, and what activity you were engaged in during leakage. This record alone can reveal a great deal about the cause of your incontinence and is thus extremely important. A sample voiding chart is included on pages 26–27. You can make photocopies of this chart and use them for your chart. If you go to your first appointment with a carefully kept voiding chart, you can save valuable time and aid in a speedy diagnosis.

THE TESTS NOTED HERE ARE DESCRIBED IN DETAIL IN THE INDEX OF DIAGNOSTIC TESTS, BEGINNING ON PAGE 278.

Physical Examination

Your doctor will do a thorough physical examination, including a vaginal examination for women and a rectal exam for men and women.

Laboratory Tests

Your examination will also include a *urinalysis,* a *culture and sensitivity test,* and a *urine test* to screen for bladder cancer. *Blood tests,* an *ultrasound exam,* or a *kidney X-ray* may be taken to detect kidney or other medical problems.

Bladder Stress Tests

If your doctor suspects that you have stress incontinence, he or she will want to observe how your leakage occurs in a test called a *full-bladder provocative stress test.* While you are lying down, a thin rubber tube, called a catheter, is inserted into the urethra and when the bladder is filled with sterile water the catheter is removed. Then you will be asked to cough. If you experience no leakage, you will be asked to stand and cough again. If no leakage occurs while you are standing and you have experienced incontinence at other times, other tests may be ordered.

Cotton Swab Test

If you have stress incontinence, it is usually because your bladder has slipped out of its normal position. A long-handled cotton swab is inserted into the urethra and the position of the handle provides a rough estimate of how much slippage has occurred.

Cystoscopy and Urethroscopy

Your doctor will look into your urethra and bladder with a long, thin instrument called a *cystoscope* to check their general condition and look for any problems. This exam will show if there is anything obstructing the urethra or any malformation that might cause inefficient emptying, or if there is infection, inflammation, or a tumor in the bladder.

Cystourethrogram

Another test for stress incontinence involves using a catheter to fill the bladder with a solution that shows up on an X-ray and taking an X-ray of the bladder while you are urinating in a standing position and straining to urinate. Also called an *incontinence cystogram,* this test shows how much abnormal slippage of the bladder neck (the area where the bladder and urethra join) occurs. It can also show how well the urethral sphincters function to prevent leakage. This test usually includes X-rays done while you are urinating (called a *voiding cystourethrogram*).

Urodynamic Studies

Urodynamic tests are designed to evaluate how the bladder and urethra function as the bladder fills, stores, and releases urine. The tests attempt to reproduce your symptoms and help determine what type of incontinence you have. These tests include:

- the *cystometrogram,* which shows how well the bladder stores urine as it fills and empties, whether the storage occurs at a normal pressure, and whether any abnormal contractions or increases in pressure occur;
- the *uroflow test,* which shows the speed and force of the urinary stream during voiding;
- the *urethral pressure profile,* which gives some idea of how well the urethral sphincter muscles function;
- the *electromyogram,* which measures the coordination between the bladder and the urethra and gives some idea of the tone of the sphincter muscles of the urethra;
- the *residual urine test,* which will show how much urine is left in the bladder after emptying.

Videourodynamics

If you have complicated incontinence, your doctor may want you to have this highly specialized test, which is usually available only at incontinence centers or major university teaching hospitals. This technique combines the visual capabilities of video technology with the urodynamic procedures described above, to provide instantaneous visualization of the urinary tract at the same time urodynamic tests are being done—kind of like a moving X-ray.

When Hillary saw Kristene for evaluation, she had most of the tests described above and it was confirmed that she had moderate (Type II) stress incontinence. Because her incontinence was moderate, Kristene thought that there was a good likelihood that she could be cured, or that her leakage could be improved dramatically with a program combining biofeedback and electrical stimulation. Hillary was very anxious to try the program. "I just thought there was no cure for leakage and that I was going to have to spend the rest of my life this way. I was willing to try anything!"

TREATMENT

Since incontinence is not a life-threatening condition, there is no compelling reason to begin treatment with heavy-duty drugs or surgery. For many people, incontinence can be improved significantly by simply going to the toilet on a regular schedule, by eliminating foods or liquids that irritate the bladder, by doing pelvic muscle exercises or a biofeedback program, by discontinuing or changing the dosage or the time drugs are taken. (Be sure to consult your doctor before changing or stopping any medication.) All drugs have side effects, some of which may be worse than the incontinence. For example, you may take a drug designed to tighten your sphincter muscle, only to find that it makes you feel nervous or jittery, raises your blood pressure, or causes urinary retention. Others may cause dry mouth. Yet when they are used correctly, drugs play an important role in treating incontinence.

Surgery can be very effective for certain people, literally freeing them from the "prison" imposed by severe incontinence, but incontinence support groups are filled with people who have failed surgery, not once, but numerous times. And any urological surgeon will point out to you—or should—that each succeeding surgery gets more difficult to perform. Given the problems and difficulties with drugs and surgery, the panel of experts convened by the National Institutes of Health for the Consensus Development Conference on Incontinence in 1988 recommended, "As a general rule, the least invasive or dangerous procedures should be tried first." This seems to be a very reasonable recommendation.

Changes in Diet

For urge or mixed incontinence

If you are suffering from incontinence, the first thing you should do is to check your daily food and liquid intake for possible dietary culprits. Many foods are known to precipitate or increase incontinence, especially urge incontinence where bladder irritation plays a significant role (doctors call this "sensory urge incontinence"). If you find any of the following classic bladder irritants listed below, you might try eliminating them from your diet for a few weeks and see if you improve:

- alcohol: liquor, wine, wine coolers, beer.
- caffeine: coffee, tea, dark sodas, some darker herb teas (including decaffeinated versions of all of these), chocolate, many cough medicines and other over-the-counter medications (check the labels).
- very acid fruit or fruit juices: orange, grapefruit, lemon, lime, mango, pineapple.
- tomatoes: tomato juice, red spaghetti sauce, pizza, barbecue sauces, chili.
- spicy foods: Mexican, Thai, Indian, Cajun, "southwest" cooking.
- milk products: milk, cheese, cottage cheese, yogurt, ice cream.
- sugar: corn sweeteners, honey, fructose, sucrose, lactose (these ingredients are added to many packaged foods).

Keeping a food diary for several days in conjunction with a voiding chart (see pages 26–27) might help you to see if there is a pattern to incontinence. Compare the two charts to see if you seem to have more frequent episodes of incontinence at a certain time of the day, i.e., after having two or three cups of coffee or after taking a morning diuretic. Or is incontinence worse after having a soda and cookies in the afternoon? If you can't see any distinct pattern, take your food diary and voiding chart to a nutritionist, nurse, or a doctor and ask if they can see things you might avoid. Anne Smith-Young, codirector of Continence Restored, points out that many people mistakenly believe that tea (hot or iced) has less caffeine than coffee. "In certain parts of the country, especially the South and the Midwest, iced tea is consumed in large quantities and people may be unaware that it can affect the bladder. In addition, iced tea is often sweetened with sugar. It's not clear what effect sugar has on the bladder, but it is excreted in the urine. Many people find that cutting out sugar reduces bladder irritability."

There are suitable substitutes for many of the above items: warm broth (watch the salt content of packaged varieties), herb tea, or cereal beverages instead of coffee; white chocolate instead of regular chocolate; low-acid tomatoes (check a seed catalog); grapes, apples, pears, and papayas instead of acid fruits.

Constipation is also one of the prominent transient causes of incontinence. As the rectum becomes impacted with stool, it's harder to use the urethral muscles. If you suffer from constipation, increasing fluid intake or using stool softeners or laxatives can help to regulate bowel function. In any event, a regular bowel regime is important for this and other health reasons.

Bladder Training

For urge, reflex, or overflow incontinence

For people who have unpredictable patterns of urination, caused by a hyperactive bladder muscle (urge incontinence), or those who urinate without any warning (reflex or overflow incontinence), bladder-training exercises can be quite effective. Bladder training focuses on establishing a predictable pattern of urination and "retraining" the bladder to adapt to this schedule. The basis for bladder training is the voiding chart (see sample on pages 26–27). Once the pattern can be observed—often in two or three days —bladder-training exercises can be instituted. Sometimes, the voiding chart alone can identify the cause of incontinence, showing that it typically occurs after taking medications such as diuretics, or after drinking coffee or alcoholic beverages. If there is no obvious cause of incontinence, your voiding chart will show the shortest interval between episodes of leakage, and bladder training can be instituted.

When Florence came to Kristene's office, she was diagnosed with urge incontinence. Her voiding chart showed that she could go for at least an hour and a half before having the urge to urinate. Kristene instructed her to use the toilet every hour and a half, whether she felt an urge or not. After three days, if she was able to maintain total dryness, she was told to add one half hour to each interval. After she was able to maintain three consecutive days without leakage, she was to add another half hour. Kristene also taught her to do pelvic muscle exercises, which were designed to help her suppress the urge when it occurred. With the combination of these techniques, Florence progressed very rapidly, adding one half hour each week. "In a little more than five weeks, I could go for four hours without having an accident. You can't imagine how happy I was with that. Now I can play nine holes of golf without fear of wetting my pants."

Timed Toileting

For reflex and overflow incontinence

Timed toileting is one very useful way to manage reflex and overflow incontinence, when urination occurs without any warning.

Reuben's daughter Helena brought him to see Kristene as a last resort before putting him into a nursing home. He was getting too frail to live alone, and he frequently leaked urine without warning. Helena had just had her house recarpeted and was afraid it would be ruined if Reuben moved in. Kristene discovered that Reuben had involuntary bladder contractions as the result of a mild stroke. Reuben's voiding chart showed that he could reliably go for two to three hours without having any leakage. She suggested trying a timed toileting program, which would help Reuben empty his bladder regularly before leakage occurred. She urged Helena to buy Reuben a watch that could be set to beep on the hour to help him remember to go to the toilet every two hours. Reuben was upset about the prospect of going to a nursing home, and was very motivated to make the timed toileting program work. He undertook the program himself for two weeks, and brought another voiding chart to Kristene which showed that he was having no accidents during the day. He began using snugly fitting rubber pants with an extra-absorbent gel pad at night and woke himself up around 2:00 a.m. to go to the toilet. Usually his pad was not wet.

This technique can be used either at home or in a nursing home. In Reuben's case, he was able to successfully carry out the program largely on his own. In cases where a person is more frail or forgetful, the help of a family member or nursing home attendant is absolutely essential for the program to be successful.

Pelvic Muscle Exercises/Kegel Exercises

For stress and urge incontinence

Exercises to strengthen the supporting muscles of the bladder and urethra after childbirth have been used in many cultures throughout history. In modern times—the late 1940s and early

1950s—Dr. Arnold Kegel (pronounced Kaý-gul), a respected Los Angeles gynecologist and professor at the University of Southern California School of Medicine, popularized these simple exercises to help women regain voluntary control over urination. Kegel initially began working with older women who suffered severe incontinence and was surprised when many reported not only a decrease in urinary leakage but dramatic improvements in sexual pleasure as well—some saying that they had experienced orgasm for the very first time. Kegel's advocacy of the technique was so enthusiastic that the exercises have come to bear his name. These are also called pelvic floor exercises, because they exercise the sling, or hammock, of muscles that serve as the "floor," or support, for the bladder, urethra, uterus, and other pelvic organs (see page 38 for a description of these muscles.)

The non-invasive nature of the exercises and the potential for restoring normal or near-normal bladder function is very appealing. If you are highly motivated, you can do the exercises on your own effectively and monitor your progress by keeping a chart of incontinent episodes. However, many people need considerable support and fairly intensive supervision to achieve results. Most people begin to see results in a few weeks, but for those whose muscles are extremely weak or who have moderate or extensive damage from childbirth or surgery, results may not be apparent for several months. These people tend to get discouraged and drop out before they make significant progress.

If you suffer from uncomplicated stress incontinence, and you can readily stop the flow of urine when you try, these exercises will probably help you a great deal. Strengthening your pelvic muscles can also help urge incontinence by enabling you to hold urine in the bladder until the urge passes so that you can then get to the toilet before leakage occurs.

Controversies Over Pelvic Muscle Exercises

Among practitioners who work with pelvic muscle exercises, there is considerable controversy about how many repetitions you ought to do, how long you need to hold each contraction, and how many times a day you need to do the exercises. The recommendation varies from "periodic exercise" to 400 contractions a day, holding each muscle contraction from 1 to 10 seconds.[10] Kegel himself advocated that the exercises be done for 20 minutes three times a day and recommended putting little reminder notes up in every part of the house.[11] Help for Incontinent People (HIP), Inc., recommends doing the exercises for 2 minutes three times a day, which should equal at least 100 repetitions.

Perhaps one of the reasons for the high failure rate of pelvic muscle exercises is that the recommended contraction time is far too short. If you hold each contraction for 4 seconds, that is probably all you will be able to hold it for when you sneeze or cough. Some practitioners now feel that contractions lasting 10 seconds or more are required to establish sufficient muscle strength.

How to Do Pelvic Muscle Exercises

In order to do pelvic muscle exercises, you must first identify the specific muscles that are responsible for stopping the flow of urine. You might want to refer to the description of these muscles and the illustration on pages 38–39 in Chapter 3 to help you visualize these muscles better. While sitting on the toilet, tighten your muscles and stop the flow of urine. If you can't stop it, try again. If your bladder empties very quickly and you run out of urine, wait until the next time you urinate and try again. If you have any muscle tone at all, and you are working the correct muscles, you should be able to stop the flow of urine. A common mistake both women and men make in doing the pelvic muscle exercises is tightening the abdominal, thigh, or buttock muscles instead of, or in addition to, tightening the muscles of the pelvic floor. Women can place a finger in the vagina and feel the muscles tighten around it, while keeping the other hand over the lower abdomen to ensure that it is relaxed. Your doctor or other practitioner can also help you identify the muscles by putting a finger in your vagina and asking you to tighten the muscles you would use to stop urination.

If you cannot stop the flow of urine, you still have a muscle, but it may be exceptionally weak and you will have to work a lot harder and considerably longer to get results. If this is the case, perhaps you might want to investigate one of the biofeedback techniques described below. Having established times to do the exercises is probably best. You can do them before you get out of bed in the morning. Then you can do them at some specific time during the day—say after lunch. And if you watch TV, you can do them during your favorite program.

HANDY GUIDE TO PELVIC MUSCLE EXERCISES*

1. *Identify the lower abdominal muscles.* Lying on the floor or bed, place your hand on your abdomen.
   - Cough. Notice that your hand moves.
   - Now tighten all of the muscles in your pelvis and the abdominal muscles. Your hand will move.
   - Now relax your muscles. When exercising the pelvic muscles, the abdominal muscles must be completely relaxed. Your hand should be perfectly still.
2. *Identify the pelvic muscles.*
   - Tighten the ring of muscles around the anus, as if you wanted to stop a bowel movement.
   - Tighten the ring of muscles around the vagina and urethra, as if you were going to stop the flow of urine. If you are not sure where these muscles are, practice while urinating, actually stopping the flow of urine. When you can stop the flow, keep it stopped for a few seconds. Stop and start the flow several times if you can.
3. *Do the basic pelvic muscle exercise.* Lying on the floor or bed, breathe deeply (don't hold your breath) and
   - Tighten the anal muscle, pulling inward and upward.
   - Tighten the vaginal muscle, pulling inward and upward.
   - Hold these muscles tight, slowly counting "one and two and three . . . ten," breathing deeply and evenly. Then relax.
   - Keep your hand on your abdomen and check to see that it is not moving while you are contracting the pelvic muscles.

   Do this exercise in "sets" of five to ten contractions at a time, several times a day. After doing the exercises for 3 or 4 weeks, increase the number of contractions in each set and hold each one longer, up to the count of ten. After you can comfortably hold the contractions for 10 seconds, you might consider gradually increasing the length up to 20 seconds.

   NOTE: You might want to photocopy this page and keep it in a convenient place.

* Adapted from *Pelvic Training Manual* and audio tape produced by HIP, Inc. The tape, which also provides a set of more advanced exercises, can be ordered for $6 from HIP, Inc., P.O. Box 544, Union, SC 29379.

Most practitioners focus only on the front part of the muscle, the part that encircles the vagina and urethra in women and the base of the penis and urethra in men. But the pelvic muscles encircle the anus as well. Tightening both muscles can help you get a stronger contraction and will offer the double benefit of improving the strength of your anal sphincter muscle as well. (Many older people who have urinary incontinence also suffer from fecal incontinence.)

Once you find that pelvic muscle exercises have cured or improved your incontinence, don't stop doing them. You should look at these exercises as a lifetime commitment to maintaining good muscle tone. *These are muscles that don't get exercised any other way,* except during sexual activity, and most people don't have sex often enough to keep these muscles in shape. Overall physical fitness may have some impact on the tone of your pelvic muscles, but because of their placement and specialized use, these muscles need special attention.

Vaginal Weight Lifting: Using Weighted Cones

For stress and urge incontinence (in women)

If you want to learn about muscle development, ask a body builder. They know better than anyone what you have to do to get the maximum performance out of a muscle. The principles of body building are simple. You progressively work out a muscle, gradually increasing the amount of weight you are using. If you work out regularly, the muscle will grow and become stronger.

This principle, which might be thought of as "pelvic weight lifting," has been applied to pelvic muscle training, utilizing a series of weighted plastic cones, weighing from 5 grams (about an ounce and a half) to 95 grams (about 2 pounds). The cones are inserted into the vagina like a tampon, and are kept in place while you walk around for 15 minutes, two times a day. If the cone is too light, it will stay without much effort and won't exercise anything. If it is too heavy, it will fall out (watch for bruised toes!). Therefore, your doctor must help you select the one that you should use at first. Cones could be a boon to those who have a tendency to "cheat" by using the wrong muscles—if the correct muscles aren't used, the cone will simply fall out.

In one English study, the cones were given to women who were waiting for incontinence surgery (which on England's overburdened National Health Service can take up to a year). To the great surprise of the doctors who did the study, and no doubt to the study participants as well, one half of the women were cured of incontinence before their surgery dates arrived.[12]

The cones are currently being studied by Dacomed, a company in Minneapolis that markets urological products. Dacomed plans to distribute the cones commercially upon approval by the Food and Drug Administration, but does not have an estimate of when they might be available.

Biofeedback

For stress and urge incontinence

Biofeedback makes use of electrical monitoring devices to record progress in exercises that condition or influence certain involuntary processes such as blood pressure or anxiety, as well as voluntary processes such as relaxation of muscle tension or improvement in muscle strength. In terms of bladder dysfunction, biofeedback machines monitor progress in strengthening the pelvic muscles. Some machines, which can be used only by women, have a sensing device like a little electronic tampon that is inserted directly into the vagina, where it can be in close contact with the pelvic muscles. Other machines have sensing devices that can be inserted into the rectum and may be used by men and women. Most machines have patches containing electrodes that are placed on the abdomen to make sure that the abdominal muscles are relaxed when you contract the pelvic muscles.

One of the biofeedback machines currently being promoted is the EMG "Perineometer."* This device consists of a vaginal probe that looks like a small, unequally weighted dumbbell about 3½ inches long and an electronic sensor box with a circle of lights on its face that light up in sequence to show the strength of muscular contractions. When you contract your pelvic muscles, the vaginal sensor monitors their strength and the lights on the box come on in sequence, showing you how well you are doing. The EMG device

---

* EMG stands for electromyograph, a machine that monitors and records muscle contractions. (See definition of electromyography in the Index of Diagnostic Tests).

also comes with a rectal probe that can be used by men, or by women who are unable to use the vaginal probe. The designers of the device report an astounding 98 percent cure (defined as "symptom-free") after an average of five weekly or bi-weekly office visits and twice daily use of the device at home. Long-term results are not yet available, and other practitioners have been unable to duplicate this extraordinary success rate. Because of the lack of convincing studies, many experts remain skeptical about the glowing success rates claimed by the device's promoters. More realistic figures probably range somewhere between 20 and 70 percent. But, even taking the rock-bottom figure of 20 percent, if that many people can avoid surgery by successfully completing a biofeedback program, then it is probably worth it for everybody to have a try.

In one biofeedback study conducted by Kathryn Burgio, a leading biofeedback researcher at the University of Pittsburgh School of Medicine, 82 percent of the participants experienced a reduction in stress incontinence.[13] Burgio did an identical study on men who had either urge or stress incontinence after prostate surgery. The men with urge incontinence had a decrease in leakage of 80 percent and those with stress incontinence had a 78 percent reduction in incontinent episodes. These statistics are difficult to duplicate, but some urologists with expertise in treating incontinence with biofeedback have observed at least a 55 percent improvement in people who completed such a course of treatment.

One of the drawbacks to biofeedback is that it generally requires a one-on-one supervision and is therefore fairly labor-intensive. It also requires that you find a clinic or therapist knowledgeable about the equipment and techniques required. Unless you are fairly well heeled, it requires that you have insurance that will pay for three or more months of training. You also have to have time to go to a clinic at least once a week. In addition, you have to be pretty motivated to keep up with the program and do your own exercises *twice a day, every day*. Nevertheless, for many people who complete biofeedback programs, the rewards can be enormous!

Combined Biofeedback and Electrical Stimulation

For stress and urge incontinence
Electrical stimulation of muscles, also called interferential therapy, has long been used by physical therapists to help return injured muscles to fitness, and it has received a recent surge in

popularity as a "passive" way to get exercise. When a low-grade electric current is applied to a specific muscle, the muscle will contract passively without any effort on your part. By gradually increasing the current, stronger contractions can be obtained, and eventually the muscle will become stronger. This type of "workout" is especially useful for people who have trouble identifying the pelvic muscles or whose muscles are extremely weak.

Currently several centers in the United States and Canada are participating in a study of the Physiostim, a device that combines biofeedback with electrical stimulation. To date, well over 10,000 women have used the Physiostim in Europe, and it has been reported that 75 percent of those who tried it experienced improvement or a cure. The Physiostim, manufactured by R. L. Medical, has a tampon-like vaginal probe for women and an anal probe for men that delivers pulsating low-grade electrical current to the pelvic muscles. In the ongoing studies, each treatment consists of about 10 minutes of biofeedback monitoring of pelvic muscle exercises and up to 20 minutes of electrical stimulation. The strength of your muscle contractions is recorded by a computer and displayed on a screen. The computer compares the strength of your contractions with the intensity of the desired contractions selected with the aid of a computerized program. As a part of the program, you are required to do 5 minutes of pelvic exercises twice daily at home during and after the treatment period that consists of two treatments a week for 4 weeks, followed by one treatment a week for 2 to 4 weeks.

These exercises and devices have an intriguing potential in the treatment of incontinence. For people who are good candidates for this type of treatment, they offer the possibility of a complete cure or significant improvement without any unwanted physical effects. And if you fail, you won't have lost anything but a little bit of time and the cost of the program.

Hillary, whose story introduced this chapter, had excellent success using pelvic muscle exercises and a combination of biofeedback and electrical stimulation. At first she did the exercises for about six weeks. By the end of that time, she was doing 15 contractions 5 times a day, holding each contraction for 5 seconds. Using only the exercises, she was able to prevent urinary leakage during her normal daily activities. For example, when she picked up her baby, she consciously contracted her pelvic muscles and was able to prevent leakage in most instances. She was unhappy, however, that she still experienced leakage when she played tennis. Kristene suspected that Hillary was having some trouble isolating her pelvic muscles, so she prescribed a combined program of biofeedback and electrical stimulation. Hillary came to the Incontinence Center for an hour twice a week for four weeks and then once a week for four more weeks. In each session, she inserted the sensor into her vagina for 20 minutes, and the stimulator contracted her pelvic muscles for her. Then she attempted to duplicate the activity of the stimulator, watching a computer screen, which showed her how much to contract her muscles and how long to hold each contraction. After two months she found that the strength of her pelvic muscles had improved enormously. "I still have some leakage, but the amount is much less and it occurs much less frequently," Hillary comments. "When I'm playing tennis, I just wear a pad that gels when it gets wet. Otherwise, I don't have to worry."

If you are diagnosed with Type I or II stress incontinence and your doctor recommends surgery, ask why biofeedback would not be effective for you. If your doctor says that it's not very effective and not worth trying, then you might consider getting a second opinion.

Drugs

If bladder training, exercises, or biofeedback techniques don't cure your incontinence or lessen it significantly, then there are a number of drugs that can be tried. There are drugs that can either increase or decrease the activity of the bladder muscle and there are drugs to increase the closure of the bladder's sphincters or relax them. Because of differing responses to various drugs, the dosage may have to be adjusted at first to find what will work and be tolerable for you. All of these drugs can have significant side effects and some may interact negatively with other drugs—either prescription or over-the-counter. There are also certain reasons, called "contraindications," why people with certain conditions should not take them, or should be carefully monitored by their doctors if they do. These conditions can cause serious problems if you take certain drugs, and in some rare instances even be fatal. So, it's important for you to be aware of what they are. The Drug

Glossary beginning on page 295 contains information on benefits, side effects, drug interactions, and contraindications for the drugs that are most commonly used for treating bladder disorders.

It is important to remember that drugs affect certain people very differently. Any one drug may cure one person, effect some improvement in another, and make still another person worse. Taking drugs, then, is really something of an experiment—to see if it will cure or cause improvement, or if it will make you worse, and to see if you can tolerate the side effects as well. Dr. Alan Wein, an acknowledged expert in the drugs used to treat urologic disorders, cautions that "a perfect result (restoration to normal status) is seldom achieved, even with the most rational pharmacologic [drug] therapy,"[14] implying that it is perhaps best not to look at any particular drug as a magic bullet, but rather as an aid to achieving continence.

One important fact to keep in mind about the drugs that are used for incontinence is that they only work for the time that they are taken, and the beneficial effects are likely to disappear when you stop taking them. Yet drugs can be very helpful in a variety of circumstances, and careful use of them can often provide temporary or long-term relief from incontinence. In the list of drugs given below, the generic name is given first and the brand names follow in parentheses. A detailed description of these drugs, including how they work and side effects, appears in the Drug Glossary.

Drugs to Improve Urine Storage

For urge and reflex incontinence

Propantheline bromide (Pro-banthine) and *glycopyrollate (Robinal)* help increase bladder capacity by suppressing involuntary contractions of the detrusor muscle.

Oxybutynin chloride (Ditropan), flavoxate hydrochloride (Urispas), hyoscyamine (Cystospaz), dicyclomine hydrochloride (Bentyl), and *Urised (a combination of drugs)* are smooth-muscle relaxants that help suppress uninhibited bladder contractions and may also decrease symptoms of frequency and urgency. Urised also has an anesthetic property.

Imipramine hydrochloride (Tofranil) is a tricyclic antidepressant that has been found to also inhibit bladder contractions and increase muscle tone in the urethra. The doses for incontinence are usually less than that given for depression.

Drugs to Improve Bladder Emptying

For overflow incontinence (to improve urine flow)
Prazosin hydrochloride (Minipress) and *terazosin hydrochloride (Hytrin)* block certain nerve receptors in the urethra to promote relaxation. They can help relax the smooth muscle of the bladder to increase urine storage.

Phenoxybenzamine (Dibenzyline) was formerly the drug of choice for relaxing the urethra, and it is quite effective. But since this drug has been found to cause stomach and bowel cancer in laboratory animals, prazosin is now preferred.

Drugs to Increase Sphincter Closure

For stress incontinence
Ephedrine and *pseudoephedrine (Sudafed and others)* can help tighten the sphincter muscles to help relieve mild stress incontinence.

Phenylpropanolamine hydrochloride (Dexatrim) is similar to ephedrine in action and is found in most over-the-counter diet pills. If this form of therapy is recommended, make sure that the drug you take contains no caffeine, since it provides unnecessary stimulation and may irritate your bladder.

Drugs to Relax Sphincter Muscle

For overflow incontinence
Diazepam (Valium) and *buspirone hydrochloride (Buspar)* are anti-anxiety agents occasionally used to relax the external sphincter muscle and the pelvic muscles in cases where partial urinary retention is caused by stress or muscle spasm. Withdrawal from these drugs should be gradual.

Hormonal Replacement Therapy (HRT)

For urge, stress, and overflow incontinence
In women, the urethra and, to a lesser extent, the bladder are "estrogen-dependent," that is, they require estrogen to function properly. Therefore, a reduced supply of estrogen is thought to be a factor in the development of both urge and stress incontinence and urinary retention. A number of studies have noted substantial

improvements in stress and urge incontinence, as well as in urinary urgency, frequency, and urinary retention, in women who take hormone replacement therapy, but these reports have been difficult to verify with urodynamic studies.[15] There are, however, many reports of improvement either by using vaginal estrogen or estrogen/progesterone cream, pills, or a small plastic patch impregnated with estrogen placed on the skin.

At this point, both the therapeutic function and the potential long-term effects of estrogen in treating incontinence remain highly controversial and many questions have still to be answered. However, if you have a history of breast cancer, uterine cancer, blood clots, or stroke among your close female relatives, you should probably avoid hormone replacement therapy if you have any other options. In any event, a yearly mammogram and PAP smear should be obtained both before and during hormonal replacement therapy. Before beginning hormone replacement therapy, you and your doctor should carefully assess your need for the drug, your medical history, and your physical condition. You might also want to do some reading on your own regarding HRT, before you decide to accept the potential risks.

Pessaries

Pessaries are vaginal inserts, similar in design to the diaphragm but heavier, which can be placed in the vagina to help support the bladder and uterus if they have slipped out of their normal positions. These simple devices were widely used before surgical techniques were developed to treat incontinence. They are still occasionally used today for women whose incontinence has not responded to treatment with exercises or drugs, but who cannot or do not want to have surgery.

Like a diaphragm, a pessary is fitted by a doctor. It can be left in place for several months, and should be removed and cleaned periodically. Women using pessaries need to be aware of the possibility of infection, and should be careful to note any unusual discharge or odor coming from the vagina. Kristene occasionally prescribes pessaries, but some of her patients have reported that their male partners can feel the device during intercourse and find it uncomfortable. Some pessaries are large and boxlike and actually prohibit intercourse. However, some are more compact (about the size of a diaphragm without the dome) and do not interfere with intercourse. Such devices may not present a problem for lesbians or women who are celibate.

If You Are Contemplating Surgery

Of all the treatments for incontinence, surgery is surely the most problematic. If you read medical articles, you will find spectacular success rates reported, usually in excess of 90 percent, and may well ask, "Why waste my time doing exercises for the rest of my life when I can be cured by surgery?" Those successes may be genuine, but they are achieved by highly skilled surgeons operating on highly selected patients. Of course, there are many competent surgeons across the country, but you need to assess their skills carefully. You might want to review Choosing a Surgeon on page 22 before you decide on surgery.

At the Consensus Development Conference in Washington, D.C., Dr. Stuart Stanton, a well-known British incontinence specialist, pointed out the difficulties even doctors have in evaluating studies on incontinence surgery.[16] Results, he noted, are usually based on patient questionnaires rather than on objective laboratory tests. The focus of the questionnaires is usually on the cure or decrease in stress incontinence symptoms, and questions about urge incontinence, frequency and urgency, or difficulties in urination that may manifest themselves for the first time after surgery are often not asked. Typically, follow-up time is less than one year.

One recent U.S. study tested women before having the modified Pereyra bladder neck suspension procedure for stress incontinence and followed them for three to four years—much longer than most other reports.[17] The study found that *only 50 percent of the women in the study were completely continent.* An additional 25 percent were improved and relatively happy with their improvement. In addition to the longer follow-ups of this study, two very significant points are noted: One is that at least 25 percent of the women studied developed incontinence at least two years *after* surgery; and the other is that quite a few women also developed urinary urgency after the surgery. This is a far cry from the 90 percent success rates reported by most surgeons. Other studies have also found that about half of the women who have surgery for stess incontinence cannot empty the bladder completely for some time afterward (usually because of too much correction) and have to empty the bladder mechanically with self-catheterization. (See page 87 for information on this procedure.)

In her own practice, Kristene teaches some of her patients to do self-catheterization *before* the decision for surgery is firmly made, so that they can better assess whether they are willing to accept the risk of having to empty the bladder mechanically on a permanent basis. If your surgeon does not offer to teach you how to catheterize yourself, you should at least discuss the issue carefully before you proceed with surgery.

Guidelines for Surgery

Kristene has some general guidelines that she uses to help determine if surgery is warranted. She looks at the severity of the symptoms, noting the number of episodes of incontinence per day, number of pads or undergarments used each day, and the degree to which they are saturated before changing them. Most important, she wants to know what kind of impact these symptoms have had on the quality of a patient's life. In evaluating test results, she reviews the outcome of urodynamic studies, bladder X-rays, and cystoscopy to see what type of incontinence you have and how severe it is. She wants to know if the incontinence experienced during urodynamic tests is similar to what you might normally experience. She also wants to know if you have failed non-surgical forms of therapy and if you have had previous incontinence surgery or other pelvic surgeries. Finally, she needs to evaluate whether you are healthy enough to undergo anesthesia and the physical stresses of surgery. Like many other urologists, Kristene feels that you should not undertake surgery until all of these factors have been considered and, generally, until other, less invasive remedies have been tried.

Bladder Neck Suspension Procedures

For stress incontinence

Although there are a number of different surgeries for stress incontinence, they are all variations on a single theme: lifting the urethra and the bladder neck (the place where the bladder and urethra join) as close to their original positions as possible to prevent slippage during straining or sudden movement. The procedures noted below accomplish this goal in a variety of ways.

Of all the procedures that are commonly used, Kristene prefers *the modified Pereyra* (pronounced pa-ref-ra) *bladder neck suspension.* She finds that operations for stress incontinence such as this one that are done through the vagina (as opposed to an abdominal incision) are preferable, because they are easier to do, have a shorter hospitalization, and if done properly, have a good success rate.

In the modified Pereyra procedure, an incision is made in the vagina and a surgical string, or suture, is placed at each side of the urethra at the neck of the bladder. The ends of the string are then pulled up through a separate small incision in the lower abdomen above the pubic bone. The two strands are adjusted, lifting the bladder neck to a more normal position; the strands are then tied over the abdominal muscles. Finally, your surgeon will look inside the bladder with a cystoscope to make sure that the stitches have not pierced the bladder wall, that the bladder neck is in the desired position (see illustration), and that there is no obstruction of the ureters.

After adequate healing (several days to several weeks), the bladder begins to function normally. The most common complication of this procedure, which usually occurs in the first six months after surgery, is the failure of the suspension threads to hold. If only one breaks or comes loose, continence may be maintained or it may not. If both strands come loose, incontinence generally returns.

For a long time, the *Marshall-Marchetti-Kranz (MMK) procedure* and the slightly different *Burch variation* were the favored bladder neck suspension procedures. Many surgeons still prefer these procedures because they are done entirely through an abdominal incision, which provides easier access to the tissues that they need to work on. Suspension of the bladder neck is accomplished by making an incision above the pubic bone and sewing the tissue surrounding the bladder neck to the fascia—strong fibrous tissue in the space behind the pubic bone near the bladder—or to the outer covering of the pubic bone itself. The MMK procedure is also often used when operations that utilize the vaginal approach have failed.

The most common problem with the MMK and Burch procedures is scarring around the urethra, which, over time, may cause it to function inefficiently. After surgery, you can expect to be in the hospital for about five days and can usually go back to work in

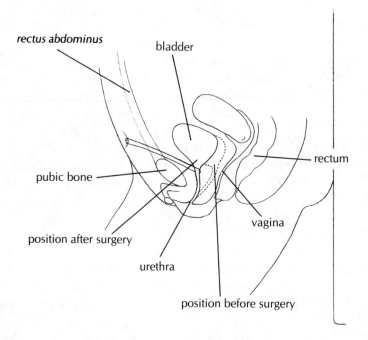

rectus abdominus

bladder

rectum

pubic bone

position after surgery

vagina

urethra

position before surgery

8. Surgery for stress incontinence. From an incision in the abdomen, stitches are run through the abdominal muscles and connective tissue that surrounds the urethra and brought up on the other side. A vaginal incision allows the surgeon to locate the position for the stitches and to guide the needle with his or her finger. The stitches encircling the urethra are pulled taut and are anchored just below the surface of the skin in the tissue of the abdominal muscles.

about three weeks, with some limitations on lifting for a few months.

Cystocele Repair

A cystocele occurs when the vaginal muscles are weakened and a portion of the bladder presses against the vaginal wall, forming a little pouch (see illustration on page 53). The main problem with a cystocele is that urine tends to get trapped in the pouch, where it can stagnate and become infected. If you are going to have a bladder neck suspension operation, and have a significant cystocele, it generally needs to be repaired at the same time to prevent urinary retention. The cystocele repair is done by bringing the fascia (connective tissue) of the muscles that lie on each side of the bladder together and sewing it securely so the bladder no longer protrudes into the vagina.

Surgery for Severe Stress Incontinence

Repair of severe (Type III) stress urinary incontinence requires more extensive surgery than for Types I and II, because regardless of which position the urethra is in, it is frequently non-functional. In addition, there is usually abundant scar tissue present, causing the tissues around the urethra to be stiff and difficult to work with.

With *sling procedures,* a piece of connective tissue, muscle, vaginal wall, or synthetic material is used to form a sling to compress the urethra. This will place the urethra in a more normal position and will also help keep it closed when the bladder is filling. Such surgery is often successful in preventing incontinence, but from 5 to 20 percent of women who have it may have to catheterize themselves because they cannot empty their bladders completely. (See information on self-catheterization on page 87.)

Many men suffer from severe incontinence following surgery to remove benign prostate enlargement or a radical prostatectomy to remove a cancer of the prostate. If non-surgical therapy fails, most doctors will recommend the insertion of an *artificial sphincter,* made by American Medical Systems. The AMS 800 Sphincter, the device that is currently in use, consists of three parts: (1) a balloon-like reservoir that is surgically implanted under the muscle tissue adjacent to the bladder; (2) a pump with a release mechanism that is placed in the scrotum; and (3) a soft, inflatable silicone cuff that encircles the mid-portion of the urethra. While the bladder is filling, the cuff is filled with fluid, which causes it to compress the urethra. The cuff and the reservoir are connected by surgical tubing. When you want to urinate, you press the pump located in the scrotum and the fluid drains out of the cuff and into the reservoir, allowing the urethra to open and the urine to drain. The fluid water is transferred back into the cuff over a three- to four-minute period and the urethra again closes.

To date, about 5,000 artificial sphincters have been implanted. Doctors implanting the devices report that between 75 and 85 percent of their patients are "satisfied" with the procedure. In about 10 to 15 percent of the men who have an artificial sphincter implanted, mechanical failures and tissue degeneration in the area of the implants have occurred. Like most mechanical devices, the artificial sphincter may break or wear out after a while and may need to be replaced; so before you decide to get a sphincter implanted, you should be aware that you may need a second surgery to remove or replace it. An artificial sphincter has also been designed for women and children, with the pump placed in the genital area underneath the large lips *(labia)*. Because of its close location to the sexual organs and urethra, this procedure should only be considered in carefully selected cases and should only be done by a surgeon with a great deal of expertise in implanting the device.

Teflon or Collagen Injections to Compress the Urethra

Another method to aid in the closing of a non-functioning urethra, used primarily in women, is the injection of Teflon (yes, it's the same stuff that covers non-stick pans) or collagen, the fibrous part of connective tissue, into the tissue surrounding the urethra. This procedure is often done when the urethra has been damaged by prior surgeries for stress incontinence, by scar tissue caused by infection, or by radiation treatments for cancer. The injections take about half an hour and can be done under a local anesthetic with intravenous sedation. About 60 percent of people require several injections, which are done several months apart.

The most common complications of Teflon injections are urinary retention, urethral erosion through contact with the Teflon, infection, and the migration of the Teflon particles to lymph nodes in other parts of the body, raising the possibility of adverse reactions and the development of tumors.

Collagen, fibrous protein material derived from cowhide, has recently been tried as a substitute for Teflon, but its use is still investigational. The potential advantages of collagen over Teflon are that the procedure can be done under local anesthesia, thus is less risky, and that the particles do not tend to migrate, as the Teflon particles sometimes do. Because of these advantages, there is a great deal of research interest in this form of treatment.

One possible disadvantage is that collagen tends to be absorbed by the body and repeated injections are often necessary, sometimes within six months. In addition, some people have immune systems that may identify the collagen as a foreign substance, produce antibodies, and possibly develop a skin rash near the site of the injections.

This treatment is most suitable for elderly people who have had several unsuccessful surgical procedures to correct incontinence; people who have had radiation therapy for cancer in the pelvic area; or people who are too frail to undergo the rigors of extensive surgery.

Urinary Diversion

In certain rare circumstances, when incontinence is very severe and has become an intolerable burden, the problem may be solved with a *continent reservoir,* by diverting the urine from the bladder to an artificially constructed reservoir in the abdomen with an outlet called a *stoma* on the skin of the lower abdomen. The urine collects in the reservoir and you have to empty it by inserting a catheter through the stoma four to six times a day. In another version of this procedure, the urine drains continuously through an artificially constructed tube of bowel through a stoma into a plastic pouch attached to your abdomen. This procedure, called an ileal conduit, is discussed in detail on page 167.

Long-term catheterization often causes the urethral tissues to wither or the sphincter muscle to stretch, causing leakage around the catheter. *A permanent suprapubic tube with closure of the bladder neck* may be the method to avoid this. In order to maintain dryness, the catheter is removed and the bladder neck is sewn shut. Then a permanent catheter, called a suprapubic tube (meaning *above the pubic bone*), is run from the bladder through the abdominal skin near the pubic bone. The end of the tube that is in the bladder has a balloon (similar to the Foley catheter) or a tip that is shaped like a mushroom so it will not easily pull out. The urine runs out into a drainage bag. The disadvantages of a suprapubic tube are infection and irritation around the tube; and if you are not careful, the tube can be pulled out.

People with severe reflex incontinence, scarring, or fibrosis in the bladder wall may only be able to accommodate small amounts of urine at a time and may have to urinate very frequently. If all else fails, *bladder augmentation,* in which the bladder is enlarged or "augmented" with a piece of intestine, can be done. The main risk of this procedure is the potential necessity of permanent self-catheterization. This procedure is discussed in more detail on page 87.

INCONTINENCE IN NURSING HOMES

Today, there are more than 1 million people in nursing homes, and more than half of them are incontinent. In fact, incontinence is the main reason for admission to a nursing home in at least 20 percent of cases. Because of staff shortages and the overall lack of training, many nursing homes rely on diapering and catheterization, which can foster dependence and loss of self-esteem, which in turn contribute to depression and possibly a rapid decline. Unfortunately, the remedies that could help the most—timed toileting, bladder training, pelvic muscle exercises, and biofeedback/electrical stimulation programs—are time-consuming and relatively expensive when done correctly, and are therefore not often implemented. At as much as $2 a day, diapering is exceedingly expensive also.

Catheterization

If urine cannot be emptied from the bladder voluntarily, it can be drained mechanically by insertion of one end of a small rubber tube—called a catheter—into the bladder. The other end of the tube is attached to a plastic bag that is strapped around the leg to collect the urine as it constantly drains. Catheters are routinely used during and after surgery on the bladder and prostate and other types of surgery as well. This type of short-term catheterization is usually not very uncomfortable and there is little risk associated with its use.

Hospitals and nursing homes rely heavily on the use of long-term (also called indwelling) catheters, which offer some measure of independence but may lead to repeated infections. The Foley catheter (see illustration) is the type that is almost universally used for this purpose. The Foley has two channels, one for the outflow of urine and one with a balloon on the interior end that is inflated once it is inserted to keep the tube from slipping out. Urine drains continuously into a plastic bag attached to the leg.

The primary risks of long-term catheterization are urinary tract infections and damage to the urethra. Because of the necessity of using a leg bag, certain types of activities may be limited.

It has been estimated that up to 90 percent of indwelling catheters are unnecessary. If one is prescribed for you or a family mem-

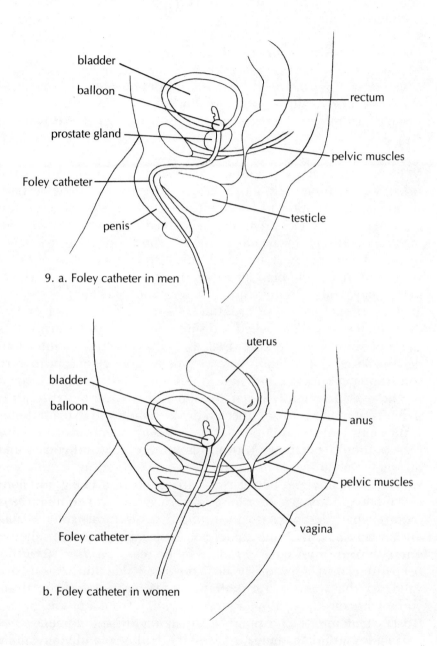

bladder
balloon
prostate gland
Foley catheter
penis
rectum
pelvic muscles
testicle

9. a. Foley catheter in men

uterus
bladder
balloon
anus
pelvic muscles
vagina
Foley catheter

b. Foley catheter in women

9. a. **Foley catheter in men.** b. **Foley catheter in women.** A Foley catheter, with a balloon on its tip, is inserted into the bladder. The inflated balloon prevents the catheter from slipping out. Urine drains continuously.

ber, ask why it is necessary. The accepted medical indications for catheterization are:

- when there is an otherwise untreatable blockage of urine;
- when there is an acute illness such as heart failure;
- when the physician needs to monitor fluid output before or after an operation or during a severe illness;
- when incontinence is exacerbating pressure sores that will not heal.

The use of a catheter in other circumstances presents substantial risks. For example, for a person who already has some urinary frequency in addition to leakage caused by an unstable bladder, inserting a catheter can irritate the bladder even further and make it contract even more. When the bladder is irritated, urinary frequency will increase, the bladder will hold a lower volume of urine, and bladder spasms might also occur. In this case, urine may leak around the catheter, and leakage may occur anyway. If spasms are severe, the balloon on the interior end of the catheter may be expelled, causing damage to the urethra. Because of these considerable risks, as well as the risk of infection, doctors should be hesitant to prescribe a catheter except in very compelling circumstances.

The most frequently given "reason" for the use of catheters is that incontinence is to be expected in old people and that a catheter is the only available solution. If your doctor mentions the above reason, then the catheter is probably unnecessary and you should do what you can to see if alternatives can be used instead. If you yourself—or a friend or relative—are faced with being admitted to a nursing home or other long-term-care facility, you might first inquire what the policy is concerning the use of catheters. If you are already in a nursing home, you or a family member should question your physician carefully as to the reason your catheter has been prescribed. If you are not convinced that the reasons are valid, ask that the catheter be removed. If this request is refused, you might consider getting a second opinion from a physician you trust or look into the possibility of changing nursing homes.

If an indwelling catheter is necessary, both you and your family members need to learn about the care and use of the leg bag which collects urine as it drains from the catheter. Essentially, the bag must be emptied several times a day, cleansed periodically, and should be replaced every three to six weeks under normal circumstances.

Intermittent Self-Catheterization

For people who are unable to empty their bladders normally because of disease or injury, intermittent self-catheterization is the most desirable alternative. It can also be useful on a temporary basis after certain types of surgery until bladder muscle tone and sensation return to normal. Most people can learn the technique and do the procedure on their own, provided they have adequate eyesight, manual dexterity, and no significant mental impairment —even children can be taught to catheterize themselves by the age of six or seven. Young or old, doing self-catheterization provides a measure of independence for those who would otherwise have to rely on the help of family members or nursing home personnel every time they need to empty their bladders. Many urologists have someone in their office who teaches patients how to do self-catheterization; many rehabilitation centers teach it as well. Although there are some variations in how the technique is taught, the basic instructions are quite similar.

Procedures for Emptying Retained Urine

Urinary retention—the inability to empty urine from the bladder completely—is the flip side of incontinence. Temporary or permanent retention often occurs after surgery, and may also be caused by prostate enlargement or scarring of the urethra from surgical procedures. Retention also occurs in some people who have interstitial cystitis, urethral syndrome, and prostatodynia. Often, indwelling catheters are used to treat urinary retention, but there are also several simple non-invasive techniques that you might want to try before you resort to invasive measures.

The *Credé maneuver* is one technique to help empty the bladder. After as much urine as possible has drained from the bladder, place your thumbs at the edge of each hip bone and spread your hands over the lower abdomen just above the pubic bone, with the fingers touching or slightly overlapped at the end. Then press firmly on the bladder. You should avoid additional straining with your abdominal muscles, since this will force the bladder upward, counteracting the force of the downward pressure. Two variations of the two-handed Credé maneuver are the closed-hand method, using one fist instead of two hands, or using a rolled-up towel to apply external pressure to the bladder.

The *Valsalva maneuver* is another widely used method of voiding retained urine. While sitting on the toilet, bend forward until your abdomen is resting on your thighs, and strain. Like the Credé maneuver, the Valsalva mechanically exerts increased pressure on the bladder, and if there is not too much urethral obstruction, retained urine can be voided.

Double voiding is yet another simple and often-used technique to increase bladder emptying. After you finish urination, wait several minutes, keeping your pelvic muscles relaxed, and attempt to void again. This procedure works for many people whose sphincter muscles don't relax readily.

If urine backs up into your kidneys (vesicoureteral reflux), your doctor may recommend that you avoid using either the Credé or Valsalva maneuver. These procedures increase pressure all over the bladder, and urine could be pushed up into the ureters. In this case, double voiding is more effective and safer.

CHILDHOOD INCONTINENCE (ENURESIS)

Because we set such a high priority on toilet training, many children experience enormous guilt, even at the tender age of three or four, whenever they lose control. By the time children reach the age of three, parents are anxious to be done with diapers and clammy bedclothes and children are expected to have achieved control over their bladders. Yet some amount of bedwetting and occasional daytime incontinence ought to be considered normal at least through age six, and for some children, even beyond that. For older children, the humiliation of a daytime accident or wet sheets at a friend's house can be intense, resulting in feelings of inadequacy, low self-esteem, and a poor body image. The anger or frustration of parents and insensitive teasing by siblings and peers can reinforce these feelings, causing painful emotional conflicts in an incontinent child.

After the age of six, incontinence becomes a social issue for both the child and the parents, and soiled mattresses, wet sheets and pajamas, and the ever-present smell of urine become a burden to the household. By this time, children can understand the consequences of incontinence, both for themselves and for others, and may be very motivated to stop involuntary wetting. Parents are motivated too, but they are often at a loss as to how to deal with repetitive episodes of wetness.

Who Wets the Bed?

After two or three years of age, the number of children who have daytime "accidents" and wet the bed decreases sharply until age six, when only about 10 percent still wet on a regular basis. Each year about 15 percent of these achieve continence, until age fifteen, when 1 to 3 percent still have some problems. For some unknown reason, boys are twice as likely as girls to suffer from enuresis. Overall, 5 to 7 million children between the ages of six and eighteen have some amount of incontinence, and unless they receive help, may carry this trait into adulthood.

Myths About Bedwetting

The most enduring myth about bedwetting is that it is essentially a psychological problem. It is also widely believed that it is the result of a sleep disorder, occurring when children sleep too deeply. While it is true that many children sleep so soundly that they fail to respond to signals from the bladder, it now appears that deep sleep is not the underlying cause for the vast majority of children. Many people also erroneously believe that there is no effective treatment for bedwetting and that waiting until the problem eventually resolves itself is the only prudent approach. But quite the opposite is true. Several approaches to treatment have been developed, including behavior modification, hypnosis, nightly waking, wetness alarms, and medications. Information on these techniques, some of which are highly effective, will be provided in the section on Treatment for Bedwetting.

Why Do Children Wet the Bed?

The causes of enuresis can be separated into two categories: *primary bedwetting*, in which the child has never achieved dry periods, and *secondary bedwetting*, when he or she has had periods of continence. In primary bedwetting, the overriding cause is most likely a lag in development of the central nervous system, whereas in secondary bedwetting, there is an identifiable medical or psychological condition that is causing incontinence. About 90 percent of the children who have problems with bedwetting have the primary type. Often these children's bodies simply mature faster than their bladders and the nerves that are connected to it. The bladder may be small, overactive, or irritable, causing frequent urination. Or the urge to urinate may simply not be as noticeable for some children as it should be. The remaining 10 percent of bedwetters have secondary enuresis, in which there may be extended periods of dryness, with reversion to wetting because of psychological stresses or certain medical conditions.

If daytime incontinence is a persistent problem, a complete evaluation of the urinary tract (see page 291) is recommended to make sure that there is no abnormality of the kidneys, ureters, or bladder, and to detect neurological problems. Food allergies, which are the cause of numerous childhood afflictions, may also be the cause of enuresis in some cases.

Although bedwetting usually does not cause serious medical problems, parents, having nowhere else to turn, frequently consult a pediatrician. If you do seek medical help, your child will probably be given a number of tests, but they usually turn out negative. NOTE: *Elaborate tests such as kidney and bladder X-rays, voiding studies (urodynamics), and cystoscopy should only be performed when there is a suspected urological abnormality based on the child's medical history, physical examination, and urine tests.* If your pediatrician thinks there is a need for these tests, he or she will probably recommend that you see a pediatric urologist. If you do consult a specialist, make sure that he or she explains the necessity of such tests to your satisfaction.

Treatment for Bedwetting

Since most bedwetting resolves spontaneously at some point, many pediatricians advise parents to take a wait-and-see approach. Nevertheless, if the parents are quite upset, or the child is very unhappy, some physicians may feel pressured into a solution and opt for *drug treatment.*

The primary drugs used to treat enuresis are oxybutynin chloride (Ditropan) and imipramine (Tofranil), an antidepressant. Both of these drugs are used to treat adult incontinence. In addition to elevating mood, imipramine blocks certain nerve impulses and decreases irritable bladder symptoms. Many children don't like to take drugs, however, especially over the long term, and even at low doses some may experience disagreeable side effects, especially urinary retention. Ditropan comes in a liquid form, which might be more palatable. Imipramine may greatly reduce or entirely eliminate incontinence, but it will do nothing toward "curing" the condition. A small percentage of children, perhaps 5 to 10 percent, may benefit from the drug, but most will wet the bed again as soon as the drug is stopped—often worse than before. For these reasons, drug treatment of bedwetting is not the treatment of choice, except when other treatments have failed.

A newer form of drug treatment is to use DDAVP (a synthetic hormone that decreases urine production by the kidneys) before bed. Side effects appear to be minimal and significant improvement has been seen in children who have taken the drug; but, as with most drug therapies, symptoms return after the drug is discontinued.

In the absence of a ready cure for bedwetting, there are also several non-medical remedies that have been employed more or less successfully by parents and children, under the term *behavioral therapy:* bladder retraining, alarm clocks to wake the child at night, wetness alarms, behavior modification, and hypnosis. But until recently these techniques have not been employed to cure bedwetting in any systematic way. Several years ago, Dr. Martin Scharf, a sleep clinician at Mercy Hospital of Hamilton/Fairfield in Cincinnati, Ohio, treated and cured an eighteen-year-old woman who had been a bedwetter all of her life. After this success, Scharf researched the conventional therapies used for bedwetting and began developing a practical supportive program, focusing on children who had failed other treatments. Scharf was amazed at the number of children who responded who had not succeeded elsewhere, and began writing a book on the subject.

The treatment plan recommended by Scharf in his popular book *Waking Up Dry* is a highly structured, goal-oriented program that requires the full cooperation of the child, as well as a lot of hard work and patience from parents, brothers and sisters, and other family members.[18] The program focuses on helping children become more aware of the need to urinate, increasing the child's bladder capacity, and strengthening the sphincter muscle to increase voluntary control. Even working with difficult cases, Dr. Scharf reports a 91 percent success rate.

COMPONENTS OF A PROGRAM TO END BEDWETTING*

- *a voiding chart,* designed to identify a pattern in bedwetting and daytime incontinence;
- *a dietary chart,* useful in identifying bladder irritants in meals and snacks such as milk products, chocolate, caffeinated sodas, highly salted foods, etc.;
- *measurement of bladder capacity,* to determine if the capacity is below normal, and to monitor progress;
- *bladder-stretching exercises* to increase bladder capacity. Once a day, the child is asked to hold his or her urine as long as possible. This exercise is timed and progress is recorded on a chart. Capacity can usually be increased by about 1 ounce a month;
- *midstream interruption exercises,* designed to strengthen the sphincter muscle;
- *a wetness alarm,* a fluid-sensitive bed pad or underpants attached to an alarm that will go off when the pad is wet. This can help improve a child's responsiveness to bladder signals at night;†
- *paired-association exercises,* practicing interrupting urination in response to a wetness alarm;
- *visualization,* conditioning and reinforcing bladder control.

* Adapted from Martin B. Scharf, *Waking Up Dry* (Cincinnati: Writer's Digest Books, 1986).
† A number of different models of wetness alarms are listed in the HIP *Resource Guide of Continence Products and Services,* P.O. Box 544, Union, SC 29739.

A study done at Johns Hopkins University[19] has shown that 30 percent of children will achieve continence just by doing the midstream interruption and bladder-stretching exercises. About 60 percent, however, appear to need the full program and most achieve continence in about three months.

Waking Up Dry takes you through every step of the program, providing information on how to support and motivate your child and what to expect at each stage of treatment. As this successful program indicates, children and parents do not need to suffer indefinitely from bedwetting. In most cases, the chances for a cure or significant improvement are very high and should be well worth the effort.

HOW TO STAY OUT OF THE UROLOGIST'S OFFICE

The surest preventive measures you can take to lessen the chances of becoming incontinent are to stay in excellent physical and mental condition and to do your pelvic muscle exercises several times a day—*always!*

Some childbirth educators have pointed out that the standard recommendation of beginning to exercise the pelvic muscles just six weeks before the anticipated due date is useless for many women. Presumably, these exercises are initiated late so prospective mothers won't get tired of doing them. But six weeks may not be nearly long enough to establish good muscle tone. To make sure your pelvic muscles are in excellent shape, you might consider initiating pelvic muscle exercises at least three months prior to expected delivery and continue for at least that long afterward. One reason it is a good idea to begin your exercises early is that if your delivery date is miscalculated, or you deliver, say, three weeks early, then you will have only done these essential exercises for three weeks—hardly enough time to put your pelvic muscles in tip-top condition to meet their biggest challenge.

Since hysterectomy has been identified as a significant cause of incontinence, unnecessary hysterectomies should be avoided. If a hysterectomy is recommended to you, ask your surgeon to justify his or her recommendation, and then get a second opinion.

One of the causes of incontinence in the elderly is the overuse of catheters in nursing homes. If you are in a nursing home, or are the primary caregiver of someone who is, make sure the catheter is medically indicated (see page 86).

If incontinence has become a significant factor in your life and is preventing you from being active, you should now be more confident about asking for help. In spite of the fact that many doctors are not informed about the causes, diagnosis, and treatment of involuntary urine loss, there are many excellent doctors who *do* understand it and know how to help you. If you have already had several treatments for incontinence, reading this chapter may have given you some clues as to why your treatment might have failed and you might be encouraged to try a new one. Coupled with the information in Chapter 2 on becoming more assertive about your medical needs and finding a good doctor, you should now be ready to take some positive action! The first thing you might do is to contact one or more of the excellent educational organizations that provide information and advice on incontinence.

EDUCATIONAL ORGANIZATIONS AND SELF-HELP GROUPS

Help for Incontinent People (HIP), Inc.

In the 1960s, Dr. Katherine Jeter worked with people who have ostomies, artificially constructed outlets for bodily wastes. Dr. Jeter found that working with children who have loss of bowel and bladder control because of birth defects gave her a special appreciation for the limitations that can be imposed by both urinary and fecal incontinence. In 1981 she decided to publish an incontinence newsletter and founded Help for Incontinent People (HIP), Inc., in Union, South Carolina. The next year, a mention of HIP, Inc., appeared in the "Dear Abby" advice column. "In one day, 19,000 letters came in," Jeter recalls. "In six weeks, we had twice that many." Later, an Ann Landers column brought 60,000 letters. The people of Union pitched in to handle the unanticipated crunch of mail. A local company donated an electric letter opener and a church opened its doors to a group of volunteers, many of them senior citizens. "Thanks to them, we answered every letter," Jeter reports.

Today, HIP has two full-time paid staff members, one part-time worker, and two volunteers, and the newsletter has an active mailing list of nearly 50,000. HIP, Inc., also provides an audio tape of how to do pelvic muscle exercises to improve continence and has an exhaustive catalog of absorbent products, garments, and devices that can help make life easier if you are coping with urine loss. Jeter, who has a doctorate in counseling and human development, organized the National Agenda to Promote Urinary Continence in 1983—a meeting devoted to identifying the most pressing problems associated with incontinence and to encouraging health professionals to address these issues. She now travels widely, talking about incontinence to public forums, professional conferences, doctors, and other health providers. "The people on our mailing list are only the tip of the iceberg," says Dr. Jeter. "We need to reach so many more."

You can write to HIP, Inc., at P.O. Box 544, Union, SC 29379 or call (803) 579-7900. The organization provides *The HIP Report,* a quarterly newsletter; an audio tape and booklet on pelvic muscle exercises; a ½" VHS video entitled *Incontinence: Cure and Comfort;* and a *Resource Guide of Continence Products and Services,* a comprehensive catalog of incontinence devices and absorbent products, plus about twenty-five articles on various aspects of incontinence reprinted from *The HIP Report.*

The Simon Foundation for Continence

In the late 1970s, Cheryle Gartley had embarked on a promising career in banking. But her advancement was interrupted by a mysterious spinal tumor that was difficult to diagnose and treat, which caused many problems including incontinence. Her doctors didn't have any solutions for her incontinence and there were no self-help organizations to turn to, so she researched the subject on her own and found that there were answers to many of her questions. Gartley gave up banking and started an educational organization, the Simon Foundation for Continence. "I wanted to see that other people didn't have to go through the same struggle I went through to find information and help," she says.

The Simon Foundation struck a raw nerve when it was mentioned in Ann Landers' column in 1983: in one day, 20,000 letters flooded in. The foundation's office, in Wilmette, Illinois, is staffed by a roster of dedicated volunteers. Gartley travels the world, attending conferences and lecturing on incontinence. You can write to the Simon Foundation at P.O. Box 835, Wilmette, IL 60091 or call 1-800-23S-IMON. The organization distributes *Managing Incontinence: A Guide to Living with the Loss of Bladder Control,* edited by Cheryle B. Gartley. This book, the first devoted entirely to the subject of incontinence, is filled with frank, inspirational personal accounts about triumphs and disasters in dealing with the problem. The Simon Foundation also provides a quarterly newsletter, called *The Informer,* a reprint series, a video/film entitled *The Solution Starts with You,* detailed information on organizing local support groups called "I Will Manage," and a set of seven videos by Dr. John C. Brocklehurst, a well-known British incontinence specialist, intended for medical professionals.

Continence Restored, Inc.

After attending the National Agenda to Promote Urinary Continence in 1984, Dr. E. Douglas Whitehead, a New York urologist, and Anne Smith-Young, a certified urology technician, formed Continence Restored, Inc., a national organization dedicated to disseminating information on bladder control and to providing support to people who have incontinence, to their families and friends, as well as to medical manufacturers and pharmaceutical firms. The organization also encourages and promotes the formation of a growing network of Continence Restored support groups throughout the United States, providing detailed information on how to start a group in your community. As of January 1990, there were eight chapters with support groups around the country and there are plans to start other groups in the near future. Each meeting has a speaker who is an expert in the field on some aspect of incontinence. The Manhattan group, for example, has been ongoing since 1985, with attendance of forty or fifty people between the ages of twenty and eighty. You can reach Continence Restored through co-directors Anne Smith-Young, C.U.T., and Dr. E. Douglas Whitehead, M.D., at the Association for Urinary Continence Control, 785 Park Avenue, New York, NY 10021.

INCONTINENCE REMINDERS

- Incontinence is a *symptom,* not a disease.
- Incontinence is *not* a normal part of aging, although age may predispose people to factors that may cause it.
- Your doctor must look for the *underlying cause* of incontinence in order to treat it properly.
- Transient causes of incontinence may be easily reversed after they are identified.
- There are a number of treatments for incontinence.
- Do not agree to surgery for incontinence until you have tried other treatments.
- Do not agree to using a catheter unless it is medically indicated.

RESOURCES

The HIP Report, Dr. Katherine F. Jeter, ed. Published by Help for Incontinent People (HIP), Inc., P.O. Box 544, Union, SC 29379. For a complimentary copy, send a long (#10) self-addressed stamped envelope to this address.

The Informer, Cheryle B. Gartley, ed. Published by the Simon Foundation for Continence, P.O. Box 835, Wilmette, IL 60091 (1-800-23S-IMON). You can receive a free information packet including a copy of *The Informer* by sending a long (#10) self-addressed stamped envelope to this address.

Managing Incontinence: A Guide to Living with the Loss of Bladder Control, Cheryle B. Gartley, ed. Ottawa, IL: Jameson Books, 1985. Now distributed by the Simon Foundation, P.O. Box 835, Wilmette IL 60091 (1-800-23S-IMON).

Ourselves Growing Older: Women Aging with Knowledge and Power, Paula Brown Doress and Diana Laskin Siegal and Midlife and Older Women Book Project. New York: Simon & Schuster, 1987. This is an essential wide-ranging resource manual for women, including information on menopause, diet, sexuality, and common medical problems. The chapter on incontinence is concise and clear and offers some insights to why bladder problems are so difficult to deal with.

Staying Dry: A Practical Guide to Bladder Control, Kathryn L. Burgio, K. Lynette Pearce, and Angelo J. Lucco, M.D. Baltimore: The Johns Hopkins University Press, 1989. Based on a highly successful program developed at the National Institute of Aging, this clearly written workbook focuses on curing incontinence with pelvic muscle exercises.

Urinary Incontinence in Adults. This free 32-page pamphlet succinctly summarizes the outcome of the Consensus Development Conference on Urinary Incontinence in Adults, October 3–5, 1988. Available from the Office of Medical Applications of Research, Building 1, Room 260, Bethesda, MD 20892 (free).

Waking Up Dry: How to End Bedwetting Forever, Martin B. Scharf, Ph.D. This definitive handbook provides a supportive program to end bedwetting. Available from Writer's Digest Books, 9933 Alliance Road, Cincinnati, OH 45242.

CHAPTER 5

Cystitis and Urethritis

LIZ GOT HER FIRST JOB AS A NEWSPAPER REPORTER and her first bladder infection in the same year, when she was twenty-one. "I kept them both for quite a long time," she remarks. After about ten years, Liz wrote a bestselling book and quit reporting, but the bladder infections continued to recur every few months. Eventually, she began to notice that sex or too much alcohol were guaranteed to set off an infection. "I must have gone to twenty doctors, but it was always the same old story," she says. "I would drown myself in cranberry juice and eat antibiotics like popcorn, but the symptoms would come back just as soon as I had sex again." Finally Liz got tired of the antibiotics and doctor bills and decided to make some changes. "While I was in college, I helped to start a women's clinic, so I was familiar with the traditional self-help remedies," she says. "I began taking vitamin C regularly and learned to flush my bladder routinely after sex. I definitely had fewer infections." Other changes were also helpful. Liz switched from the diaphragm to the cervical cap and after beginning to use it, she had only about one infection a year. Then because she was dating several men at one period, she began asking them to use condoms instead. "I found that I didn't mind them that much, and that I got infections even less frequently—about once every two years."

Annie is a thirty-five-year-old computer analyst. "I was fine until I reached eighteen," she recalls. When she was about eighteen, she started getting bladder infections. "I was using the diaphragm and a lot of the flare-ups seemed related to sex," she remembers. In her mid-twenties Annie decided to switch to the Pill, hoping that giving up the diaphragm would be helpful, but it wasn't. "Having these infections all the time made me fearful of sex," she says. "I was beginning to think it just might be easier to give it up altogether. Then I got mad about not being able to have sex when I wanted to and got into this weird mental game of alternating guilt and anger." Finally, Annie was hospitalized with a severe kidney infection and was referred to Kristene, who was on staff at the hospital. "She really changed my life," Annie reports. After doing tests to rule out more serious disorders, Kristene prescribed suppressive antibiotic therapy. "I haven't had an infection in more than a year," Annie says happily. "It's really a relief to know I wasn't crazy."

Until they found ways to control recurrences, Liz and Annie lived from crisis to crisis, drowning themselves in cranberry juice and taking endless rounds of antibiotics, always dreading that creepy-crawly feeling in the bladder heralding yet another visit from an old nemesis. Like Annie, many women feel guilty or embarrassed about frequent attacks of cystitis, as if there is something they are doing wrong that causes recurrences. Perhaps you, like Liz, have ended up doctor-shopping, always searching for a new antibiotic, always hoping for a cure. After many years, Liz and Annie both found solutions to recurrent cystitis. Liz changed her contraceptive method and now has only an occasional infection. Annie found that taking one pill at the first sign of an infection keeps her bladder infections under control. If you answer "yes" to several of the questions in the Self-Evaluation Checklist below, you should begin to look for the cause of your recurrences, and either on your own or with the help of a sympathetic doctor, develop a plan to reduce or eliminate them.

SELF-EVALUATION CHECKLIST

____ Have you had more than two bladder infections in the past six months or more than three in the last year?

____ Have you been to several doctors in an attempt to stop recurrent bladder infections?

____ Do bladder symptoms flare up routinely after sex?

____ Do you use a diaphragm?

___ Does your doctor prescribe antibiotics over the phone when you get a recurrence of cystitis without asking for a urine culture?

___ Do you feel guilty—as if you've done something wrong—when another bladder infection strikes?

___ Have you been referred to a psychotherapist because your infections may be "all in your head"?

___ Did you have bladder infections as a child?

___ Does another female relative in your family have a history of bladder infections?

___ If you are pregnant, have you been checked for any "silent" infections?

___ Do you have diabetes, obesity, a neurologic disorder, or other long-standing medical illness?

___ Do you, or does a relative whom you are caring for, have an indwelling catheter?

___ Have you been diagnosed with urethritis?

WHAT THIS CHAPTER CAN DO FOR YOU

No one knows why some women are plagued with recurrent bouts of cystitis, but recent research has yielded some intriguing clues. This chapter will help you understand what is going on in your bladder: why you may be susceptible when your best friend isn't, how bacteria get into the bladder, and how they may behave once they are there. Knowing that there are specific physiological processes involved in bladder infections can be very helpful in dispelling the feelings of guilt, anger, or frustration that you may experience when cystitis attacks occur without apparent explanation. It should also help you to feel less guilty about getting recurrent infections and motivate you to develop a plan of action. We will review new diagnostic guidelines that have been developed by urologists and methods of treatment that have been successful in breaking the cycle of recurrent cystitis. Over the years, alternative practitioners and women themselves have discovered a host of self-help strategies that can help reduce recurrences. Rebecca has reviewed these and provided a number of suggestions for integrating them into your daily routine.

WHAT IS CYSTITIS?

Our understanding of cystitis, like that of the common cold, has lagged far behind the many advances of medical science. Although there is still no magic bullet that is guaranteed to stop recurrent bladder infections, intensive research in the past decade has begun to yield some clues as to why certain bladders are so susceptible to bacterial infections and why recurrences are so difficult to control.

Compounded from the Greek word *kistis,* meaning bladder, and *itis,* meaning inflammation, the term *cystitis* literally means an inflammation in the bladder, which is generally the result of a bacterial infection. The term *urethritis* is used when the condition is limited to the urethra. When both the bladder and urethra are involved, the term *cystourethritis* is sometimes used. In the past, flare-ups of symptoms associated with sexual activity were often referred to somewhat disparagingly as "honeymoon cystitis," but it might be more descriptive and accurate to refer to this condition as "sex-related cystitis." Sometimes, you may have intense, cystitis-like symptoms but a urinalysis will reveal no bacteria in your urine. In this case, you may be told that you have the "frequency-dysuria syndrome" or "acute urethral syndrome" or perhaps even "interstitial cystitis." These conditions are quite different from cystitis and their treatments are quite different as well. (See Chapter 6.)

The term *urinary tract infection (UTI)* is often used interchangeably with cystitis, but technically it refers to an infection anywhere in the urinary system, including the kidneys, ureters, bladder, or urethra. Untreated bladder infections can sometimes travel up into the kidneys and cause severe, even life-threatening infections. This condition is referred to as "pyelonephritis" (*pyelo* referring to a part of the kidney called the renal pelvis, and *nephros,* the Greek word for kidney). We will not deal with kidney infections in detail in this book, but because the kidneys are connected to the bladder and can affect and be affected by what happens there, we will mention them briefly where relevant.

WHO HAS CYSTITIS?

If you have had more than one bout of cystitis in the last year, you are not alone. Cystitis accounts for more than 5 million doctor's visits annually, exceeded only by visits for upper respiratory infections (bad colds, flu, bronchitis, and the like). In fact, cystitis is so prevalent that one out of every five women in the United States can count on being initiated into the painful, unpredictable rites of cystitis during her lifetime. About 75 percent of those who have one episode will never have a recurrence, or will have fewer than three in one year. The unfortunate remainder, up to 25 percent, will experience more than three episodes a year. Some will have even more.

The incidence of urinary tract infections seesaws between the sexes. As babies, males are far more susceptible than females, the cause is often congenital, and most involve the kidneys. Boys quickly outgrow their susceptibility, but after the age of five, about 5 percent of schoolgirls will have at least one infection. The onset of sexual activity increases the chances of developing cystitis for women,[1] and 5 to 10 percent of pregnant women will develop an infection but may not have any symptoms. Women, in fact, are about thirty times more likely to develop cystitis than men,[2] but after the age of sixty the score evens out somewhat. Because enlargement of the prostate gland may cause urinary retention, older men are more susceptible to UTIs than younger men; in addition, prostatic secretions may lose their antiseptic properties in old age. More than one third of women over the age of seventy have bladder infections, 20 percent of which are "silent," i.e., you have no symptoms even though bacteria is present in the urine, and may go undetected for a long time.[3] The elderly are particularly at risk for urinary tract infections because of routine catheterization, which results in over half a million infections each year, and they can be fatal to the elderly and infirm. Many of these infections could be prevented by reducing unnecessary indwelling catheterization (see page 84).

SYMPTOMS

The first bladder infection is usually a shock. The symptoms arise abruptly, and they can be painful, relentless, and even frightening in their intensity. Such infections seem to have a propensity for striking at the most inopportune times: major events like weddings or graduations, vacations or business trips, exams, performances, starting a new job, or establishing a new relationship. To the sufferer, it seems that the symptoms won't get better on their own, and both business and pleasure must be put aside until they are brought under control. Sometimes you can "drown" an incipient infection with water or cranberry juice, but once bacteria get firmly established, antibiotics must be used to do the job.

When a bacterial infection develops in the bladder, you may experience some combination of the following symptoms, especially the first three, which are considered by many physicians to be the "classic triad" of cystitis symptoms:

- burning or stinging during urination *(dysuria)*
- urgent need to urinate
- frequency of urination
- voiding small amounts of urine
- frequent waking at night to urinate *(nocturia)*

Kidney Involvement

People who suffer from recurrent cystitis soon learn to recognize the characteristic tickle in the bladder that usually precedes a flare-up. If you have a history of bladder infections, there is a 40 percent chance that you will develop a kidney infection at some point. Such infections can cause scarring of the delicate kidney tissue and ultimately kidney failure if left untreated. Typically, kidney infections are accompanied by chills, high fever, nausea or vomiting, and pain in the flanks (under the ribcage on the back) which may radiate to the groin. Therefore, *if you notice these symptoms in addition to the usual cystitis symptoms, be sure to mention them to your doctor so that he or she can perform appropriate tests and start antibiotic treatment immediately.*

HOW BLADDER INFECTIONS OCCUR

The way in which bacteria invade the bladder is relatively straightforward. In the bowel, many species of bacteria live quietly, carrying out their assigned task of breaking down the food you have eaten—and sometimes eating each other. But outside of the bowel, especially in the urinary tract, they can become unruly troublemakers.

Bowel bacteria emerge in the stool, and no matter how excellent your hygiene is, some may stick to your skin and begin to multiply.

103

In women, these bacteria cross the *perineum,* the short bridge of flesh between the anus and vagina, and can then settle in the *introitus,* the entrance to the vagina. The introitus provides a cozy shelter where these bacteria can grow and multiply. Normally, the body's abundant natural defenses render such errant bacteria harmless. However, it appears that some women's natural defense mechanisms may be deficient, making them more prone to adventurous bacteria setting up housekeeping in the vaginal opening. From there, they can easily move into the vagina or into the urethra and on into the bladder. Some studies have clearly shown that bacteria frequently enter the bladder, but they are quickly disposed of by the bladder's most important defense mechanism—normal voiding, which washes the bacteria out of the bladder. Deficiencies in other bladder defenses, such as lowered estrogen levels or damage to the bladder lining, may also make it easier for bacteria to attach themselves to the bladder lining.

Researchers are now convinced that whether or not bacteria take hold and reproduce in the bladder depends upon three factors: the number of bacteria in the initial invasion, the ability of the bacteria to adhere to the bladder lining, and the strength of the bladder's inherent defenses. It appears that the last factor is the most significant.[4]

E. coli (Escherichia coli), the most populous of the many species of bacteria in the bowel, has been identified as the causative agent in 75 to 85 percent of uncomplicated bladder infections. There are more than 150 different types of *E. coli,* but only five or six of its subtypes consistently cause bladder infections (see illustration). Other species of bacteria that can cause cystitis are *Proteus, Klebsiella, Pseudomonas, Enterococcus, Enterobacter,* and rarely, *Streptococcus* or *Staphylococcus.*

Sex and Cystitis—A Contributing Cause

The association between sex and cystitis has long been assumed; hence the origin of the phrase "honeymoon cystitis." It is clear that for many women, the precipitation of cystitis does indeed occur during the "honeymoon,"[5] i.e., the initiation of a new sexual relationship, and that frequency of intercourse plays a role as well.[6] It has also been suggested that repeated thrusts of the penis, penetration of the vagina with fingers or objects, or manual stimulation of the clitoris may "massage" bacteria into the urethral opening that

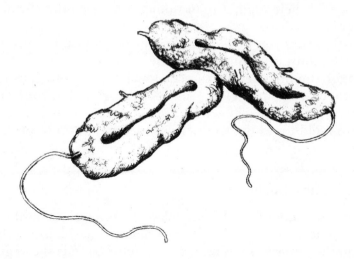

10. **E. coli bacteria.** *Escherichia coli,* the most common cause of urinary tract infections, as seen under an electron microscope. The whiplike tails help the bacteria to move.

ultimately travel up into the bladder.[7] In addition, bruising of the urethra during vigorous intercourse can cause swelling and inflammation and, perhaps, an increased susceptibility to infection. Nuns have been found to have a very low incidence of cystitis compared to sexually active women, corroborating this supposition.

The Diaphragm Connection

Long before the connection between cystitis and the diaphragm was noted in urological journals, gynecologists and urologists who saw women on a daily basis were well aware of the association. Now studies have been done by urologists and it appears that women who use the diaphragm are *more than twice as likely* to get urinary tract infections as are other sexually active women.[8] In fact, one study found the incidence to be *more than four times as high.*[9] Several reasons for this significantly higher incidence have been suggested. For one, the vaginas of women who use the diaphragm appear to become more alkaline. (Acidity normally inhibits the growth of bacteria. Conversely, alkalinity may promote its growth. Indeed, diaphragm users seem to have heavier growths of bacteria, espe-

105

cially *E. coli,* in their vaginas than women who use other forms of contraception.) [10]

The stiff spring rim of the diaphragm presses on the urethral sponge, the body of spongy tissue that surrounds the urethra. Even though the rim does not directly touch the urethra, it can put a great deal of pressure on it, causing "bruising" and inflammation and possibly obstructing the free flow of urine. This may allow bacteria to build up in the bladder, a situation known to promote infection.

Defenses Against Infection

The environment of the healthy bladder is normally sterile and there are some elementary but elegant defense mechanisms which ensure that it remains so. The first and most basic is the regular flushing that occurs during urination from four to eight times a day. Generous fluid intake, defined by most urologists as eight full glasses of fluid per day, ensures efficient flushing, washing out bacterial intruders in the process. Drinking plenty of fluid also dilutes the urine, lowering the concentration of bacteria that might have gained access to the bladder. Many people who have urinary urgency and frequency often restrict their fluid intake to avoid living in the bathroom, but this practice can increase the concentration of urine and, thus, of irritants in the bladder. It also poses the risk of dehydration, which can be extremely dangerous.

Another basic defense mechanism of the bladder is its natural acidity (pH 5.5 to 7.0), which helps to control bacterial proliferation. (See page 162 for an explanation of the pH scale.) Women appear to be naturally more susceptible to bladder infections than men, and this may be partly due to the fact that the urine of women has a higher, or less acidic, pH reading. In fact, one study found that the urinary pH of infection-prone women was even more alkaline than that of women who did not have infections. [11]

In addition to current knowledge about the bladder's mechanical defenses, we are beginning to get a glimmer of more sophisticated phenomena that may operate within the bladder to protect it from repeated bacterial invasion. Current research efforts are now being directed toward finding clues related to how the bladder lining interacts with bacteria and various substances.

Although the exact mechanism is not yet well understood, the lining of the normal bladder appears to repel bacteria. This may explain why so many people never get bladder infections, or get them only on rare occasions. But it is now thought that some people may have a defect in the bladder lining that allows bacteria to adhere more easily. Certain bacteria, especially many strains of *E. coli,* have hairy, fingerlike projections, called *pili* or *fimbriae,* that can insert themselves into receptive cells on the bladder surface in a sort of lock-and-key fashion.[12] Once they are attached, they can't be washed out, even by industrial-strength flushing. They have to be killed. In addition, there may be more attachment sites in some people's bladders. Immune, hormonal, and genetic factors, including blood type, may also play roles in preventing or allowing bacteria to thrive in the bladder, but thus far, these are exceedingly complex issues that may take years of research to unravel.

DIAGNOSIS

The diagnosis of cystitis is not a complicated business, but it is often done incorrectly. All too frequently, this is the scenario at the doctor's office: you urinate into a cup and five minutes later, the nurse tells you that you do or don't have any bacteria in your urine. If you have bacteria, and sometimes when you don't, you will quickly be given a prescription for antibiotics and perhaps a drug to soothe your irritated bladder. This is a case of underdiagnosis. Or your doctor puts you through a series of urodynamic tests, to see how well you can urinate, and a kidney X-ray, to see what your urinary tract looks like. If you can't urinate up to speed (which you might not be able to do if you are recovering from the trauma of an infection), your doctor may dilate the urethra in an attempt to help you urinate better. This is a case of diagnostic overkill and is unlikely to help control or reduce the frequency of episodes. In either case, you are left at the mercy of your next infection.[13]

The correct diagnosis of recurrent cystitis focuses not only on discovering if bacteria are indeed causing the symptoms, but also upon the type of bacteria that are present, the pattern of recurrences, and whether they seem related to factors in your life such as use of the diaphragm, sexual activity, or your diet. A simple urinalysis, physical examination, and a careful medical history should provide some important clues as to what is causing repeated recurrences and enough information to choose the appropriate treatment.

Finding a Doctor

Like women who are plagued with cystitis, many doctors are frustrated by their inability to stop recurrences, sometimes resorting to elaborate tests, looking for something—anything—to explain repeated attacks. But they usually end up back at square one: plain old garden-variety cystitis. Chapter 2 provides some general guidelines for finding a doctor who understands your type of bladder disorder and is interested in helping you overcome it. In the case of cystitis, most women will probably initially turn to their gynecologist, internist, or family practice physician. Because the diagnosis of uncomplicated cystitis requires no special training, these doctors should be able to help you—if they are willing to look for the cause of repeated infections and to help you develop a plan for preventing further recurrences. The only way to find out if this is the case is to be very specific about what you want.

Tell any doctor that you see that you are not interested in being prescribed antibiotics on an episode-by-episode basis; that instead, you are interested in finding out why you are having repeated bouts of cystitis and in figuring out how to keep them from recurring.

Make it clear that, until you have gotten recurrences under control, you want your urine analyzed each time you have symptoms, to make sure that bacterial infection is indeed what is causing your symptoms. If you are having episodes of infections *without* bacteria, then your treatment would be quite different. (See page 173 for information on the painful bladder syndrome.)

If your doctor does not think that the above goals are important, or achievable, then you might consider looking for another doctor. If you are a member of an HMO and your doctor is not responsive, you should request to be referred to an outside specialist.

Preparing for Your Doctor's Visit

Chapter 2 also makes some suggestions for helpful things to do before you go to your doctor's visit (see page 24). Whether you have a long-standing relationship with a doctor or are seeing a new one, a thorough medical history can provide a lot of essential information about what might be causing recurrent infections. Before your visit, it might be useful for you to compile an accurate medical history, including:

- When you had your first bladder (or kidney) infection.
- How many infections you have had each year since then.
- When you had your last infection.
- How many of these infections were documented, i.e., if you had a urinalysis and if each was positive or negative. (If you are unsure about this, you might want to request your medical records from any doctor you saw for an extended period.)
- Other than urinalyses, what type of diagnostic tests you have had and what their results were, such as kidney X-rays, urodynamic tests (see the Index of Diagnostic Tests for a list of these), or cystoscopy. (If your memory is fuzzy, your past medical records should show any tests you have had.)
- What types of drugs you have taken for bladder infections in the past and any medications you are currently taking (both prescription *and* over-the-counter drugs).
- If you are sexually active. If so, how frequently you have sex, if you have more than one partner, or if you have a new partner.
- If you use a diaphragm. If so, when you started using it and if you have noticed any correlation of diaphragm use with recurrences of cystitis.
- How many times you have been pregnant, and whether the pregnancies ended in abortion, miscarriage, or childbirth.
- If you had cystitis during any of your pregnancies.
- What surgeries you have had, if any, especially a hysterectomy or other pelvic surgery.
- If you have any other health problems.

It is now clear that about 90 percent of urinary tract infections (UTIs) are *uncomplicated* infections with no underlying physical abnormality, and hence do not call for invasive tests or elaborate treatments. In the other 10 percent—the *complicated* infections— an underlying cause can usually be found. These conditions must be treated before recurrent cystitis can be brought under control. For uncomplicated cystitis, the diagnosis is very straightforward. It consists of a careful *medical history,* which will offer clues as to the possible cause of your infections; a thorough *physical examination,* which might reveal other conditions or physical abnormalities that might be causing repeated infections; a *urinalysis,* which will reveal whether or not there is bacteria in your urine; and a *culture and sensitivity (C&S) test,* which will identify the specific type of bacteria and note which drugs will kill it. Further details on these tests can be found in the Index of Diagnostic Tests on page 278.

Until recently, the culture and sensitivity (C&S) test was considered the cornerstone of the cystitis diagnosis. But today, with better knowledge about bacteria and the drugs that will eradicate them, many doctors feel that the information gained from a urinalysis (that bacteria is present and a general count of the numbers) is enough to begin treatment. Now, in many cases the C&S test is used primarily to confirm the diagnosis, and does not often change the chosen course of treatment.[14] The test is important, however, in determining the specific bacteria that are causing repeated attacks, and it provides useful information in developing an effective treatment program.

Other Tests

If you take one or two courses of antibiotics and continue to have frequent recurrences, then your doctor may decide to do some further tests, including:

- *blood tests* to screen for diabetes and kidney problems;
- a *cystoscope examination,* in which your doctor will look inside your bladder with a cystoscope to see if there are any tumors, stones, obstructions, or other abnormalities;
- an *intravenous pyelogram (IVP)* or kidney *ultrasound (US)* to aid in identifying the condition and function of the kidneys, ureters, and bladder. If a growth or other abnormality is found, more extensive testing such as a *CT (Computed Tomography) scan* or *magnetic resonance imaging (MRI)* may need to be done;
- a *voiding cystourethrogram (VCUG)* to show how efficiently you urinate, to see whether there is any back-up *(reflux)* of urine from the bladder to the kidneys, and to reveal any *urethral* or *bladder diverticula* (tiny pouches that can trap urine and become a home for bacteria);
- *urodynamic testing,* to see how efficiently the bladder functions.

Further information on all of these tests can be found in the Index of Diagnostic Tests on page 278.

What Constitutes a Genuine Infection?

In the not-so-distant past, urine cultures that grew less than 100,000 (10^5) bacteria per milliliter of urine were considered to be "negative." The rationale for this principle rested on the assumption that lower bacterial counts were nearly always caused by "contaminants" such as yeast, lactobacilli, and other organisms that normally inhabit the vagina but do not usually survive in the bladder. These vaginal bacteria are relatively easy to distinguish from bowel bacteria like *E. coli* that typically cause cystitis. It is now thought that up to 20 percent of the women with "acute dysuria," that is, burning with urination, may have less than 1,000 (10^3) bacteria per milliliter of urine.[15] Most laboratories have revised their standards slightly and classify a urine specimen as "positive" if 10,000 (10^4) bacteria are visible, but may not routinely report lower counts. If you persist in having cystitis symptoms but your urine culture shows "no bacteria" in the urine, your doctor can request a report on *any bacteria present.*

If you are sexually active and your urine culture is "negative," ask your doctor about testing for *Chlamydia.* A Chlamydia infection in the urethra can mimic the symptons of a bladder infection, but usually does not respond to the same medication. (See page 127 for more information on Chlamydia.)

Several studies have revealed that up to 30 percent of women who have cystitis-like symptoms have genuinely sterile urine.[16] Nevertheless, these women are often treated as if they have bacterial cystitis. If you have persistent symptoms of cystitis after two or three days of antibiotics but have genuinely sterile urine, i.e., no bacteria at all can be found in your bladder, you may have "urethral syndrome" or interstitial cystitis. Both these conditions, which are just beginning to be dealt with by urologists, mimic the symptoms of cystitis, but their management and treatment are radically different. Chapter 6 explains what is known about these conditions.

Classification of Bacterial Infections

Until recently, doctors tended to look at each bladder infection as a separate entity and did not make much attempt to look at the pattern of recurrence. But it now seems that recurrent bladder

111

infections often have an observable pattern that can provide important information in terms of treatment.

Dr. Thomas Stamey, a well-known urologist who has worked with cystitis for many years, has devised a simple but very useful system for classification of bacterial infections that has become a standard for diagnosis,[17] helping doctors to make an educated guess as to whether your infection will respond to certain treatment regimens. According to this system of classification, *most people have only one infection, or only an occasional infection,* i.e., less than three a year. Those who have recurrent infections either have *a persistent infection with the same organism* that is for some reason difficult to eradicate, in which there is usually only a short period before infection recurs; or *three or more reinfections a year with a different organism,* which appear in clusters usually separated by intervals of six months or longer.

By distinguishing between these three patterns of recurrence, your doctor can better determine which drug might work for you. The types of drugs that are generally used to treat cystitis, and some guidelines for their use, are listed in the next section.

TREATMENT

Antibiotics have been, and remain, the standard medical treatment for cystitis. There are some very solid reasons for this. For one, within hours, they can kill enough bacteria to reduce the urgency, frequency, and painful urination associated with bacterial infections, and in many cases can eradicate most of them in just a few days. But antibiotics, especially if they must be relied on over the long term, have drawbacks as well. Some have uncomfortable physical side effects such as nausea, loss of appetite, diarrhea, dizziness, fatigue, and an increase in vaginal yeast infections. With the exception of yeast infections, all of these effects are transient, and disappear as soon as you stop taking the medication. Many women find that vaginal yeast infections can be difficult to get rid of, and often may be almost as bothersome as the cystitis symptoms themselves. Before you embark on another round of antibiotics, you might want to read the section beginning on page 122 on Alternative Remedies, to see if there are non-medical approaches that you have not yet tried.

There is a bewildering array of antibiotics on the market: their names seem incomprehensible, many make you feel lousy, and they can be shockingly expensive—another reason for investigating alternative remedies first. It is therefore useful to have a working knowledge of the drugs you are likely to encounter. As you will see, this is not such a tall order.

As we mentioned earlier, the choice of appropriate antibiotics for treating cystitis has mostly been empiric, that is, an educated guess based on a doctor's clinical experience. In a high percentage of cases, this therapy works—at least for the current infection. If you have an infection, or one is strongly suspected, your doctor will choose a drug that

- can achieve a high concentration in the urine;
- is not likely to influence the development of bacteria that are resistant to the drug;
- is not likely to kill off friendly bacteria in the bowel which would result in a yeast infection;
- is effective in treating most of the bacteria that cause UTIs; and
- is low in cost.

Drugs that fulfill these criteria should be the first choice for treatment unless otherwise indicated—for example, if you are allergic to certain medications or classes of drugs or if you have developed a strain of bacteria that is resistant to a specific drug.

Dr. Lowell Parsons, from the University of California School of Medicine in San Diego, has exhaustively reviewed the literature on antibiotic treatment, and coupled with his own experience in studying and treating cystitis, has developed a helpful classification of the antibiotics commonly used to treat cystitis.[18] The following drugs are listed in order of preference for treating cystitis:

Nitrofurantoin: This drug closely fulfills the requirements listed above and is usually a first choice for treatment unless otherwise indicated. Nitrofurantoin macrocrystals can be taken with meals and may therefore have fewer side effects than generic forms, although many people experience digestive problems when taking this drug.

Sulfa drugs: Sulfa drugs are very effective against *E. coli*, but many types of bacteria are resistant to them. Carbenicillin, a member of the penicillin family, also works well against *E. coli*, *enterococci*, and *Proteus mirabilis*, but it is expensive.

Amoxicillin: This antibiotic is effective against most bladder bacteria, but it causes yeast infections in about 25 percent of the women who use it and is fairly expensive. Amoxicillin is a member of the penicillin family, so if you are allergic to penicillin, you should not use it.

Trimethoprim-sulfamethoxazole (TMP-SMX) and cephalosporin: These drugs are very effective against most bacteria that cause UTIs, but cephalosporin causes vaginal yeast infections in 30 percent of cases.

Ampicillin and tetracycline: These old standbys for cystitis treatment work well but have significant side effects, including gastric distress and yeast infections, which can be severe in some people. Their use is recommended only for someone who experiences side effects to other oral medications. Norfloxacin and Cipro, two newer drugs in this group, are effective but very expensive.

More complete information on all of these antibiotics and on drugs that should not be taken during pregnancy is available in the Drug Glossary at the back of the book.

NOTE: If you are prescribed a course of antibiotics, it is important that you take them *exactly as directed.* Otherwise, you run the risk of killing off the weaker bacteria only, or setting the stage for a worse infection or for the development of a resistant strain of bacteria.

Types of Antibiotic Treatment

In the past the standard antibiotic treatment was anywhere from ten to fourteen days, but it now appears that treatment for this length of time is, in most cases, medical overkill. In routine cases, drug treatment for three days, or in many cases, a single megadose, is effective. In addition, many doctors are now willing to be more flexible in the use of antibiotics, prescribing them to prevent recurrences (prophylactic treatment) or to eradicate persistent infections (suppressive therapy). Some doctors will even help you work out a program of self-administered antibiotics to be taken at the first sign of infection.

If you are able to identify a specific factor that tends to precipitate episodes of cystitis, such as sexual activity, you might want to consider *prophylactic, or preventive, antibiotic therapy.* Lynne, who suffered with sex-related flare-ups for years, finally found a doctor who encouraged her to try preventive therapy. "My anxiety about post-sex recurrences was so great that I began to dread it. Now I take a single pill either just before or just after sex, and haven't had a recurrence in more than two years." If you feel that recurrences are related to intercourse, ask your doctor about giving you a prescription for this method of treatment.

If you find prophylactic antibiotic therapy appealing, there are several points you might want to consider:

- There may be a tendency for bacteria to develop a resistance to the drug that you are taking, so you should have periodic urine cultures to make sure the drug is still effective.
- Since infections tend to occur in clusters, separated by symptom-free periods, it is recommended that you try prophylactic therapy for a few months, then discontinue the drug for a while and see what happens. If infections recur, you can restart the drug, or a different one, again.
- From an economic standpoint, this method is much cheaper than going to the doctor for repeated occurrences.

For persistent infections, some doctors prescribe *suppressive antibiotic therapy,* using a very low dose of a particular antibiotic for three to six months or perhaps longer. The goal of this type of treatment is simply to wear down the bacteria over time. You may take one pill a day in the very beginning, and then drop down to one every other day. A urine culture should be done after three to six months of therapy to see if the infection has cleared. The goal of suppressive therapy is to keep the lower urinary tract sterile (infection-free) over a long period of time to allow the bladder and urethral defense mechanisms to replenish themselves and get as strong as possible.

Annie, whose story appeared at the beginning of this chapter, had repeated attacks of cystitis until Kristene suggested that she try suppressive antibiotic therapy. "I take half a pill if I feel *any* signs of an infection," Annie says. "If the symptoms continue the next day, I take one or two pills. If they go beyond that, I go in for a urine culture." Since starting this type of treatment, Annie has not had to go to call Kristene or go to the emergency room in over a year.

If you are doing intermittent self-start antibiotic therapy, it is important for you to check your urine for signs of infection before you begin taking antibiotics.[19] This can easily be done with chemically treated dipsticks, which do not test for bacteria but confirm the presence of white blood cells (indicating that the body is fighting infection) and nitrites, by-products of bacterial invasion. To find out if you have an infection, urinate into a sterile cup and immerse the dipsitck in the urine for a few seconds. The chemically treated sticks will turn certain colors and can be compared to a color scale on the container. Dipsticks are manufactured by Boehringer Mannheim Diagnostics (9115 Hague Rd., Indianapolis, IN 46250) and by the Ames Co. (P.O. Box 3100, Elkhart, IN 46515), and can be purchased in most pharmacies.

Self-Administered Single-Dose Antibiotic Therapy

For women who have more than the occasional infection (one or two a year) that are not predictably associated with some precipitating event, such as sexual activity, taking a single megadose antibiotic at the first sign of infection can be useful. If your doctor is very familiar with your case and knows that there is nothing unusual about it, he or she might consider this type of treatment. It can work very well and is quite convenient and economical.

Geraldine, a financial consultant, often has recurrences of cystitis when she travels. "I travel a lot and it's difficult to see a doctor when I am away from home," she says. "And in my line of work, I can't afford to let an infection get out of hand—I'd be running to the toilet every few minutes at meetings." Because Geraldine is often out of town when recurrences happen, Kristene recommended that she use a home urine test. At the first sign of symptoms, Geraldine tests her urine and begins a three-day course of antibiotics, which she always carries with her. Your doctor can order the home test kits and give you several at one time. (See the Index of Diagnostic Tests for information on where to order and how to use the home urine test.)

Some women, like Phyllis, rely on a combination of prophylactic and self-start therapy. She takes one antibiotic tablet right after she has sex, which usually prevents a recurrence. But occasionally she will still get symptoms. Then she uses self-start therapy, taking antibiotics at the dose recommended to treat the actual infection.

If you do decide to try self-administered antibiotic therapy and are not using the home urine test, you might want to drop off a clean-catch urine sample (see page 288) at your doctor's office, or go in for a urinalysis before and after therapy to make sure that the single-dose regimen is effective in killing all of the bacteria in your bladder.

Regardless of what type of antibiotic therapy you use, you may also be given a prescription for bladder analgesics, such as *Pyridium* or *Urised,* that can help lessen the symptoms. These drugs will not kill bacteria, but they do help alleviate—often very quickly—the burning and stinging you get along with the infection.

Used in the ways described above, antibiotics can be very helpful in controlling the recurrence of urinary tract infections. But most of them have annoying or unpleasant side effects and can ultimately be expensive, so the idea of taking them off and on forever is not very appealing. It would seem, then, that prevention—if it were possible—would be a very high priority. The following section reviews an array of preventive techniques that are known to be very useful in the management of recurrent cystitis.

PREVENTION

Based on our current knowledge about bladder infections, there is a substantial array of common-sense preventive measures that can be undertaken either by themselves or in conjunction with antibiotic therapy and alternative remedies (see page 122). Essentially, these are alterations in contraception, sexual activity, personal habits, diet, and stress level that remove or reduce factors that often seem to precipitate attacks of cystitis. These techniques are, in general, easy to do, have no side effects, and are cheap or free. And even if they don't help reduce cystitis attacks, they won't hurt you—even in large doses. Liz, whose story opened this chapter, is an excellent example of someone who employed preventive measures with great success. Here are things you can do on a routine basis:

Drink a generous amount of fluid, especially water. Drinking dilutes the urine and therefore lowers the bacterial count. Above all, **avoid getting dehydrated.** Dehydration prevents the regular wash-out of bacteria and may make you more susceptible to bladder infections.

Urinate frequently and completely. Do not keep urine in your bladder beyond the point where it feels uncomfortable. When urinating, take time to relax completely so that the bladder has time to empty completely.

117

Drink lots of cranberry juice. Cranberry juice has always been the true-blue home remedy for bladder infections—and not without reason. In the bladder, cranberry juice breaks down into hippuric acid, a compound that has natural bactericidal properties. Unfortunately, you would have to drink an enormous amount of cranberry juice a day to make a significant impact on a developing infection. Nevertheless, many women say that if they begin drinking cranberry juice as soon as symptoms become noticeable, it often nips an infection in the bud. At the very least, drinking large amounts of cranberry juice or water will flush the bladder, which in some cases may be enough to get rid of the bacteria. Another positive property of cranberry juice is that its acidity can amplify the effectiveness of nitrofurantoin, one of the drugs most frequently used to eradicate bladder bacteria. However, certain antibiotics, especially erythromycin, are more effective at a more alkaline pH. Therefore, if you are taking erythromycin, drinking cranberry juice in large quantities would be contraindicated. You might want to take some baking soda instead (one half to one teaspoon in water).

If you use cranberry juice in a self-help program to control cystitis, you might want to consider the following. The "juice" you buy in the supermarket is no more than 10 to 25 percent cranberry juice, and has quite a bit of added sugar. On the other hand, the unsweetened concentrate you buy in health food stores is so tart that it may be unpalatable to all but the hardy few. Some people have found that the tartness of concentrated cranberry juice can be ameliorated somewhat by cutting the concentrate to half-and-half with plain or sparkling water and sweetening it with a little honey. However, the real thing may still not be delicious enough to drink glass after glass, which is what you would need.

Vitamin C (ascorbic acid) is another substance that can be used to intensify the natural acidity of the urine and perhaps help inhibit the growth of bacteria. Many people erroneously think that orange juice will also acidify the urine, but because of the way it breaks down in the body, it will not. (See page 161 for more information on how vitamin C works in the bladder.) People with interstitial cystitis or urethral syndrome or just plain "touchy bladders" should avoid vitamin C in its acid form as well as certain other substances that specifically acidify the urine, such as cranberry and citrus juices, since acid may further irritate an inflamed bladder.

NOTE: You can't tell if your urine is acid or alkaline (the pH reading) by just looking at it, nor can you tell what effect whatever you put in your mouth (food, liquid, or vitamins) is having on it. But you can check urine pH by using chemically treated nitrazine strips (a sort of glorified litmus paper available at many pharmacies). (See page 162 for more information on urine pH.)

Do not drink, or drink only in moderation, known bladder irritants such as alcohol, coffee, tea (both caffeinated and some herbal teas as well), sodas, and acidic fruit juices.

Avoid foods that typically irritate the bladder such as chocolate (contains caffeine) and spicy foods, especially Mexican, Indian, and Thai, and Cajun cuisines. You might also want to look at the section on diet in the chapter on interstitial cystitis (beginning on page 158) for a more detailed discussion of foods that may irritate the bladder.

Stop using the diaphragm. As mentioned earlier, diaphragms have been identified as one of the causes of repeated bladder infections. The standard for diaphragm fitting in the United States is "the largest size that is comfortable for the patient."[20] But this means "comfortable" in the clinic, and may not accurately reflect what you may feel after several hours of wear.

If you or your doctor believes that the diaphragm is causing cystitis, then changing your birth control method might be very beneficial. Until recently, diaphragm users had few realistic alternatives. But now, the cervical cap offers an extremely attractive barrier method of contraception for the 50 to 75 percent of women who can be fitted with it. As yet, no scientific study has looked at whether or not the cervical cap actually lessens the incidence of bladder infections, but there is a mountain of anecdotal evidence that suggests that it does. The cap is not available everywhere, so getting one involves more than simply deciding to try it. You can get a list of providers from the National Women's Health Network, 1325 G Street N.W., Washington, DC 20005 (202-347-1140).

If you think your diaphragm is causing repeated UTIs, try switching to condoms for a while, as Liz did, and see if you get as many infections. You could also try having sex without putting the penis into the vagina. Many people, especially men, don't see this as "real" sex, but it is a valid and often highly erotic alternative.

Drink water or other liquid both before and after sex, so that you can void a reasonable amount of urine afterward. The idea is not just to squeeze out a few tablespoons of urine, but to get a good flush. Therefore, it is advisable to wait until you can void a normal amount of urine.

Make some changes in sexual activity. For most women, orgasms are difficult to achieve without direct stimulation of the clitoris, immediately above the urethral opening. If intercourse has the effect of "massaging" bacteria into the urethra, vigorous clitoral stimulation with the fingers, either by your partner or through masturbation, may provide even more specific pressure on the urethra. If you don't use a diaphragm but cystitis recurrences are clearly sexually related, you might try to make some changes in your usual pattern of sexual activity and see if it helps. Avoiding certain sexual positions may be helpful, but in the end, for most women, no clitoral stimulation equals no orgasm. Short of forgoing orgasms, the best you may be able to do is to try to identify what is, for you, "non-essential" stimulation around the vaginal opening and try to avoid that as much as possible. You might also try avoiding intercourse for a while and see if it helps. Read Chapter 9, Staying Sexual, and try experimenting with alternative ways to have orgasms.

Perhaps your mother didn't warn you, but all sex-education materials offer a standard caution to **avoid vaginal penetration after anal intercourse.** This is very common-sense advice. If you are susceptible to bladder infections, the direct introduction of bacteria from the anus, containing the dreaded *E. coli,* is definitely not a good idea. And bacteria can be tracked from the anus to the vagina by hands and fingers as well. If you do engage in anal activity, keeping condoms and finger cots handy can help avoid the direct transfer of bacteria.

NOTE: If you think there is even a remote risk of AIDS, you should always use condoms for anal intercourse.

At the very least, **communicate.** Making your partner aware of your problem, and thus giving him or her some responsibility in the matter, can be extremely useful. Certainly it can make you feel better to share the responsibility for making sex good for both partners.

Wear loose clothing. Tight pants can irritate the soft tissues surrounding the vaginal opening and make them more susceptible to infection. They also hold in heat, which helps to incubate bacteria.

For women, **wipe from front to back,** especially after a bowel movement. The assumption is that wiping from back to front or not wiping carefully can help bacteria move from the anus to the vaginal opening.

NOTE: A few scattered studies have looked at the standard advice that is invariably offered when bladder infections flare up: drink lots of cranberry juice, wipe from front to back, wear loose clothing. Surprisingly, these studies challenge some of our most cherished assumptions about the causes, and thus the prevention, of cystitis. In one study, 56 percent of the women in the group that consistently got urinary tract infections said that they wiped from front to back, while only 38 percent of the women who *did not* get UTIs said that they usually wiped in the prescribed way.[21] In another study done at the University of Utah, researchers looked at the diets, clothing, and urination habits of female students and found no correlation between frequency of infection and drinking cranberry juice, wearing tight clothing, or wiping from front to back.[22]

Change tampons and sanitary pads frequently. Tampon strings and warm, moist napkins provide great nesting places for bacteria. Tampons may also alter the normal flora of the vagina in some way, just as the diaphragm apparently does. Therefore, regular changes of these menstrual products would seem to make sense. On the other hand, there has been some suggestion that changing tampons too often can cause drying of vaginal tissues, because each tampon is most absorbent when it is first inserted.

Increase the amount of lactobacillus in your vagina (commonly known as the "yogurt remedy" because yogurt is a source of lactobacilli). Women with repeated urinary tract infections seem to have more alkaline pH and lower levels of lactobacillus in their vaginas.[23] Lactobacillus is a "friendly" bacteria that lives in both the bowel and vagina. Its presence appears to inhibit the growth of yeast and to interfere with the proliferation of *E. coli,* as well as with its adherence to the bladder wall.[24] Many people advise eating yogurt, which contains lactobacillus acidophilus. This may increase the lactobacillus and thus lower the concentration of both yeast and *E. coli* in your bowel, which could potentially be helpful. However, the most direct ways of increasing the population of lactobacillus in your vagina are: (1) douche with it; (2) using a plastic speculum, pour an ounce or two in and let it stay for three or four minutes; or (3) insert a few gelatin capsules containing acidophilus crystals into the vagina. How you do it isn't that important. The critical point is to make sure that the culture is *alive and kicking* when you insert it. Lactobacilli are not very hardy little organisms, so because of over-pasteurization most of the bacteria in store-bought yogurt may be dead. The same goes for many of the capsules you can purchase in a health food store. The surest bet for getting a live culture is to get liquid or crystal preparations that are kept in the refrigerator at health food stores.

Try to reduce stress. The role of stress in the precipitation of bladder infections is quite controversial. Although there is little documentation on the subject, self-care advocates, alternative practitioners, and many cystitis sufferers have long contended that stress can play a role in precipitating bouts of cystitis. It is commonly known that stress influences the production of hormones and brain chemicals, called neurotransmitters, that stimulate or inhibit nerve transmission. Stress may also have a negative impact on the immune system, which may affect systems of the body and perhaps the bladder as well. Given these factors, it is conceivable that stress could make you more vulnerable to cystitis attacks. Check page 163 for information on stress reduction.

Like Liz, a number of people find that making some of the changes suggested above can greatly reduce or even eliminate recurrent bacterial infections. But others try all of these alterations and still have infections. If you find yourself in this situation, you might want to try some of the alternative remedies described in the following section.

ALTERNATIVE REMEDIES

Before the age of antibiotics, cystitis was treated with an array of traditional remedies and some of the more helpful ones are still being used today, especially herbal and homeopathic remedies. People who have severe side effects from antibiotics or do not want to take them often rely on these time-honored remedies.

Herbal Remedies

Herbs have been employed for 2,000 years in Chinese medicine and are still the basis for quite a number of prescription and over-the-counter drugs today. In terms of urology, the herbal apothecary is brimming over with preparations that are said to purge, soothe, or help heal the bladder, but these potions can be quite bewildering for the uninitiated. Even if you are fairly conversant with medicinal plants and their properties, before using them to treat cystitis or other bladder conditions, it is advisable to consult an herbalist who can help you select appropriate preparations for use with bladder conditions. You might also want to look at one of the standard herbal reference guides listed in the Resources at the end of this chapter.

Numerous herbs have properties that can directly affect the bladder. Some are disinfectant (can kill bacteria), analgesic (are soothing), diuretic (can increase the output of urine), or narcotic (reduce or relieve pain). Herbs are usually taken as teas, tinctures, or powders, but people with bladder problems should avoid taking tinctures, since these preparations are alcohol-based, and alcohol is well known to be one of the prime bladder irritants. You might also want to avoid the many herbs with a high tannic acid content, since tannin is excreted in the urine as gallic acid—another known bladder irritant. (Tannic acid, commonly found in roots, leaves, and bark, is the substance that gives coffee and tea, including many herb teas, their characteristic dark color.)

The herbs that are most commonly recommended for prevention and/or treatment of cystitis are goldenseal, horsetail, shave-grass, cornsilk, cleavers, comfrey, lemon balm, and marshmallow. Goldenseal *(Hydrastis canadensis)*, long used in medicinal herbal preparations by Native Americans, has documented antibiotic and anti-inflammatory properties. Berberine, one of the constituents of this herb, has been shown to have antimicrobial effects against *E. coli* and other less common organisms that cause bladder infections.[25]

Like drugs, herbs have both risks and benefits which ought to be evaluated before they are taken. In normal doses, herbs work slower and more gently than drugs and therefore have far fewer unwanted physical effects. But in high doses, they can also be toxic. In evaluating various herbs, you might want to ask the following questions (which are essentially what you might ask about any prescription or over-the-counter medication):

- What are its properties, i.e., is it acidic or basic, analgesic or narcotic?
- What is it traditionally used as: a disinfectant, a diuretic, an anesthetic, or an emetic, et cetera?
- Is there a known toxic dose?

- Does it contain tannic acid?
- What are the side effects at normal dosage?

Homeopathic Remedies

Homeopathy is a school of healing based on the principle of "like cures like," founded by Dr. Samuel Hahnemann, a physician who lived in Philadelphia in the 1790s. Hahnemann believed symptoms are a direct manifestation of an illness and that by introducing small amounts of substances that would cause similar symptoms, the body would be stimulated to react to the substances and to the illness as well. Today, homeopaths practice throughout the country and many medium-sized cities will have a homeopathic pharmacy. In England homeopathic remedies are available by prescription from the National Health Service. Many homeopaths report excellent results in treating cystitis with apis mellifica, cantharis, belladonna, and other homeopathic remedies. If you are interested in trying any of these, your best bet is to consult an experienced homeopath.

CYSTITIS DURING PREGNANCY

The effect of the hormonal changes of pregnancy on susceptibility to cystitis remains unclear. During pregnancy, when dramatic hormonal changes occur, the kidneys produce more urine, the ureters relax somewhat, and the bladder empties less efficiently. As a result of these and other factors, from 5 to 10 percent of pregnant women develop bladder infections, many of which will be silent or asymptomatic (an infection without any symptoms).

A urinalysis is a standard part of every prenatal visit and will help to identify silent infections, but in women who do not get early prenatal care, infections may go undetected. Up to 40 percent of these women will develop kidney infections, usually in the third trimester. It is strongly suspected that such infections can cause or contribute to premature births and low-birth-weight babies.[26] Therefore, routine screening for bacteria in the urine during pregnancy, especially the third trimester, is recommended. For women who have bacteria in their urine, monthly cultures need to be done and antibiotics can be prescribed when needed. Because of the high incidence of false positive tests, *two* urinalyses showing bacteria and a positive culture should be obtained before antibiotic treatment begins. This avoids exposing the fetus to unnecessary antibiotics.

Because of danger to either the mother or the fetus, many antibiotics are unsafe for use during pregnancy. Some, like tetracycline, can prevent proper development of the enamel on the baby's teeth. If a drug's safety during pregnancy has not been established, then it is best avoided.

CATHETER-ASSOCIATED INFECTIONS

A catheter (a rubber tube about the size of a soda straw) is frequently inserted into the bladder to provide urinary drainage after surgery or injuries, during chronic illness, or when someone is unable to control the bladder due to depression, disorientation, or neurological problems. In spite of elaborate precautions to maintain sterility, catheter-induced infections occur in almost everybody who has one continuously in place for more than ten days. These infections are difficult to eradicate because of the continual presence of a foreign body in the bladder (see illustration on page 85) and the evolution of resistant strains of bacteria following repeated courses of antibiotics. Catheter-related infections are a significant cause of illness and even death among the elderly as their health declines, but for short-term catheterization the incidence of infection is relatively low.

Given the seriousness of catheter-associated infections, it would seem that preventive measures are important, and many have been tried with varying results. One technique that has been somewhat successful is the use of a "closed-drainage" catheter system that prevents the entrance of bacteria into the catheter from the tubing and urine collection bag. The most important preventive measure is the frequent cleansing of the opening of the urethra to help prevent the migration of bacteria on the outside of the catheter from the urethra into the bladder.

Because of the difficulties in preventing and treating bladder infections with indwelling catheters, it is best to avoid their use if at all possible. Today, many urologists and gerontologists believe that up to 90 percent of indwelling catheters are unnecessary. If a long-term catheter is recommended for yourself, or for a friend or relative, ask your doctor or a nursing supervisor if there are any possible alternatives. The section on catheter use on page 84 provides some guidelines for when such use is necessary, and some suggestions for avoiding it whenever possible.

CYSTITIS IN CHILDREN

Cystitis in adults tends to be dramatically symptomatic, but in babies (most commonly boys with congenital abnormalities), the symptoms can be much more generalized and less easily recognized. Typical signs of a bladder infection in children include low-grade fever, loss of appetite, malaise, and a general failure to thrive. Because the symptoms are so non-specific, infections may endure for some time before a diagnosis is made. The danger of undetected bacteria in the urine is that infection will ascend into the kidneys where it can cause scarring and lead to kidney problems later in life, or that it will spread into the bloodstream and can cause severe illness. Because of the high likelihood of kidney involvement, childhood cystitis should not be treated lightly.

Vesicoureteral reflux, in which urine backs up from the bladder into the kidneys, is the cause of up to half of childhood kidney infections. In this condition, the normal *peristaltic* action of the ureters is impaired, and if infected urine backs up into the kidneys it can cause permanent scarring of the kidney's tissues.

Diagnosis of childhood UTIs begins with a urine culture. Special collecting containers may be used for babies. If it is difficult to get enough urine to analyze, your pediatrician may take a suprapubic aspiration. A thorough physical examination followed by an *ultrasound* test of the kidneys is often helpful in identifying congenital abnormalities that may cause urinary tract infections. A *renal scan* —a kidney function test that does not require the injection of dye —can also be useful. A *voiding cystourethrogram (VCUG)* is the main test used to diagnose the severity of vesicoureteral reflux. (See the Index of Diagnostic Tests for information on these tests.)

Pediatric urologists usually recommend ten days of antibiotics followed by a lesser dose for up to three to six months or longer depending upon follow-up urine cultures. Most children will outgrow vesicoureteral reflux as the urinary system matures. However, if the child continues to have infections while on antibiotic therapy, surgical repair usually results in a cure.

URETHRITIS

Infection or inflammation of the urethra, *urethritis*, causes about 100,000 office visits each year and is usually sexually transmitted. For diagnostic purposes, urethritis is divided into two basic categories:

- urethral infections caused by gonorrhea *(gonococcal urethritis or GU)* and
- infections caused by other organisms *(non-gonococcal urethritis or NGU)*, including *Chlamydia trachomatis,* which accounts for far more cases of urethritis than gonorrhea, *ureaplasma urealyticum,* a bacteria that also causes pneumonia, *herpes viruses, trichomonas,* and *venereal warts,* caused by *human papilloma virus (HPV).*

Up to 40 percent of people who get urethritis have both GU and NGU at the same time. Therefore, it is important to make sure that you are checked for each type of infection if you have symptoms, or if you think you have been exposed.

The symptoms for GU and NGU are essentially the same in both men and women. They include a milky or clear discharge from the urethra (which is easier for men to detect), and the surrounding tissues are often swollen and tender. The swelling can be accompanied by painful, slow, or difficult urination, and sometimes even urinary retention. If you are exposed to gonorrhea and an infection takes hold, the symptoms can appear as soon as one or two days after exposure. The incubation period for other non-gonococcal urethral infections can be anywhere from one to five weeks. Both men and, more commonly, women can be asymptomatic, that is, they will have no symptoms at all. This is especially dangerous in the case of gonorrhea and Chlamydia, which are very likely to cause pelvic inflammatory disease and possibly infertility in women or can spread to the prostate and testicles in men with similar consequences.

The diagnosis of urethritis is made by identifying pus in the first few drops of urine or from a *urethral smear,* cells obtained by inserting a swab into the urethral opening. Since there are a number of organisms that can cause NGU, several different tests may be required to make an accurate diagnosis. The results of these tests are normally ready in about three days. Cultures to show the presence of Chlamydia used to take several days, but a new test, called an *immune assay,* can show the presence of Chlamydia by the activity of antibodies that are produced in response and can be done in your doctor's office. The results can be ready in as little as 45 minutes. If you have not been sexually active for a while and your symptoms recur, or the symptoms persist after therapy, additional tests such as wet mount slides, herpes cultures, or Pap smears may be done.

Your doctor may also check your urethra for venereal warts, caused by the human papilloma virus (HPV), especially if you have had them before, or if you currently have visible warts on or near the genital area. Some subtypes of the HPV have been associated with changes in the cells on the face of the cervix that may be precancerous. If you have HPV and get a normal Pap smear, you should get several follow-ups to check for any recurrence of the warts after treatment, including a follow-up Pap smear. If you have warts *and* an abnormal Pap smear, your doctor may decide to do a biopsy to rule out cervical cancer. Visible venereal warts in men are treated and do not require special post-treatment check-ups and tests. Men whose female sexual partners have abnormal Pap smears should be followed more frequently, and smears from any suspicious lesions visible to the naked eye or when stained with a 5 percent solution of acetic acid should be sent for HPV typing. In women with normal Pap smears who have visible lesions, podophyllum, a caustic herbal preparation, is applied; this usually kills warts with one or two applications.

Urethritis is not as clear-cut in women as it is in men; therefore, misdiagnosis is fairly common. Women who have urethral tenderness but negative urinalysis and cultures of urethral smears, i.e., *no substantial reason can be found for their symptoms,* are sometimes told that they have "urethritis." If no evidence of infection can be found but you still have urethral discomfort, you might want to read the section on urethral syndrome (for women) on page 173 or on prostatodynia (for men) on page 193.

Treatment

Urethritis can be difficult to identify and treat because there are various possible causes and because two types may exist simultaneously, and the condition may be asymptomatic.

Gonococcal Urethritis (GU):

Penicillin was formerly the preferred treatment for GU. But today cefotexime (Rocephin) is favored because gonorrhea is less resistant to it, and the injections are not as painful. If you are allergic to penicillin, gonorrhea can also be treated orally with tetracycline or doxycycline for five days, or with a single megadose of Spectinomycin. Five days of ampicillin or amoxicillin may also be used.

A follow-up urethral smear or urinalysis using the first urine of the day should be obtained three to seven days after therapy to make sure that your infection was not caused by a resistant strain of gonorrhea, or that you did not also have an infection with another organism as well.

Non-Gonococcal Urethritis (NGU):

- *Chlamydia:* oral tetracycline or doxycycline for one to two weeks. In women, these drugs are likely to cause a vaginal yeast infection.
- *Trichomonas:* A seven-day regimen of metronidazole (Flagyl) is the standard treatment for trichomonas infections. However, this is a very strong drug with numerous side effects. The side effects can be minimized by taking a single megadose, two smaller doses taken in one day, or four doses taken one half hour apart.
- *Herpes:* There is no drug available that can eradicate this virus, which lives in nerve roots and is likely to recur without repeat exposure. However, acyclovir (Zovivax) cream can be applied to herpes sores during flare-ups of an active infection or can be taken orally for up to six months, which may reduce the frequency and severity of infections. Acyclovir pills may lessen the severity of the initial outbreak of herpes, but it is often less effective for recurrent episodes.
- *Venereal warts* or *human papilloma virus (HPV):* Visible warts can be treated topically with podophyllum, trichloroacetic acid, or with 5-fluorouracil, a drug that inhibits viral replication by interfering with protein synthesis, or warts can be burned off with electrical current or with a CO_2 laser beam. Condoms should be used for at least three months following therapy to avoid reinfection.

As with gonococcal urethritis, one of the most important keys to treatment for NGU is getting a follow-up exam and appropriate tests or cultures to make sure that the organism that caused the infection is eradicated.

Prevention of Urethritis

The incidence of urethritis is definitely associated with the number of sexual partners you have. Therefore, the principles of safer sex that have been developed to slow the spread of AIDS would also be helpful in preventing urethritis:

- having only one sexual partner at a time;
- knowing the recent sexual history of a new partner;
- using condoms for vaginal or anal intercourse.

If there is any question as to whether you or a potential partner might have been exposed to any of the sexually transmissible diseases, it would be a good idea to be checked for the ones mentioned in this chapter, as well as for the HIV (AIDS) virus, before engaging in vaginal or anal intercourse. If there is some question that one of you might have any of the conditions that cause urethritis, you might consider taking antibiotics.

Because the organisms that cause urethritis are almost always sexually transmitted, diagnosing and treating your sexual partners at the same time is another extremely important preventive measure. If you learn that you have any of the conditions that can cause urethritis, you should immediately notify all of your sexual partners and suggest that they go in for treatment. In the case of gonorrhea, federal health regulations require that you give the names of all your sexual partners to your doctor or to the clinic where you receive a diagnosis.

REMEMBER: Using condoms in *all* non-monogamous situations could prevent most cases of urethritis!

Both cystitis and urethritis can be frustrating conditions to deal with. But they need not wreck your life. Instead of waiting in dread for the next episode of cystitis, you should now be able to identify some of the factors that may be precipitating recurrences. And by asking the right questions, you should now be able to find a doctor whom you can work with and formulate a plan of care aimed at liberating you from the pain and unpredictability that recurrent episodes of cystitis impose.

CYSTITIS REMINDERS

• When cystitis symptoms flare up, a urinalysis (or at least a urine dipstick test at home) should always be done to make sure that bacteria are present.
• If you have more than three episodes of cystitis a year, you should begin looking for the cause.
• A single megadose of antibiotics or a short three-day course may be as effective as seven- to fourteen-day regimens.
• Changing contraception, sexual practices, and personal habits may help reduce cystitis flare-ups without medication.

RESOURCES

SELF-HELP RESOURCES

The Herb Book, John Lust. New York: Bantam Books, 1974. This is one of the most popular and accessible guides to medicinal herbs.
Overcoming Cystitis: A Practical Self-Help Guide for Women, Wendy Smith. New York: Bantam Books, 1987. This excellent guide is written by a woman who brought her own chronic cystitis under control using self-help strategies and occasional prophylactic antibiotic therapy.
Understanding Cystitis, Angela Kilmartin. New York: Warner Books, 1986. This was the first book to address the issue of cystitis and was the only available resource for many years. Written by an Englishwoman who had severe cystitis herself, the book is very sympathetic and contains some excellent common-sense self-help advice on dealing with chronic cystitis, but makes little reference to scientific literature. Some of the recommendations (for example, to flush the bladder with coffee at the first sign of infection) may actually be harmful. This book does not mention interstitial cystitis or urethral syndrome.
The Way of Herbs, Michael Tierra. New York: Washington Square Press/ Pocket Books, 1980. This herbal guide combines Eastern, European, and Native American healing traditions.

The Woman Doctor's Guide to Overcoming Cystitis, Kathryn Schroetenboer-Cox and Sue Berkman. New York: New American Library, 1989. This book, written from a doctor's perspective, reviews the standard information on cystitis in a clear and readable fashion.

MEDICAL RESOURCES

Detection, Prevention and Management of Urinary Tract Infections, 4th ed., C. M. Kunin, ed. Philadelphia: Lea & Febiger, 1987.
Urinary Infection and Inflammation, Jackson E. Fowler, Jr., ed. Chicago: Year Book Medical Publishers, 1989.

CHAPTER 6

The Painful Bladder Syndrome: Interstitial Cystitis and Urethral Syndrome

KATHY, A FORTY-SEVEN-YEAR-OLD ADVERTISING EX-ecutive, has to urinate about twenty-five times a day and has dark circles under her eyes because she usually wakes up three or four more times a night to empty her bladder. She had her first bladder infection when she was seventeen and had periodic recurrences after that. About six years ago, she had an unusually bad attack. "This time the pain was really intense. It felt different—like razor blades in my bladder," she remembers. Kathy's gynecologist could find no bacteria in her urine but gave her antibiotics, suggesting that she lower her stress level and maybe take a vacation. "I was willing to do anything, so my husband made arrangements and we went to Florida for a week. As soon as we got off the plane my symptoms got so bad that I had to go to the hospital. They found nothing wrong and gave me a lot of tranquilizers," she says. When Kathy returned home, she went to a urologist. "He said that I had 'urethral syndrome,' and dilated my urethra. That really set things off. I was urinating about every half hour and had a constant burn in my bladder." She saw a neurologist, who found nothing wrong but referred her to a psychiatrist. "Finally, about two years ago, my mother sent me an article from the newspaper about a woman who had interstitial cystitis. It described my symptoms exactly."

Kathy's experience is typical of many people who have interstitial cystitis. She saw five doctors before she found out what was wrong with her, and then she essentially diagnosed herself. When

she came to see Kristene, she said, "I think I have interstitial cystitis. Can you help me?" Kristene did the appropriate diagnostic tests
and found that Kathy had a moderate form of the disease. Then,
together, they planned Kathy's course of treatment.

Until recently, interstitial cystitis (IC) was thought to be a rare
disorder, and many doctors still believe this. But things are beginning to change. Thanks to the efforts of the Interstitial Cystitis
Association and a small group of concerned physicians, doctors are
becoming more aware of the procedures that are necessary to diagnose the disease, and people who may have it are more aware
that help is available.

HOW THIS CHAPTER CAN HELP YOU

The Self-Evaluation Checklist below notes the symptoms and
typical experiences of people who have interstitial cystitis and "urethral syndrome." If you check several of the items on the list, then
the information in this chapter may be of help to you. If you have
not yet seen a doctor, or if you have been to several with unsatis-
factory results, this information can help you ask the appropriate
questions to get a correct diagnosis and realistic treatment. If you
are a long-time interstitial cystitis patient, you may already know a
great deal about many aspects of the disease. In that case, it may
be instructive to compare your experiences, symptoms, and treatments with those of the other IC patients whose experiences are
used to illustrate the information in the chapter. If you have IC
and are considering getting pregnant, you may want to know how
other women who have this condition have fared during their
pregnancies. If you have not had good results with other forms of
therapy and are considering having your bladder removed, you
may find the section Major Surgery (page 164) particularly rele-
vant. The section What It's Like to Have Interstitial Cystitis is a
composite of thoughts and feelings of many people who have the
disease. If you have IC, you may be able to identify with many of
these experiences. Or if you know someone who has the disease,
this section may help you gain a deeper appreciation of their daily
struggles. If you have been diagnosed with "urethral syndrome,"
or you have repeated episodes of cystitis-like symptoms but have

no bacteria in your urine, then you might find the section on this common but little-understood disorder helpful.

____ Do you have urgent, frequent urination, but consistently get negative urine cultures?

____ Do you have continual pain in your bladder, urethra, or vagina that is relieved briefly by urination?

____ Do you consistently wake up two or more times at night to urinate?

____ Does your doctor treat you over the phone for cystitis without checking your urine for bacteria?

____ Have you been given antibiotics as a treatment for cystitis symptoms even though there are no bacteria in your urine?

____ Have you tried many treatments for interstitial cystitis and still have pain and frequency?

____ Are you taking medications for interstitial cystitis that don't seem to help?

____ Are you contemplating surgery for interstitial cystitis?

____ Have you seen several doctors and gotten no relief?

____ Have you had repeated urethral dilations, but still have the same symptoms?

____ Have you been told that you have "urethral syndrome," urethritis, non-bacterial prostatitis, or prostatodynia?

____ Have you been told nothing can be done to help you?

____ Have you been referred to a psychiatrist and been told "it's all in your head"?

WHAT IS INTERSTITIAL CYSTITIS?

Interstitial cystitis literally means cystitis, or inflammation, in the bladder wall. In this case, however, the inflammation does not appear to come from an invasion of bacteria. Its cause is unknown. Because the symptoms vary so much from person to person, and response to treatment is so unpredictable, doctors specializing in IC are beginning to think about it as a "symptom complex" with a number of possible causes.[1]

Since it is difficult to say exactly what interstitial cystitis is, it is perhaps easier to describe the symptoms that you might experience and its signs—objective evidence of disease. (A sore throat is a *symptom*; the reddened mucous lining of the throat is a *sign*.)

In 1987, the Urban Institute, a social policy research organization in Washington, D.C., conducted a survey which provided the first in-depth look at the lives of people with interstitial cystitis.*[2]

The respondents noted the following symptoms:

- waking at night two or more times to urinate (85%)
- urgency of urination (84%)
- frequency of urination—15–50 times in 24 hours (80%)
- pain in the bladder, urethra, or vagina (78%)
- pain relieved by voiding (57%)
- painful intercourse (57%)
- difficulty in emptying the bladder (51%)
- difficulty in starting flow (47%)

For many people, especially those with milder cases, the symptoms may wax and wane, and unpredictable flare-ups can be difficult to bring under control. Some people with severe cases perceive pain as pressure, burning, "electric shocks," spasms, or stabbing pain that is present almost continually. "Some days may be better than others, but the pain is always there," says Constance, who has had IC symptoms for twenty-seven years but was only diagnosed in 1984. In addition, many of the women who answered our survey said that their symptoms usually or always flare up with ovulation and are usually worse from midcycle until one to three days after menstrual bleeding begins. Many people also reported that their symptoms are exacerbated by physical or emotional stress, acid foods, travel, and intercourse.

In 1915, Dr. G. L. Hunner published a paper on rare bladder ulcers in women who had urgent urination, extreme frequency, and sleep disruption due to the constant need to urinate. Most of

* This landmark survey was directed by Dr. Philip Held of the Urban Institute, the National Institutes of Health, the Interstitial Cystitis Association, Dr. Mark Pauly of the Wharton School, and Drs. Alan Wein and Philip Hanno of the University of Pennsylvania School of Medicine in conjunction with the Interstitial Cystitis Association. Randomized questionnaires were sent to more than 400 urologists and some of their patients, more than 900 female members of the ICA who had been diagnosed with IC, and more than 100 members of the general population.

these women were post-menopausal and had been experiencing dire symptoms for an average of seventeen years.[3] Hunner identified large bleeding ulcers or sores in the bladders of many of them, and soon the presence of ulcers became the hallmark of the disease. With the rather primitive equipment available at the time, Hunner was probably seeing only the most prominent of many small, superficial hemorrhages that dot the bladders of many IC patients. Today, with instruments that provide clear visualization of the interior of the bladder, small hemorrhages can readily be seen. The ulcers that Hunner described bear his name today, but their frequency is quite rare, even in severe cases, and their presence or absence is no longer essential to a diagnosis of interstitial cystitis.

While the signs of interstitial cystitis can't be seen with the naked eye, in many cases dramatic changes occur in the bladder, which can be seen through a cystoscope when the bladder has been overdistended (stretched to its full capacity) with water. Tiny pinpoint hemorrhages dot the bladder surface and blood may be seen in the urine. These *petechial* hemorrhages are now considered to be the hallmark of interstitial cystitis. In the worst cases, perhaps about 10 percent, the bladder lining becomes scarred from the ulcers and the bladder may shrink, becoming hard and fibrotic. Such bladders may hold only 1 or 2 ounces of urine at a time, as compared to 8 to 12 ounces for a normal bladder. "My urethra just doesn't function very efficiently," says David, who has had interstitial cystitis for eight years. "Sometimes I just stand there for two or three minutes before anything happens, and a lot of times, it isn't worth the effort."

Although it is a singular disease in many respects, interstitial cystitis has some striking similarities with certain other diseases in which inflammatory processes predominate: lupus erythematosus, rheumatoid arthritis, asthma, irritable bowel syndrome, allergic rhinitis (nasal congestion due to allergies), and polyarteritis (inflammation of the smaller arteries). While many IC patients have no other major diseases, it is not uncommon for people with IC to have a constellation of these conditions. Liza is typical of this group. In addition to IC, she also suffers from inflammatory bowel disease, chronic low back pain, and allergic rhinitis.

Although there is no known correlation between interstitial cystitis and bladder cancer, many people with IC worry that they may be at higher risk for developing bladder cancer. At this time, there is absolutely no evidence that the chronic inflammation of interstitial cystitis stimulates the growth of bladder cancer.

Contrary to a widely held myth, *there does not appear to be any psychological cause for interstitial cystitis.* However, persistent symptoms can ultimately have severe psychological and emotional consequences. In cases of long duration, sleep deprivation and chronic pain may cause addiction to painkillers. The inability to work productively and to enjoy normal pleasures may cause feelings of personal failure, a poor self-image, and ultimately, depression—even thoughts of suicide. In general, interstitial cystitis is not a life-threatening condition and many people have learned to cope with it successfully. However, numerous IC patients report having suicidal thoughts three to four times more frequently than the general population, and there have been many reports of actual suicides.

One of the supreme ironies of this very peculiar disease is that, except for eyes that are puffy from lack of sleep or from tears of frustration, this enormous suffering is largely hidden, with none of the usual outward signs of illness such as pallor, a limp, palsy, or a noticeable fading of vitality. Interstitial cystitis has no outward, visible signs. In fact, many people have found that this is a significant disadvantage. "Friends don't really seem to understand that even though I might look okay, I get tired easily and can't do everything that they can do," reports Ida. Other people remarked that their friends thought them "undisciplined" or "neurotic" because they appeared to be in apparent good health.

Pregnancy and Interstitial Cystitis

In 1989, the Interstitial Cystitis Association did a survey on how women who have mild, moderate, and severe forms of the disease and became pregnant fared. The survey revealed that women who had mild symptoms often got worse and their symptoms remained worse for up to six months after delivery. Women with severe symptoms often seemed to improve, and remained that way for up to six months after delivery. Women with moderate symptoms appeared to remain much the same. As for pregnancy outcome, there was no significant difference in the number of Cesarean deliveries and the disease did not appear to have any impact on the general health of the infant.

WHO HAS INTERSTITIAL CYSTITIS?

Because underdiagnosis of interstitial cystitis has been the norm for so long, it is difficult to say exactly how many people have the disease. The responses revealed some fascinating, if disturbing, data and dismissed, as well, some widely held myths about the disease.

According to the Urban Institute survey, there are somewhere between 20,000 and 90,000 *diagnosed* cases of interstitial cystitis in the United States. Doctors responding to the survey acknowledged having an average of five patients with some form of the painful bladder syndrome for every one who was diagnosed with IC, so perhaps five times as many people have the disease as have been reported—somewhere in the range of 100,000 to 450,000. Even if the lower figure is considered, IC is far more common than such well-known diseases as sickle cell anemia (30,000), cystic fibrosis (50,000), and hemophilia (20,000). Because of the tendency toward underdiagnosis, the Urban Institute data suggest that the number of people who have interstitial cystitis approaches the higher figure of 450,000.

Ninety percent of interstitial cystitis patients are women. Prior to this survey, IC was thought to be primarily a post-menopausal disease. This may have been because it took people so long to get diagnosed. However, the survey found that quite the opposite was true. The average age of the onset of symptoms in this study was forty, and 25 percent of the diagnosed respondents were under thirty years of age. Earlier medical literature tells us that a small number of teenagers and children have also been diagnosed with the condition.[4] The Urban Institute survey found few black women and even fewer black men with IC. But until more extensive research is done, we cannot make the assumption that the incidence of IC is necessarily lower in blacks or other minorities. The dramatically lower figures may be a reflection of minorities' lack of access to health care.

POSSIBLE CAUSES OF INTERSTITIAL CYSTITIS

Doctors who work closely with interstitial cystitis are baffled by the peculiarities of the disease and, to date, do not have any concrete information on its causes. But until we understand the poten-

139

tial causes, we cannot develop reliable, effective treatments. A number of intriguing theories regarding possible causes have been proposed, but so far there is little concrete evidence to support any of them:

- *A history of urinary tract infections.* Childhood bladder problems are ten times more common in people with IC than in the general population, and adults were ten to twelve times as likely to have had one or more UTIs.[5]
- *Bacteria, virus, or fungus.* One early theory held that interstitial cystitis was caused by some type of infection, such as *Streptococcus*, but so far no evidence has been found to support this idea.
- *Antibiotics.* Since an overwhelming majority of IC patients have been treated with antibiotics for UTIs, it has been suggested that these drugs might somehow damage the bladder lining. One study has shown that nitrofurantoin, an antibiotic commonly used to treat UTIs, does not damage the rabbit bladder,[6] but it is not clear how this antibiotic interacts with the human bladder lining.
- *Autoimmune disorder.* The chronic inflammation in the bladder characteristic of IC resembles an autoimmune disorder in which antibodies (substances that form in the bloodstream in response to invasion from a foreign substance) act on the bladder wall in some way. To date, no bladder antibodies have been found.[7]
- *Deficiency in the bladder lining.* The bladder lining is coated with a thin layer of a sugar-based substance called *mucin* by some researchers and *glycosaminoglycans* (*GAGs* for short) by others. The filmy layer coats the bladder somewhat as Pepto-Bismol coats the stomach, preventing toxins or bacteria in the urine from gaining access to the delicate inner layers of the bladder wall. The positive response of many IC patients to Elmiron, a drug that acts as a synthetic GAG layer, has provided some support for the idea that the bladder lining may be defective in some way.[8] Yet no substantial difference in the GAG layer of people with IC and those with normal bladders has been found.[9]
- *Toxic substances in the urine.* Some doctors who work closely with IC have speculated that there may be toxic substances in the urine that might irritate or injure the bladder lining. The fact that severe IC symptoms disappear completely in most cases when the urine is diverted from the bladder to an interior

"pouch" or to an outside collection bag suggests that the urine may contain some substance that sets off an inflammatory process.[10]

- *Abnormal numbers of mast cells.* A good bit of research interest has focused on mast cells, commonly found in connective tissues throughout the body, which release histamine and other substances when they break up or degranulate. Some studies have suggested that mast cells are found in higher concentrations in the bladders of about one half of all IC patients.[11] However, a recent study found elevated levels of mast cells in higher concentrations in non-IC patients who had other bladder disorders than in those who had been diagnosed with the disease.[12] Until further research is done, it is not clear what this means. It does suggest, however, that elevated levels of mast cells in the bladder wall can't be used as a definite sign or "marker" in the diagnosis of interstitial cystitis.

- *Abnormal metabolism of tryptophane and serotonin.* Some question has been raised about the role of serotonin and its precursor, tryptophane, in the disease process of interstitial cystitis. These potent chemicals, found in the brain and nervous system, affect sensory perception, sleep patterns, the transmission of nerve impulses, and the constriction of blood vessels—all areas in which people with IC have problems. Not much research has been done in this field, but there has been a lot of speculation about whether foods containing tryptophane increase IC symptoms. (See page 159 for more discussion on tryptophane in the diet.)

- *Hormonal factors.* The fact that 90 percent of interstitial cystitis patients are women has led researchers to speculate about the possible role of hormones in the disorder; which hormones, and how they affect the bladder, is still a mystery.

- *Pelvic surgery.* The fact that about one third of IC patients had a hysterectomy, Cesarean delivery, or some other type of pelvic surgery prior to coming down with the disease has prompted some speculation about the role of surgery or perhaps anesthesia in the development of the disorder.

This review of the possible causes of interstitial cystitis raises many questions but provides few answers. Clearly, a great deal of painstaking research will need to be done before we begin to get a more complete picture of the disease. There are a number of pilot studies now under way that should give us a better understanding of basic bladder function. Hopefully, this research will help uncover the cause of interstitial cystitis and lead to a cure.

PREPARING FOR YOUR DOCTOR'S VISIT

Because there is no specific test for interstitial cystitis, your symptoms and your medical history are very important in evaluating whether or not you have the condition. Therefore, it would be helpful for you to prepare carefully for your visit, using the guidelines begining on page 24. In addition, one of the most useful things you can do is to take a voiding chart to your first visit, showing how much and what kind of liquid you drink each day, how frequently you urinate, both day and night, and how much urine you produce each time for two or three days. If you don't do this, your doctor will probably ask for one anyway, and you will have to do it for your next visit. A sample voiding chart can be found on pages 26–27. Your doctor will also want to know:

- how long you have had your symptoms;
- if you have pain that is relieved by emptying your bladder;
- what event, if any, precipitated your symptoms;
- if you have a history of urinary tract infections;
- if anyone else in your family has bladder problems;
- if you have any allergies;
- what other medical conditions you have or had;
- if you are taking any medications; and
- if you can identify things that worsen your symptoms.

DIAGNOSIS

Until interstitial cystitis began getting some attention from prominent urologists around 1986 and 1987, when diagnostic guidelines were established, diagnosis of the disease was a hit-or-miss proposition even when the symptoms were very compelling. The Urban Institute survey found that people with IC symptoms saw an average of two to five doctors over a period of more than four years before obtaining a correct diagnosis. Indeed, it is not unusual for someone to see ten or more doctors before getting a correct diagnosis. In a letter to the Interstitial Cystitis Association, Helena described a typical series of misdiagnoses: "I have suffered from vague, painful urinary symptoms on and off for four years. I am twenty-seven and this 'reaction to stress,' 'psychosomatic problem,' 'reaction to sex,' or 'urethral syndrome' makes my life horrible when it strikes. I am losing my mind and do not know where to turn."

Rebecca's survey on interstitial cystitis revealed a wide variety of conditions with which people with interstitial cystitis have been misdiagnosed:

Psychological problems
 need to find a lover or get married
 suffering from not having a baby
 nerves/depression/nervous breakdown
 being a complainer/wanting attention
 need to get life in order
Urethral problems
 "urethral syndrome"
 small/underdeveloped urethra
 urethral stenosis/stricture of the urethra
 faulty location of urethra
 voiding problems
Bladder problems
 urinary tract infections
 trabecular (scarred) bladder
 calcium deposits in the bladder
 urinary retention
 spastic bladder
 fallen bladder
 trigonitis
Gynecological problems
 endometriosis
 uterine polyps
 embedded ovary
 fibroids
 tumor on ovary
 tubal pregnancy
 pelvic floor myalgia
 adhesions from surgery
 yeast

Miscellaneous
   appendicitis
   fatigue syndrome
   multiple sclerosis
   rectal infection

   This list of rather surprising diversity illustrates widespread confusion about interstitial cystitis on the part of doctors and enormous frustration on the part of patients, whose complaints have often not been taken seriously or who have been treated for numerous conditions that they did not have. Being aware of the many conditions that can be mistaken for interstitial cystitis should help you avoid misdiagnosis. If you have the classic symptoms of interstitial cystitis listed on page 136, and are told that you have any of the problems listed above, you should insist that your doctor carefully justify the diagnosis. If he or she cannot do this to your satisfaction, then you might do well to get a second or even third opinion.

The Key to Getting a Correct Diagnosis

   Drs. Alan Wein and Philip Hanno have noted that *the most frequent reason for misdiagnosis has been the physician's failure to consider the possibility of interstitial cystitis in the first place.* As Dr. Hanno further observes, "Many physicians do not even believe the condition exists."[13] Because there are no specific tests that can definitively identify the disease, the diagnosis of IC is essentially one of exclusion; that is, after other possible conditions have been tested for and excluded, and you still have symptoms, then you probably have IC.

   Another prominent reason for frequent misdiagnosis is that the tiny hemorrhages that are considered the hallmark of interstitial cystitis are not usually visible on a cystoscope examination done in the doctor's office. They can only be seen when the bladder is overdistended (filled to its capacity with water) when you are under general anesthesia. Until recently, most doctors have been reluctant to subject young, apparently healthy people to the risks of general anesthesia when they did not think it was necessary. No doubt another reason for frequent misdiagnosis is a tendency on the part of many physicians not to take the symptoms of interstitial cystitis seriously, seeing many IC patients—most of whom are women—as complainers, neurotics, or psychosomatics.

One of the consequences of misdiagnosis is mistreatment, which often compounds the problem and leaves you more miserable and confused than ever. With a better understanding of the interstitial cystitis syndrome, we can hope that misdiagnosis will become the exception rather than the rule, and that the severe symptoms of the disease will be taken seriously and treated sympathetically by physicians.

Diagnostic Tests

If, on the basis of your medical history and voiding chart, your doctor suspects interstitial cystitis, he or she may order the following tests.

THE TESTS NOTED HERE ARE DESCRIBED IN DETAIL IN THE INDEX OF DIAGNOSTIC TESTS, BEGINNING ON PAGE 278.

- A *urine culture* to rule out bacterial cystitis;
- a *urine cytology* test to look for cancer cells;
- a kidney X-ray *(intravenous pyelogram or IVP)* or an *ultrasound* test to rule out abnormalities of the kidneys and ureters, and to look for other possible bladder abnormalities such as stones and tumors or pelvic masses.

Urodynamic tests may also be done to assess basic bladder and urethral function.

- A *cystometrogram (CMG)* will show if the proper nerve signals are being sent and received by the bladder; it will also show how much urine your bladder will hold normally (your *functional bladder capacity*) and whether the bladder is emptying completely.
- A *uroflow* test measures the flow of urine to see how well you urinate over a period of time.
- A *residual urine test* will show the amount of urine left in the bladder after voiding.
- The function of the pelvic muscles will be assessed by an *electromyogram (EMG)*, which tests the response of your pelvic muscles to nerve stimulation.

The most important parts of the evaluation for interstitial cystitis are the overdistention of the bladder and cystoscopic examination

145

of the bladder's interior to look for hemorrhages. The bladder overdistention is also one of the standard treatments. Because these procedures may be painful, they may be done under general anesthesia or intravenous sedation, and may or may not require an overnight hospital stay, depending on your doctor's preference. A biopsy of the bladder wall is often done at the time of the bladder distention, to rule out other obscure causes of symptoms. Like some doctors, Kristene often chooses to begin conservative therapy, such as dietary changes and oral medications, before subjecting her patients to this procedure. Dr. Magnus Fall, who has done research on IC for many years at the University of Göteborg in Sweden, feels that biopsies are not always necessary in routine cases, noting that they are probably more appropriate for research purposes.[14]

THE CLASSIFICATION OF INTERSTITIAL CYSTITIS

In the not-so-distant past, many IC specialists referred to the more severe form of interstitial cystitis as "classic" disease. Others preferred to label mild to moderate disease as "early" and the more severe form as "late" IC. But these labels imply that "early" should at some point become "late," which is an issue that is far from settled. Most urologists who are familiar with IC believe that the condition of the bladder and symptoms do not deteriorate over time. In fact, the "early" form is often referred to as "non-ulcerative" IC. Drs. Hanno and Wein have suggested[15] classifying IC patients into four categories:

- those with symptoms, *but no unusual findings* from urodynamic studies, cystoscopic investigation, or biopsy;
- those who have symptoms and *abnormalities in bladder or urethral function*, but the bladder appears normal when it is overdistended and bladder capacity and biopsy are normal;
- those who have symptoms and *the bladder cracks, bleeds, or hemorrhages* during distention and capacity is decreased;
- those who have symptoms and *the biopsy shows the increased presence of mast cells in the bladder wall.*

These criteria take into account the tremendous range in symptoms and the disease process itself. They are not highly specific, but they offer patients and physicians a general way to assess the severity of the disease and can provide some guidance in choosing appropriate treatments. As this classification illustrates, there is not a direct correlation between a person's symptoms and the condition of the bladder.

TREATMENT

Since the cause of interstitial cystitis is unknown, treatments are primarily aimed at alleviating the symptoms. People with mild symptoms may choose not to have some of the more aggressive forms of therapy, because these treatments may be quite uncomfortable for several days afterward. But even when the symptoms are very severe, a conservative approach is recommended, moving methodically from the least invasive and most likely to work, to more drastic surgical treatments designed to block pain or to divert the urine. Each of these treatments may work for a certain percentage of patients, at least for a while. But more often than not, the symptoms return. One of the most discouraging realities about interstitial cystitis is that some people have tried every type of treatment and are still in pain.

Because the chance of success with medically accepted treatments is limited, interstitial cystitis patients have been particularly inventive about improvising self-help regimens and seeking out alternative treatments. Often these have been used as adjuncts to medical treatments and in many cases, changes in diet, personal habits, or lifestyle have resulted in significant improvement.

If you are suffering from severe pain and frequency, you may be tempted to try everything at once, but this scatter-gun approach might be counterproductive. Since the results of various treatments are so unpredictable, Dr. Grannum Sant of Tufts University in Boston recommends undertaking only one type of therapy at a time, suggesting that if something works but you are trying two or three new treatments, you won't know what is working and may have to start from scratch again.[16] This seems like sound advice, unless your symptoms are very severe, in which case you may want to try anything that might bring them under control.

Endoscopic Therapy

Endoscopic procedures allow your doctor to "look within" an organ or body cavity. In urology, the endoscopy is done with a cystoscope, which allows direct visualization of the interior of the bladder and urethra. The following treatments may be performed in conjunction with endoscopy.

Distention of the bladder, also called hydraulic distention, is used in both the diagnosis and treatment of interstitial cystitis. In treatment, the bladder is filled with water for varying amounts of time, from a few minutes to several hours. About 30 to 50 percent of the people who undergo this procedure experience a lessening of symptoms for up to six months or longer.[17] After the procedure there can be some temporary bleeding or burning during urination. Some people experience a decrease in urgency and frequency quickly, but others may have to wait two weeks or longer until the irritation caused by the procedure subsides.

Some urologists believe that ulcers in the bladder may be a specific source of pain and that their removal can be helpful. In *transurethral resection (TUR) or cauterization,* a cystoscope is inserted into the bladder and through it a probe with a hot tip is inserted. The tip is used to burn away the ulcerated tissue and seal off blood vessels. Swedish researchers have had success in reducing pain in 40 and 70 percent of the cases they have treated.[18]

Laser Treatment

Many people who have relatively severe cases of interstitial cystitis have pain accompanied by bleeding from ulcers or hemorrhages in the bladder wall. A few physicians have had some success in stopping bleeding and reducing areas of inflammation (and hence reducing pain) with the neodymium-YAG contact laser, which is commonly used to remove cancerous tumors in the bladder. This type of treatment has been used for people who have not had success from other treatments such as DMSO and other bladder instillations (see below). In the only recent report on laser treatments, about two thirds of the study participants experienced relief or improvement of symptoms, although many of them had a recurrence of symptoms from six to eighteen months after treatment.[19]

The primary complications of laser treatments are the danger of bowel perforation due to "scatter" or burning through the bladder wall. These problems can be minimized by restricting the laser energy output. In laser treatments, as in surgery, the skill of the practitioner is all-important, so you should choose the doctor who does your treatments with great care. Be sure to ask how many people he or she has treated with this type of procedure, how many people have been helped, and if any serious complications have occurred. Although there have been reports of disastrous results from laser treatments, Kristene has treated about fifty patients using the neodymium-YAG laser, which eliminates the danger of "scatter," with excellent results.

Bladder Instillations

The industrial solvent DMSO has been used on everything from arthritis to sports injuries and many claims have been made for miraculous cures. Surprisingly, interstitial cystitis is one of the conditions in which some effectiveness has been documented. In fact, treatment with RIMSO-50, manufactured by Research Industries Corporation, is the only FDA-approved use of this compound.

It is not known exactly how DMSO works in the bladder, but researchers have observed it has many properties that make it a logical choice for the management of IC. In addition to being a powerful anti-inflammatory agent, DMSO may relax the bladder muscle, and appears to have analgesic properties that can soothe irritated tissues. Further, DMSO easily penetrates membranes, and if it is mixed with other drugs, it enhances drug absorption.[20]

A DMSO treatment can be done in the doctor's office in 15 to 20 minutes. In this procedure, about 2 ounces (one quarter of a cup) of DMSO, or a "cocktail" with other drugs, is placed into the bladder through a small catheter. The liquid is then held in the bladder for about 15 to 20 minutes. Some people find it difficult to retain the solution for the necessary amount of time, and that it can sting the urethra when it is released. DMSO can occasionally also cause a "chemical cystitis" (severe burning in the bladder) for several days afterward. Some people who have had this reaction find that taking Pyridium, a bladder analgesic, the day before the treatment, and drinking lots of water or taking baking soda afterward can help "cool the burn" and shorten the time of discomfort.

Another minor but less socially acceptable side effect of DMSO is a garlic-like odor on the skin and breath, which occurs for about

149

a day after the treatment. Some people find this a particularly disagreeable side effect, especially at work or on social occasions. But others, like Myra, seem to roll with the punches and refuse to let a case of industrial-strength bad breath ruin a major social occasion. On the evening of her first DMSO treatment, Myra and her husband were supposed to take their daughter and a new boyfriend whom they had not met to the Four Seasons restaurant in New York. "When I was getting dressed for dinner, my husband noticed that I smelled like garlic," she says. "He thought it was so offensive that we should break the engagement." Frantically Myra called her doctor, who assured her that the odor was perfectly normal, and advised her to drink lots of water. "I felt fine and could not smell it on myself, so I took a shower and used a lot of mouth spray. During the dinner, whenever my husband could detect the odor, he would tap me on the shoulder—more mouth spray." Myra reports that the evening went very well, and says that afterward she realized it was her first victory over interstitial cystitis.

The normal regimen is one DMSO treatment every week for four to eight weeks and then periodically as needed if the result is good. If you have not had significant improvement after six to eight treatments, however, you and your doctor should probably pursue other forms of therapy. DMSO has been found to cause deformities in animal fetuses, so its use is *not* recommended during pregnancy.

Several studies have carefully investigated the effectiveness of DMSO for mild, moderate, and severe cases of interstitial cystitis. In milder cases, from 50 to 90 percent of the study participants experienced moderate to excellent improvement.[21] In the most severe cases, 50 to 70 percent of the patients had good to excellent results. Some people, unfortunately, experience no relief at all. Because of its positive track record, and its lack of long-term side effects in most people, DMSO has become one of the standard treatments for IC.

Some doctors have begun enhancing DMSO with a combination of hydrocortisone (another anti-inflammatory agent), heparin (an anticoagulant and a major constituent of the bladder's GAG layer), and sodium bicarbonate. Kristene uses a variation of this formula, substituting an 0.5 solution of bupivacaine, a long-acting local anesthetic, for DMSO. This cocktail seems to eliminate some of the discomfort that is typically associated with bladder instillation. The regimen seems very promising, offering relief to more than half of the people who have tried it, and formal studies are pending. Because no controlled trials have been done, no data exists to support the contention that these formulas work better than plain DMSO.

Chlorpactin is another solution that has been employed in efforts to alleviate the symptoms of IC. Before administration, a bladder X-ray known as a voiding cystourethrogram (VCUG) needs to be done to make sure that the ureters will be able to prevent the solution from traveling up to the kidneys, where it could cause major damage. Because the instillation of chlorpactin is painful, some doctors have started instilling a less concentrated solution. This has the advantage of avoiding the use of general anesthesia and cutting down on side effects afterward.

The use of chlorpactin in the treatment of interstitial cystitis presents a puzzling contradiction. On the one hand, it is caustic to the delicate mucous membrane lining of the bladder. On the other hand, after the initial pain has subsided, some people have gotten long-term relief. In one study, one third of the patients treated with chlorpactin had a remission of their symptoms for longer than six months and 70 percent experienced some improvement.[22]

Silver nitrate is another solution that has been instilled into the bladder to relieve the symptoms of interstitial cystitis. Older studies suggested greater than 50 percent of IC patients experienced relief of symptoms with silver nitrate, but its use is currently not very widespread and there is no recent data on its effectiveness.

Drugs

Given the complex and sometimes overwhelming manifestations of interstitial cystitis, the IC sufferer's pharmacopeia is understandably imaginative and extensive. One drug will seem to work fairly well for a substantial number of the people who try it, while giving others no help at all. Few studies have been done on most of the medications prescribed for IC; therefore, each drug tried is something of an experiment. But given the desperate situation of many IC patients, the experiment is often worth it. The following drugs are the ones that have been most frequently employed in the treatment of IC.

Sodium pentosanpolysulfate (Elmiron) is a synthetic sugarlike substance that appears to aid in restoring the protective lining of the bladder. In studies at seven sites being done to satisfy FDA requirements for approval, more than 40 percent of the patients had a reduction in pain, nearly 40 percent had a decrease in urgency, and 65 percent experienced a significant decrease in urinary frequency. Elmiron seems to be most effective in decreasing frequency. So far the chief side effect of Elmiron appears to be diarrhea in a small percentage of people, and a few people have also experienced bleeding disorders and hair loss.

You do not have to be in a study to get Elmiron. Your doctor can obtain it on a "compassionate use" basis, by contacting the manufacturer, Medical Marketing Specialists of Boonton, New Jersey. Elmiron is currently in the final phase of clinical trials and should be approved for general use by the Food and Drug Administration sometime between the end of 1990 and 1992.

Amitriptyline (Elavil) belongs to the class of drugs known as *tricyclic antidepressants* which has long been used to treat anxiety and depression. Because it blocks central nervous system activity and has a sedative effect, Elavil has also been successfully used in treating pain syndromes. The use of this drug for interstitial cystitis was discovered quite by accident when one of Dr. Hanno's patients began taking it for depression and experienced a dramatic improvement in her IC symptoms. Elavil is the least invasive of the treatments for IC and it seems to work well for many people in whom pain and/or nocturia are the most bothersome symptoms. In one study, 40 percent of the patients had a total remission for an average of eight months.[23]

In normal tissue, histamines are released from the breakdown of mast cells, causing an inflammatory response—pain, puffiness, and ultimately fibrosis, the formation of scar tissue in the bladder wall. Both prescription and over-the-counter *antihistamines* such as Benadryl have been used to counteract the effects of histamines.

Non-steroidal anti-inflammatory agents are another logical class of drugs used in the management of interstitial cystitis. These range all the way from over-the-counter medications like aspirin and ibuprofen (Advil, Motrin or Nuprin) to prescription anti-inflammatories such as naproxen (Naprosyn, Anaprox) and piroxicam (Feldene).

Alpha blockers have been employed on a limited basis in the treatment of IC as well as urethral syndrome. These drugs interfere with nerve impulses to the smooth muscles of the bladder neck and urethra, blocking pain and relaxing the urethra. In the past, phenoxybenzamine (Dibenzyline) was widely used and is still prescribed today, but it has been found to cause cancer in laboratory animals, so its long-term use is not recommended. If your doctor prescribes Dibenzyline, ask him or her about possible alternatives. Prazosin hydrochloride (Minipress) is a newer alpha-blocking drug that can be used in place of Dibenzyline.[24] Some people find these drugs difficult to take because they relax *all* smooth muscles, including the blood vessels, and may make you feel at first as if "you stand up, your blood doesn't."

Painkillers, muscle relaxants, and sleep medications are mainstays for many IC patients. For people with very severe symptoms, these preparations may offer the only respite available from unremitting bladder pain. And for people who have trouble sleeping because of pain and severe frequency, sedatives may provide the only possibility of a few hours sleep. But the disadvantages of chronic use of the drugs in this category can be significant. Many people don't like the "drug hangover" that often occurs with narcotics and find it difficult to function normally if they take enough to kill the pain. In addition, the danger of addiction is significant. If you are taking a drug that is potentially addictive, you and your doctor should carefully monitor your intake to avoid addiction. You might try going off a drug periodically and substituting another type of drug, or try alternative pain remedies such as acupuncture and acupressure (see page 156), transcutaneous electrical nerve stimulation (TENS) (see below), or investigate the treatments provided by a pain clinic (see page 270).

TENS Unit

Many people with interstitial cystitis experience chronic pain in the bladder, urethra, clitoris, vagina, or even rectum. Drugs may mask the pain or block nerve receptors that transmit pain impulses, decrease inflammation, or reduce pelvic congestion, but they may also mask your ability to function normally and may make you feel as if you've been out drinking all night. *Transcutaneous electrical nerve stimulation (TENS)* is one non-drug method of pain control that has long been used to reduce the pain of severe back injuries. It has also been successfully used in the treatment of interstitial cystitis in Scandinavia. This small battery-powered device provides a low level of electrical current which is transmitted by one-inch-square electrodes that are taped to the skin above the bladder and/ or lower back. The unit itself is no larger than a phone beeper and can be worn on a belt or tucked into a pocket.

Some reduction in pain sensations should be felt within a few weeks, but you may not get the maximum benefit for at least a month or more. Therefore, use of TENS needs to be looked at as a long-term treatment. Scandinavian studies have suggested that people with severe symptoms seem to benefit the most from TENS therapy and have found that about 20 percent of these people could be classified as "cured."[25]

Dr. Naomi McCormick, a psychologist who has severe IC symptoms, used a TENS unit for more than a year. "I had poor results from most of the conventional treatments for IC and had side effects from pain medications, so TENS seemed a reasonable thing for me to try. I found that it was most effective with two electrodes taped over my abdomen or two over my lower back." The device causes a tickling sensation, and the intensity of the impulses can be adjusted for your own needs. McCormick points out that the electrical impulses of the TENS unit do not interfere with the transmission of pain impulse; rather, they distract you from it.

There is no danger to using the TENS device, but it is recommended that it only be used for about two hours at a time, especially if skin irritation develops. McCormick points out that you may need to be careful not to fall asleep with the unit on. "You can get skin irritation or even minor burns if you are not careful," she says. In these instances, she recommends the use of aloe vera gel to help heal irritated spots.

Using the Physiostim device (see page 72), Kristene has found that pain is markedly decreased in about one half of the patients she has treated by applying electrical stimulation directly to the vagina.

Studies on the treatments described above typically find that about half of the people who try a given treatment respond positively, at least for a while. But the hard fact about interstitial cystitis is that there is no treatment that will eradicate symptoms for everyone. Even though many people experience some relief from medical treatment, they often find it necessary to supplement these treatments with alternative forms of therapy.

ALTERNATIVE REMEDIES

Bladder Retraining

Erin had a urinary tract infection after the birth of her second child. Antibiotics killed the bacteria, but a burning sensation remained. Eventually, the pain went away, and she was symptom-free for two years. Then, in 1985, her symptoms returned and she was diagnosed with interstitial cystitis. "On good days, I go every hour," she says, "but on my worst days, I have to go all the time." Erin had DMSO treatments but didn't get any relief, then took Elmiron for nine months with no improvement in her symptoms. Finally, in desperation, she started a bladder-training program. "When I started the program, I went to the bathroom every half hour, and often it wasn't worth the trip—nothing would come out," she says. After three months of the bladder-training program, Erin increased the interval between trips to the bathroom to four hours. "It's still difficult on bad days," she says, "but it's certainly better than before."

Bladder training, also referred to as bladder *retraining,* has been successfully used to help people with incontinence increase their bladder capacity by gradually increasing the amount of time between urination. (See page 64 for more information on the use of this technique for incontinence.) Like any other muscle, the bladder muscle responds to repeated stretching by becoming larger and stronger. Nerve impulses to and from the bladder also respond to being "worked out" by firing less erratically. This technique has been adapted to use by anyone who suffers urgency and frequency, and has been especially effective with interstitial cystitis patients.

There are presently a small number of bladder-retraining programs in the United States, including one run by Susan Blaivas, a psychologist who practices in suburban New York City, and another by Paul Koprowsky, a social worker who works with Dr. Lowell Parsons in San Diego. "The goal of this program is to put people back in charge of their bladders," Blaivas says.

Blaivas runs a highly structured program that lasts for fourteen weeks. "At the end of that time, people should be voiding in response to a full bladder, rather than to ill-defined sensations," she says. Patients who enter the program fill out a detailed voiding diary (see pages 26–27 for a sample chart), noting everything they drink, how much they urinate, and a number of more subjective

155

factors, such as how much urine they *think* is going to come out. "This is an excellent consciousness-raising technique," Blaivas says.

The program may sound very easy, but for someone with interstitial cystitis who has intense urgency it can be very difficult. "If I was having a bad day, I did nothing but watch the clock," Erin says. "There were some days I thought I wouldn't make it." If the patient has a partner, Paul Koprowsky often has the partner come in so that he or she can get a clear understanding of the concepts of the program. "That kind of support is very essential," he says. Koprowski also warns that after you have successfully completed the program, it is easy to fall back into your old habits if you are not careful.

Both of these programs use 15-minute increases each week and establish an appropriate amount of fluid to be consumed. Usually symptoms of frequency and urgency begin to decrease about the fifth or sixth week, and by the end of the program, many people can reasonably go 3 to 4 hours between voids.

Koprowsky has also treated quite a number of people who have "normal" bladders. Many people with bladders that show no signs of disease suffer from urinary urgency and/or frequency, and complain that they cannot go on long car trips or to unfamiliar places because of "tiny bladders." People who work at home, where they have constant access to a toilet, or teachers and therapists, whose work day is chopped up into many short segments, often establish a pattern of frequent urination, in which their *functional* bladder capacity decreases significantly (although the true capacity remains the same). In treating interstitial cystitis, Kristene has found that once the pain is under control, bladder retraining has been very effective in decreasing frequency.

Since there are so few programs available at this time, if you want to try bladder retraining, you will either have to do it by yourself, which many people can do effectively, or convince a therapist or other health-care professional to support you through a program.

Acupuncture and Acupressure

Acupuncture has been used in China for over a thousand years and was introduced in Europe in the seventeenth century. Today, the scientific basis for acupuncture's use in anesthesia, pain control, and healing has been widely validated, and the concept is being increasingly utilized in treating a variety of conditions. Many acupuncturists supplement needle stimulation with a variety of Chinese herbs that are known to have a beneficial effect on pain and inflammation. *Acupressure* is a technique similar to acupuncture. It utilizes the same points on the body, and a steady pressure, from light to very strong, is applied with the thumb and fingers.

In acupuncture treatments, very thin needles are inserted into the muscles at specific points located along meridians, or nerve pathways, and are turned manually, or may have a mild electrical current applied to them. When used in pain control, needles are inserted at specific *acupuncture points* which stimulate the release of certain chemicals, especially endorphins (the highly touted substance that produces the "jogger's high"), monoamine (a deficiency is thought to be involved in the manic depressive syndrome), and serotonin, a chemical involved in sleep and sensory perception. Each of these chemicals, or neurotransmitters, can interfere with the transmission of pain impulses.

In terms of bladder disorders, acupuncture probably has the most specific application to interstitial cystitis, where pain is a prominent component. This technique is known to be effective in reducing inflammation and in calming muscle spasms, and in treating subsidiary conditions such as allergies and immune deficiency (which may contribute to the IC syndrome). In response to Rebecca's survey, many people with interstitial cystitis said that they had tried acupuncture, and success was quite varied. Quite a few people, like Sara Jane, found that treatments relieved pain for a while but that eventually it returned, and treatments became ineffectual. Others, like Lucinda, found that nothing, including acupuncture, was of much help in relieving the pain.

Acupuncture is frequently practiced by chiropractors, naturopaths, and osteopaths, by some MDs, and by a variety of other practitioners. If you decide to get acupuncture treatments, you might want to find a practitioner who has had some success in treating IC or other types of bladder pain.

In addition to undertaking bladder retraining (see page 155), Erin has been having acupuncture treatments for IC for about ten months and is finally beginning to get some response. "Now I have good days far more often than I did when I was on medication," she says. "I used to have almost no good days, and now I have almost no really bad days and quite a number of good days. I feel I have made substantial progress—since I stopped taking any medication." For about eight months, Erin had treatments twice a week and has now cut down to once a week since she went back to work full-time. "Each treatment lasts about an hour and a half, and I usually have between 40 and 50 needles placed at different points on my body." Erin says that the needles don't hurt but may create sensations similar to small electric shocks. "Sometimes it feels like waves traveling through my body. Not really unpleasant." She reports that during the first weeks of treatment she felt "really drained" and experienced tingling sensations where the needle points had been, but both of these reactions subsided quickly. Erin's acupuncturist also prescribes certain Chinese herbs recommended for the kidneys. He says that her case is the most difficult he has treated, but he's very pleased with her progress.

SELF-HELP STRATEGIES

Because of the constant need for relief and the lack of satisfactory treatments for interstitial cystitis, a significant body of self-help information has evolved. *Every* IC patient has her or his trusted remedies and many have shared them in support groups. Some of these strategies, such as diet and stress reduction, are aimed at eliminating factors that may cause flare-ups of symptoms, while others are intended to minimize urgency and frequency and intensity, or to take the edge off of daily pain. Here is a survey of the self-help strategies that many people have found helpful.

Diet

Many people who have interstitial cystitis say that diet is the single most important influence on their symptoms. Others don't see any apparent connection and practice no restrictions at all. Conventional wisdom tells us that you shouldn't eat things that make your symptoms flare up. Some people have found that a low-acid diet is very helpful. Dr. Larrian Gillespie recommends an acid-free diet in her book *You Don't Have to Live with Cystitis!* for interstitial cystitis patients.[26] Although it is frequently referred to as "the Gillespie diet," Gillespie did not invent the low-acid diet. Such a regimen has been used for many years for a variety of conditions.

More than one third of the people who answered Rebecca's survey said that acidic foods definitely make their symptoms worse, usually *much* worse, and some maintained that certain foods were "guaranteed to put me to bed." Foods that seemed to bother people the least were carbohydrates such as rice, pasta, and potatoes, and chicken and meat.

Of all the dietary no-no's, alcohol headed the list, with caffeinated beverages (coffee, tea, caffeinated sodas), chocolate, citrus juices, and tomatoes following close behind. People mentioned a variety of fruits that tend to escalate symptoms, especially bananas, strawberries, and pineapple. Quite a number said that spicy foods were also likely to cause symptoms to flare up. Although people tended not to be specific about *which* spicy foods bothered them, certain ethnic foods, especially Thai, Indian, and Mexican, contain pungent spices notoriously high in substances that induce the body to release histamines—a prominent factor in the interstitial cystitis disease process. A significant number of people said that they have also given up wheat and milk products. Vinegar and soy sauce seem to bother many people, raising the question of whether it is the acidity or fermentation (or perhaps both) that serve as bladder irritants. Some people said that fish or meat bothered them, while others found these items to be dependably non-irritating.

Some question has been raised about the role of the brain chemical serotonin, and its precursor tryptophane, in interstitial cystitis. Tryptophane is present in a wide variety of foods, and is found in many of the foods that seem to exacerbate IC symptoms.

Rather than being recommended by a doctor, the diets of IC patients are frequently self-imposed, and some of them are extremely stringent. "I would eat dog food for the rest of my life if I thought my symptoms would go away," says Nina. And Clarissa observes, "You sound like a fruitcake when you talk about your diet, but I feel that it's essential in controlling my symptoms."

If you think that food allergies strongly affect your IC symptoms, one way to pinpoint what you are allergic to is to go on a strict "elimination diet," cutting out all but a core group of foods that don't bother you. Or you can look for a doctor or nutritionist who specializes in treating allergies. Arlene and Karen, who both have severe IC, found a doctor who specializes in treating food and environmental allergies. "At first we had to eliminate all but about ten or fifteen foods," Arlene reports. "Then it took six grueling months to get a clear picture of which foods were the baddies. We kept making mistakes and learning, but it was worth it." Arlene says that it was helpful to do the diet with another person. "It was so much better than doing it alone," she says. "We could support each other and share our successes and failures." Doing the experiment together was also instructive. "We were sensitive to entirely different things, and clearly saw that these sensitivities are very individual."

The existence of systemic yeast or a "yeast syndrome" is extremely controversial, and not widely accepted in the scientific community, but some people with interstitial cystitis have reported improvement with the yeast-free diet that is so popular today. The theory is that yeast or other molds can inhabit many systems of the body and that overgrowth can stimulate the development of allergies and ultimately suppress immune function. What effect this would have on the bladder is unclear. Nevertheless, a diet that eliminates yeasts, cheeses, molds, alcohol, and other fermented products such as vinegar, soy sauce, and tofu provides a good basic elimination diet, leaving rice, potatoes, pasta, vegetables, meat, and chicken, the very things that our survey respondents say bother them the least.

The yeast-free diet is extremely stringent, and like Arlene and Karen, you may be on it for many months. The diet can be very difficult to maintain, especially for people who have significant attachments to food. It can also be difficult for people who cook for several others, as well as for those who eat out frequently or travel a great deal. *But it can be done,* and some people have had excellent results in reducing the symptoms of interstitial cystitis by eliminating or reducing their intake of foods containing yeast and mold. As an alternative to a strict elimination diet, some people have had excellent results with a rotation diet; that is, only eating troublesome foods every four or five days.

Vitamins and Minerals

To date, no research has been done on the positive or negative effects of vitamins on interstitial cystitis. Indeed, the role of vitamins on normal bladder function remains to be determined. One minor exception has been in the area of bladder cancer, where vitamins A, B_6, and C have been found to have a possible protective role in healing and prevention (see page 237).[27]

Many people who responded to Rebecca's survey said that they take vitamins, and a few felt that they were essential to their dietary regimens, but most said that they did not seem to have any discernable effect on IC symptoms. However, if your diet is severely restricted, taking selected vitamin supplements might be very sensible. Regrettably, we can't offer you any specific information on vitamin therapy for interstitial cystitis; no one can. In order to help you evaluate which vitamins could *potentially* be helpful and which ones could be harmful, we will review what is known about certain vitamins and amino acids and their *theoretical* relationship to the metabolic processes that are known to be involved in IC.

Vitamin A helps maintain healthy mucous membranes.

Vitamin B complex influences, among many other things, the transmission of nerve impulses and carbohydrate metabolism. With the specific exception of B_6, the B vitamins aid in the production of serotonin and its precursor, tryptophane, which some people believe may intensify IC symptoms. On the other hand, B_6 is thought to help prevent the breakdown of tryptophane into serotonin. In addition, baking soda and oral contraceptives may destroy B_6, so if you take either of these regularly, you might want to consider taking a B_6 supplement.

Vitamin C, or *ascorbic acid,* is not manufactured by the body, and must be obtained through food or vitamin supplements. Ascorbic acid may irritate the bladder, so IC patients should only take it buffered with calcium carbonate. A great deal of attention has been focused on the role of vitamin C in the synthesis and maintenance of collagen, a primary component of fibrous connective tissues. Vitamin C is also said to temper allergic responses by functioning as a natural antihistamine. Also it promotes the absorption of other vitamins, especially A and E.

Calcium is one of our most important dietary substances. In addition to promoting strong bones and teeth, it facilitates nerve transmission and muscle activity. Calcium is thought also to have a calming effect and to aid sound sleep. Both Vitamin D and magnesium, certain hormones, and especially estrogen are necessary for calcium absorption.[28] You can boost your daily calcium intake by eating antacid tablets, which are primarily calcium carbonate. Too much calcium, however, can cause urinary stones.

Vitamin E, a natural vasodilator (helps blood vessels to open up), could be helpful in reducing the pelvic congestion that is common with interstitial cystitis. This vitamin is found in leafy green vegetables, broccoli, eggs, whole wheat, and many other foods.

Maintaining Alkaline Urine

The normal pH of urine, that is, its acidity or alkalinity, is about 5 on a scale of 1 to 14:

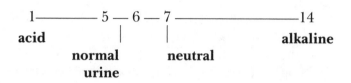

In her book *You Don't Have to Live with Cystitis!*, Dr. Larrian Gillespie reported that the urine of people with interstitial cystitis is typically alkaline (pH greater than 7) and that many of her patients found that acid foods caused symptoms to flare up. Other urologists, however, have found that the urinary pH of IC patients is extremely variable, ranging anywhere from slightly acid (pH 5 or 6) to slightly alkaline (8).

In response to Gillespie's report, many people with IC went on low-acid diets, while others have been restricting their diets for years because much of what they eat seems to have a negative effect on their bladders. But what does a "low-acid diet" really mean? Many people are confused.

Foods in their natural state are either acidic, neutral, or alkaline. When they are consumed, they are broken down into a host of chemical constituents, filtered out of the bloodstream by the kidneys, and passed out of the body in the urine. Some foods, like cranberries, are very acid in their natural state and break down into hippuric acid and other substances. On the other hand, orange juice, which is very acid when it is on the breakfast table, shows up in the urine as alkaline. There doesn't seem to be a rule about what will come out acid and what will come out alkaline.

One way to cut through the confusion is to test your own urine after eating and drinking any number of items, and see how these foods are being broken down in your body. You can buy some litmus paper or nitrazine paper (available at some pharmacies) and dip the chemically treated strips into your urine several times a day.* Soon you will begin to see if what you eat and drink has any appreciable affect on your urine.

---

* Nitrazine paper can be frightfully expensive—up to $18 for a small roll. There are cheaper brands, however. Ask your pharmacist to check several pharmaceu-

No one has studied this issue definitively, so for the present it is impossible to say what the role of pH is, if any, in interstitial cystitis. Nonetheless, some people with IC have found that drinking water that has a neutral or slightly alkaline pH is better than drinking the slightly acidic city water. Many people also take one half a teaspoon of baking soda in water before dinner to prevent a flare in symptoms if bladder irritants are to be consumed.

NOTE: Because of the high salt content, people who have heart conditions or high blood pressure should consult their doctors before taking baking soda.

Stress Reduction

In our fast-paced, success-oriented society, we are confronted by stress at every turn. Stress may be a contributing factor in recurrent cystitis and in interstitial cystitis. It may also be a factor in the development or recurrence of cancer. In response to a very obvious need, stress reduction programs have become a thriving industry with a wide variety of strategies and therapies to help us cope.

Responses to stress are highly individual and the methods for relieving it are too numerous to be covered here in detail. However, some of the stress reduction strategies that people with bladder disorders have successfully used are calming, non-competitive exercise such as walking, swimming, canoeing, bicycle riding (if you can ride in pleasant, uncrowded surroundings), yoga, massage and other types of body work, meditation, listening to music, visualization, hypnosis, and supportive psychotherapy. *The Relaxation Response* and *The Mind-Body Effect,* both by Dr. Herbert Benson, provide an excellent overview of stress reduction and relaxation techniques. These books are listed in the Resources at the end of Chapter 10.

Of course, stress arises not only from what we do but from how we react to people, situations, and various stimuli as well. These responses are complex and deeply ingrained, and sometimes very difficult to change. Yet with hard work, stress-producing responses can be controlled. You may be able to identify these responses yourself, perhaps using the books mentioned above as a guide, and

---

tical catalogs to find a cheaper brand. EM Science, 111 Woodcrest Road, Cherry Hill, NJ 08034-0395, makes *ColorpHast®* for under $10.

work successfully to modify them. If not, you might want to consult a therapist who specializes in stress reduction who can help you identify and manage specific stress factors.

As we pointed out earlier, the medical treatments typically work for about half of the people who try them—at least for a time—and responses to alternative therapies and self-help remedies are quite varied. Regrettably, nothing seems to work for about 5 to 10 percent of people with the severest symptoms and, ultimately, many of them look to surgery as a last resort.

MAJOR SURGERY

"One of the most difficult decisions both patients and their urologists confront in the management of interstitial cystitis is when to throw in the towel," Dr. Lowell Parsons observed in a talk to an Interstitial Cystitis Association support group in Los Angeles. Parsons was referring to the decision to remove the bladder. For patients, the decision is irreversible. If someone found a cure for the disease tomorrow, or more likely ten or more years from now, or if a drug was discovered that alleviated the symptoms reliably and substantially, people who have had their bladders removed would not be able to take advantage of the discovery. For both patients and their doctors, opting for surgery also means that they have lost the fight to successfully manage the disease.

As with any medical procedure, there is a range of outcomes. Some people, like Georgeanna, who is only thirty-four years old, are very happy with the results. "Before surgery, my whole life focused on my disease. Now I can date, sleep, swim, and go to movies without having to worry about my bladder."

Olivia had to endure a series of surgeries before she improved. "First, I had my bladder enlarged. The pain cleared up for a month, but came back again. Then my doctor diverted my urine to a bag outside the body, but left the bladder in. I had the same pain, plus nausea all the time." Olivia finally had her bladder removed and is pain-free, although she now has occasional urinary tract infections. Nevertheless, she is pleased with the result. "After I recovered from the surgery, my husband and I went on a trip to Georgia and we got there so much faster because we didn't have to stop every half hour."

Jill, who has a particularly nasty form of IC, is one of the people whose surgery was not successful. She got an Indiana pouch, but her doctor did not remove her bladder at the time of surgery. Three months later, she had to undergo another major operation to have her bladder out. After the surgery, Jill had difficulty in catheterizing (draining) her pouch and has been plagued by kidney infections. "I wasn't warned about the potential problems attached to this surgery," she says. "I thought that I would wake up and everything would be all right." On the bright side, Jill finds wearing a leg bag for urine drainage "no big deal" and sleeps better at night.

With the dramatic surgical advances that have been made in our lifetime—open-heart operations, reattachment of limbs, and delicate microsurgeries—we have come to look upon surgery as the ultimate quick fix. Yet the surgical procedures that are currently available for interstitial cystitis are exceedingly complex operations with a host of complications and post-surgical problems, and doctors who have done a number of these procedures are less enthusiastic than they once were about them.

In a 1989 survey on surgery, the Interstitial Cystitis Association uncovered two interesting facts: one, given the constant pain they had to endure, most people were happy with their surgeries; and two, people whose bladders were left in often had to return to surgery and have them removed in order to be pain-free.

In the case of interstitial cystitis, there are few guidelines available that can be used to predict who will do well afterward, so it's essential that you and your doctor evaluate your condition very carefully. Some surgeons have offered general guidelines for when surgery is appropriate. Dr. Parsons suggests that surgery should be considered "only when the bladder has really been destroyed by the disease" and surgery offers the sole possibility of improvement. Drs. Wein and Hanno feel that surgery should only be considered "for patients who have failed a multifaceted approach to conventional, conservative therapy."

In talking to both patients and doctors, we discovered that standards for when to perform surgery vary considerably from doctor to doctor. However, there seems to be general agreement that surgery is appropriate if the *true bladder capacity* under anesthesia is small (350 cc), pain is intolerable, and the symptoms are of long duration.

If you are contemplating surgery, it's also important to keep in mind that bodies and health histories are different, and what worked for one person may not work for you—the undesirable effects experienced by one person may not occur at all, or their impact may be much less for you. Before you decide to have surgery, you should be aware of all of the potential risks and post-surgical problems and be sure that you can live with them if the worst occurs. For example, some people who have certain procedures cannot urinate efficiently afterward and must do intermittent self-catheterization (see page 87). The hard fact is if you don't think you will be comfortable catheterizing yourself for the rest of your life, then you should not proceed with surgery.

The following surgical procedures are the ones employed in the treatment of interstitial cystitis.

Augmentation Cystoplasty

Traditionally, removing most of the bladder and replacing it with a piece of bowel, called *augmentation cystoplasty*, has been the first choice of surgery for interstitial cystitis.

In this procedure, the diseased bladder is cut away just above the base of the bladder, leaving the trigone, the area where the bladder's nerves are concentrated, and the ureters, which enter the bladder at the top of the trigone. A piece of the bowel about 8 inches long is detached from its normal position, cut open, and folded to form a parachute-shaped pouch, which is sewn securely to the trigone. The bowel-pouch, which still has its nerves and blood supply intact, forms an enlarged bladder that will store up to 3 cups (24 oz.) of urine.

The augmentation procedure has been favored, in many cases, because it is not a "last-resort" procedure, i.e., if it does not work, there is still another procedure—a urinary diversion—that can be done. An augmentation also leaves you closer to "normal" anatomically than any of the other surgeries, that is, urine is still collected in the enlarged bladder and is evacuated through the urethra. But not everyone who has this procedure can urinate normally. After augmentation, you will need to empty your bladder every three to six hours in order to prevent infection and kidney damage. Since the bowel segment does not have the same muscular structure as the bladder, your new bladder will probably have to be emptied with abdominal straining or the Credé maneuver (see page 87).

If these techniques are not sufficient, intermittent catheterization may be required. (See page 87 for information on how to do this procedure.)

Bladder augmentation works well for some people, but a few find that the frequency is relieved but pain is still a problem. In a few people, the insidious disease process of interstitial cystitis may attack the augmented bladder as well, causing the symptoms to return.[29] In this case, the bladder may need to be removed, and the urine either diverted to an external bag in a procedure called the ileal conduit, or to an internal reservoir or pouch made from a segment of bowel, called the Koch or Indiana pouch.

URINARY DIVERSIONS

Koch (Indiana) Pouch or Urinary Conduit

The *Koch* or *Indiana pouch* was developed for use when the bladder had to be removed because of invasive bladder cancer, but has now been done for a number of IC patients, many of whom had previous augmentation surgery. In this procedure, the bladder can be left in or removed, and an internal reservoir or pouch is made from a bowel segment. This is another form of urinary diversion. The ureters are attached to the closed end of the pouch, so that the urine drains into it from the kidneys, and the open end is drawn to the abdominal wall, where a nipple-like protrusion, or stoma, emerges from the skin or is attached to the urethra. The pouch is drained with a catheter four to six times a day.

Another type of urinary diversion is a *conduit,* in which the ureters are attached to a tube fashioned from a short piece of bowel, usually the *ileum,* a part of the small intestine—hence the name *ileal conduit.* The conduit in turn is attached to a stoma in the abdominal wall, and the urine drains continuously into a plastic bag attached to the stoma.

In both of these procedures, the bladder may or may not be removed. Unfortunately, some people with interstitial cystitis inexplicably continue to have pain in the bladder even though the urine has been diverted. To prevent this from happening, some doctors prefer to remove the bladder (a *cystectomy*) at the time of the diversion, to decrease the likelihood of further surgery.

The hospital stay for these procedures is usually between seven

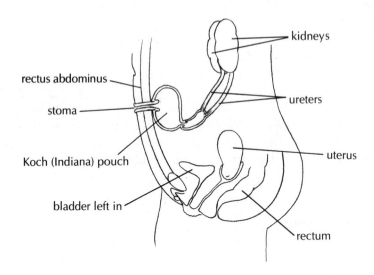

kidneys

rectus abdominus

ureters

stoma

uterus

Koch (Indiana) pouch

bladder left in

rectum

11. **Koch (Indiana) pouch.** This internal reservoir for urine is fashioned from a segment of bowel, and lies in the lower abdomen. You can see where the ureters are attached to the closed end of the bowel segment and where the pouch forms a stoma and emerges from the abdominal wall. In this procedure, the bladder can be left in or removed.

and ten days. After the surgery, you will not be able to eat solid food for three to five days. You will probably be discharged from the hospital with two catheters that will remain in place for one or two more weeks: one in the urethra and a suprapubic catheter that exits the skin above the pubic bone. These catheters help to make sure that no urine stands in the bladder until it is healed. About two to three weeks after your surgery, an X-ray will be taken to make sure the suture line has healed. As with most major surgeries, you will not feel like your old self for about a month, but most people feel relatively comfortable after about two weeks.

As with all major surgeries, these procedures have the potential for serious complications. For bladder surgery, the most common complications are bowel obstruction, bleeding, infection, urinary or fecal leakage from the suture line, problems with general anesthesia, and complications of preexisting medical problems. In order to undergo these procedures, you need to be in good physical condition and have no major bowel or kidney problems. Betty, a psychotherapist who has severe IC, is very interested in surgery but is taking a wait-and-see approach. "I'm just trying to hold out for a few more years, until surgical techniques are better," she says, "then I'm going to get rid of the damn thing."

WHAT IT'S LIKE TO HAVE INTERSTITIAL CYSTITIS

Until recently, interstitial cystitis has been an invisible disease. Many doctors did not believe that it existed. Employers were unsympathetic about decreased productivity. Insurance companies routinely denied applications for disability. In addition to revealing how widespread the disease really is, the Urban Institute survey offers for the first time a clear picture of the profound impact that interstitial cystitis has on the lives of its sufferers, finding that:

- 50 percent have pain while riding in a car;
- 63 percent have pain with intercourse;
- 50 percent are unable to work full time, and those who do work receive $3.41 an hour less than people without IC who have comparable schooling;
- between one third and one half have received no help from any treatment;
- people with IC have suicidal thoughts three to four times as often as the general population;
- people with interstitial cystitis rate the quality of their lives lower than do people on kidney dialysis, whose suffering has been widely documented.

To flesh out these statistics, Rebecca did a special survey in which she asked people with interstitial cystitis to describe how the disease has affected their lives. Many responded thoughtfully and perceptively, describing the disruption in their personal lives, careers, and leisure activities.

"Interstitial cystitis has taught me a lot about limitations—both my own and other people's," says Joni. "Unless you have lived with chronic illness yourself, or with someone who has such a condition, it is very hard to understand how complicated one's life can be." This observation echoes the feelings of many people with the disease, who expressed regret, grief, or anger at having to adjust to limitations in every aspect of their lives. Symptoms may wax and wane, but in cases where they are severe, these limitations may amount to disability. "When I was unable to attend my grandmother's funeral in a town thirty miles away, I finally had to admit to myself that I was disabled," says Alma, who has struggled with very intense IC symptoms for many years. "I play the organ at church and every Sunday I wonder if I can get through the service without having to leave to go to the bathroom," says June, who has also had severe symptoms for many years.

"IC is a disease of the entire family, not just the person diagnosed with it," says Norma, pinpointing an issue that is key for most IC sufferers. A few people reported that family members did not adapt very easily to changes required by the disease. Tanya's whole family is understanding, but sometimes they get annoyed at being inconvenienced. "It's only natural, though," she observes sympathetically, "since I get upset myself." Wilma finds that the disease has been hard on her husband, too. "He's always waiting by the bathroom."

Before much was known about interstitial cystitis, it was thought that the disease caused severe marital strain. Surprisingly, however, the Urban Institute survey found that divorce was no more common among people with IC than among the general population. In our survey, the overwhelming majority of respondents mentioned devoted spouses, and spoke with gratitude about the support and understanding they received from their families. "If anything, my boyfriend and I are closer than ever because of having to deal with this disease," Clarissa says. "He is very concerned about me, and that feels good." "I have a portable potty in the car and a saint for a husband," Fran says appreciatively. Lilianna isn't so lucky—her husband complains about how much toilet paper she uses.

Jeanette notes that the disease can also be hard on friends. "Although they understand and sympathize, at times they get annoyed at being inconvenienced," she says. When friends failed to respond sympathetically, many people turned to their support group, finding an abundance of sympathy and encouragement, and making meaningful new friendships.

Children may sometimes feel cheated and view a parent with IC as less than perfect. "My kids see me as a chronic pill taker. They don't understand that I have to have medications and treatments to keep me going," remarks Goldie. "When my children were younger, they used to think it was humorous that we stopped at every gas station in town," says Nanette. She notes, however, that they became more understanding as they grew older. "IC has certainly put a strain on my family," Emily reports. "One day when my six-year-old was leaving for school, she told me, 'Mom, you had better be standing up when I come home.' "

It's understandable that younger children have a difficult time comprehending a chronic illness like interstitial cystitis and the limitations it imposes, because they can't see anything wrong. On the other hand, many people said that their older children have been especially caring and sympathetic. "My sons, age nineteen and twenty-two, have been to support group meetings with me," says Virginia proudly. Perhaps "family night" could become an occasional support group activity to encourage involvement of spouses and children.

Some of our respondents suggested that if you tend to have difficulties with in-laws, you may not get any extra points by having IC. "My in-laws act like I'm crazy and that there is nothing really wrong with me," Trudy comments. "I am ridiculed by my husband's family," says Anjelica. "I guess they think I am lazy and just don't want to work."

In addition to strain in family relationships, limitations are also felt on the job, where responsibilities cannot be easily put off until another day. Some people, like Irene, have deliberately not sought out better jobs. "I would like to look for other work, but I know the problems my condition presents," she says. "Therefore, I just stay put." Others have been forced to give up their jobs altogether. Sheri, who is an executive secretary, describes a common situation: "My boss is not very understanding when I take time off," she says. "When I missed a week because of a bladder distention last year, it affected my merit review." After that, Sheri went to her doctor's appointments on her lunch hour and scheduled DMSO treatments late on Friday afternoon. Jobs that require working with the public were clearly the hardest on people. "I am a teacher, and frequency affects my ability to stay in the classroom for long periods," says Caroline, who has comparatively mild symptoms but still needs to urinate about every half hour. Roberta, a waitress who has had severe symptoms for nearly forty years, says she finally gave up her job because of the pain. One has to marvel at the courage and determination it must have taken to stick to such a physically demanding job for so long.

A few of the people who answered our survey expressed regret at having to give up exciting career opportunities. "I own a modeling agency and school and a ballroom-dancing operation," Lana wrote. "Each day was exciting and challenging, and I looked forward to someday franchising my operation. Now I struggle just to make it through the day without letting on that I am in pain." Mary Ellen had a dynamic career as a journalist and served as a war correspondent in Vietnam. "Because my symptoms are so severe, I can no longer work in Third World countries or in war zones," she says, explaining that the logistics of locating bathrooms in strange places were just a constant worry.

While having to slow down and accept significant limitations can be hard and frustrating, some people have found a positive side to it. "I have learned to savor the moment and enjoy the little things more," says Polly, who has had IC for eighteen years.

Missing out on recreational activities is another of the limitations that interstitial cystitis imposes on people. "My husband loves boating," says Terri, "but we don't go out when the water is rough. We have adjusted by going out only when it is calm, but it's sometimes unpredictable." "We are both golfers," Pauline says, "but I have difficulty playing nine holes without going to the bathroom, even when my symptoms are mild."

Interstititial cystitis is like incontinence in several significant respects. One of them is the strong potential for isolation. "We have no social life when my symptoms are bad," Margaret says. "I tend to do more things alone now, because it's so difficult to go to concerts, theater, or on trips," says Nancy. "And I no longer go to the opera because you are not permitted to return during an act if you need to go to the bathroom." "When the pain is bad, I hole up in my room, drink lots of water, and listen to music or sew," says Marty. "I feel condemned to meeting people in bathrooms around the world."

Some people, like Eleanor, struggle very hard to maintain their identity. "I feel very uncomfortable viewing myself as a sick person," she says. "I find I can cope with pain better if I work. If I stay home and focus on it, I get very depressed." Many other people stressed how important their work was to maintaining equilibrium.

In spite of the limitations and frustrations imposed by interstitial cystitis, quite a few of our survey respondents expressed a steadfast refusal to let the disease get the best of them. "After the initial shock of learning that we have to deal with this disease the rest of our lives, emotions even out," says Julianna. "I still continue on with life even though the pain is ever present." Like Julianna, many people with the disease have developed coping mechanisms that allow them to stay active and interested in the world around them. Many of these strategies are described in Chapter 10.

The Urethral Syndrome: The Orphan Disorder

Abby had a normal bladder until she became sexually active. After that, she began having periodic urinary tract infections. At some point, she found that she was getting cystitis-like symptoms without bacteria. "Now I get eight or ten flare-ups a year," she says. Her doctor told her that she had a small bladder and a "urethral stricture," and dilated her urethra. "When I get really bad symptoms, the dilation seems to help," Abby says. "Now my doctor is reluctant to dilate anymore. He says it's a Stone Age procedure, but he will usually do it if I ask him." Abby has a "lifetime supply" of Pyridium, and finds that it helps soothe the burn when her symptoms flare up. "Alcohol will always make my symptoms flare," she says. "But I've learned to flush my bladder well with water after drinking. Intercourse sometimes precipitates symptoms also, so I make it a point to empty my bladder right afterward. That seems to help."

Many women go to their gynecologist or urologist and complain of prickly, tingling, or burning sensations around the urethra and/or vulva with occasional episodes of urinary frequency and urgency, and sometimes painful urination. The symptoms often flare up after sex or the consumption of bladder irritants such as alcohol, coffee, or spicy foods. Applied to women only, the term *urethral syndrome* is often used in cases such as Abby's when symptoms are present but are not well defined enough to suggest interstitial cystitis. "Urethral" means focused on or around the urethra (possibly including the bladder and the vagina as well). "Syndrome" means a collection of signs and symptoms that describe a particular condition. The condition is very ill defined, and since it is neither life-threatening nor very dramatic, it has not been of much interest to researchers. What causes this condition, and which treatments are appropriate for it, constitute one of the most obscure controversies in urology.

Many doctors are baffled by these symptoms and may not be of much help to you. If you are lucky, they will tell you that they don't know what is causing your problem and treat it empirically, that is, with basically anything that experience tells them might work. If you are not so lucky, you may be told that you have any number of other conditions, not unlike the list of misdiagnoses for interstitial cystitis listed on pages 143–44. Some doctors who see a lot of women with this condition have come to think of the so-called urethral syndrome as the milder end of the painful bladder spectrum, with interstitial cystitis being at the more severe end. It is often difficult, in fact, to say just where urethral syndrome ends and interstitial cystitis begins. However, if you have episodes of frequency, urgency, and nocturia, a feeling of pressure in the bladder, or pain in the urethra after urination, you could probably benefit from some of the treatments that are used for interstitial cystitis. Until the interstitial cystitis disorder is better understood it is unlikely that its relationship to the urethral syndrome will be clarified.

It is estimated that 2 to 3 million women—perhaps as many as have bacterial cystitis[30]—have symptoms that would fall into the urethral syndrome category. Some men have similar symptoms as well, and in them the condition is referred to as prostatodynia, which means pain in the prostate. At this point, it is impossible to say just what "urethral syndrome" is. At best, we can describe it, tell you the standard tests and procedures that are used in diagnosis, give you an idea of the range of treatments that have been tried, and suggest some coping mechanisms that have worked for women with the condition.

Some of the possible causes of urethral syndrome that have been suggested are urinary tract infection, Chlamydial infection, hyperactivity of the sphincter muscle or dysfunction of the urethral nerves, pelvic surgery (especially hysterectomy), estrogen deficiency, allergies, stress, and quite a number of less common conditions. Sometimes these conditions can be identified and treated and sometimes they cannot. Many women are simply told, like Abby, that they have a small bladder or a small, damaged, or fibrotic urethra. In many cases, the functional capacity of the bladder may be diminished, but unless the bladder is distended under anesthesia it is not possible to tell what its *true* capacity is. And when a urethra is "too small" has yet to be defined. It may be that swelling from inflammation causes a diminished urinary flow and prevents the bladder from emptying completely—making the urethra *seem* smaller. Or it may be that in response to irritation or inflammation, urinary frequency develops, causing the bladder's *functional capac-*

ity to decrease—so you feel as if you need to urinate more frequently.

As with interstitial cystitis, the diagnosis of "urethral syndrome" is made by excluding other conditions. Infection needs to be ruled out, and this often involves more than the routine urinalysis and culture and sensitivity tests. Several studies have found that about half of the women who have urgency and frequency actually have some type of organism, such as Chlamydia or mycoplasma (an organism which also causes pneumonia), or a low-colony count of an infection caused by bacteria such as *Staphylococcus saprophyticus* —which does not show up on a routine urinalysis or culture and sensitivity (C&S) test. Infections caused by these organisms are generally classified as "urethritis" (see page 127) and can be treated with antibiotics. However, if you continue to have urethral symptoms after taking several rounds of antibiotics, then your condition may very well belong in the painful bladder category.

Distinguishing "urethral syndrome" from interstitial cystitis is often difficult and sometimes impossible. Without looking in your bladder when you are under anesthesia, there is no definitive way to tell whether you have what is now considered to be interstitial cystitis. In any event, preparing a voiding chart (see pages 26–27 for sample) will provide a great deal of useful information for your doctor to work with. Whether it's worthwhile to put you through the tests necessary to make a definitive diagnosis is something that you and your doctor will have to decide. If your symptoms are severe enough to require treatments such as bladder overdistension or the instillation of DMSO, then diagnostic procedures may be warranted.

Diagnosis

The onset of urethral symptoms is often spontaneous and may be associated with a particular event, such as a urinary tract infection, becoming sexually active, pelvic surgery, menopause, catheterization, getting very chilled, or stress. Tests used to diagnose this condition might include:

- *urinalysis and urine culture* to rule out urinary tract infection;
- *urethral swab* to rule out Chlamydia or non-gonococcal urethritis (see page 127);

- *urine cytology* to rule out cancer; and
- *cystoscopy* to rule out other urinary tract diseases.

Treatment

For a long time, the standard treatment was to dilate the urethra with graduated metal rods. This practice is now generally frowned upon, but it has been shown to be helpful in some cases. Occasional dilations, or two or three at spaced intervals, will probably not harm the urethra, but over-use of dilation, referred to by some urologists as "the rape of the urethra," may cause scarring or even incontinence. Some urologists also still do a meatotomy, cutting the urethral opening to enlarge it, or a urethrotomy, making a lengthwise cut in the urethra to make the urethra permanently bigger. These procedures are considered very dangerous by most urologists and are strongly discouraged. At present, no studies have been done to show that dilation, meatotomy, or urethrotomy has any medical value. Given the potential for damage and scarring that these procedures can cause, there seems little justification for them.

Based on the results of your physical examination and tests, the following treatments are commonly done for urethral syndrome. Some of the drugs used to treat interstitial cystitis are also used in the treatment of urethral syndrome, especially anti-inflammatory drugs, diazepam (Valium), and occasionally alpha blockers, and estrogen or hydrocortisone cream rubbed directly on the urethral opening. Although these drugs only treat the symptoms, some people find that their symptoms may resolve after an extended round of drugs such as these. Even though no bacteria can be found in the urine, a few women seem to respond well to long-term antibiotics.

If none of these remedies works for you, you might want to read the sections on the medical and alternative treatments for interstitial cystitis, as well as the section on self-help, and see if any of it sounds potentially helpful. Dietary changes, bladder-training programs, and bladder instillations have afforded relief for many interstitial cystitis patients, and have worked for women with urethral syndrome as well.

Urethral syndrome, and its male counterpart, prostatodynia, can be frustrating disorders for the people who have them as well as for their doctors. When symptoms first develop, they are likely to be frightening because it may be difficult to find out what is wrong. Since there are no reliable medical remedies for these orphan conditions, a combination of patience, thoughtful experimentation with diet and personal habits, and a sympathetic doctor who is willing to help you find helpful remedies may be your best solution.

THE INTERSTITIAL CYSTITIS ASSOCIATION

In 1984, Dr. Vicki Ratner, who was then in the second year of a grueling six-year residency in orthopedic surgery, appeared on "Good Morning America," ABC's popular morning news and talk show. Ratner told the story of her struggle with interstitial cystitis and talked about the fledgling Interstitial Cystitis Association (ICA) she had started with a small group of other women who also had the disease. Normally the group got five or six letters a week at their post office box. "The next time someone went to check the box after the show, we had *bags* of mail," says Judith Heller, another IC sufferer who is now treasurer of the organization. "It was too much to fit into the car. We had a hard time figuring out how to cart it all away."

Within a month, more than 10,000 letters poured in. And they continued to come. Debra Slade, who came down with the disease while she was teaching at Columbia University, gave up her job to become the organization's executive director. Slade has coordinated a highly successful congressional lobbying campaign for funding for basic research on IC and a program to increase public awareness of the disease. The ICA has more than 10,000 names on its mailing list and coordinates a nationwide network of support groups that includes at least one group in each state and several in Canada. The ICA maintains a listing of materials on interstitial cystitis, publishes the *ICA Update,* a quarterly newsletter, and sponsors an annual conference that is attended by people with IC, their families, doctors, nurses, and other health professionals. You can write to the ICA at P.O. Box 1553, Madison Square Station, New York, NY 10159. Canadian residents should also write to this address to find out the location of support groups in Canada.

CONCLUSION

In its worst form, interstitial cystitis is one of the most difficult diseases imaginable. Yet the vast majority of people do not have severe cases and have made excellent adjustments to living with the disease. And for anyone who has the disease, in the last five years the outlook has improved dramatically. It is now easier to get diagnosed, the number of doctors who are familiar with the necessary diagnostic criteria has increased, and doctors who work with the disease have had more experience with the various treatments that are available. In addition, people with the disease, support groups, and alternative practitioners have developed self-help strategies and coping mechanisms that can help lessen symptoms and give you a sense of control over your life.

The information in this chapter is complemented by Chapter 9, Staying Sexual, and Chapter 10, Coping Strategies for Everyday Survival. If you have had IC for a long time, you are no doubt adept at coping, but you might want to read these chapters to see if there are any new coping mechanisms that might be of use to you in your day-to-day struggle.

INTERSTITIAL CYSTITIS REMINDERS

- Interstitial cystitis is not "all in your head."
- Interstitial cystitis is not a life-threatening disorder.
- There is no known cause and no certain cure for interstitial cystitis.
- The most frequent reason for misdiagnosis of IC is the doctor's failure to look for it.
- In order to get a correct diagnosis, you must have a cystoscope examination under general anesthesia.
- You should try all conservative forms of therapy before considering surgery.
- Interstitial cystitis is not related to cancer.

RESOURCES

BOOKS AND NEWSLETTERS

Living with Chronic Illness: Days of Patience and Passion, Cheri Register. New York: The Free Press/Macmillan, 1987. Based on in-depth interviews with thirty people (including the author) who live on a day-by-day basis with chronic, often painful illnesses, this book shatters some myths about long-term illness and provides some penetrating insights into its impact on people's lives.

ICA Update, Debra Slade, ed. This newsletter, containing the latest information on interstitial cystitis, comes free with membership in the Interstitial Cystitis Association. Send $35 to the ICA at P.O. Box 1553, Madison Square Station, New York, NY 10159.

MEDICAL BOOKS AND ARTICLES

All of the following materials can be ordered from the Interstitial Cystitis Association, P.O. Box 1553, Madison Square Station, New York, NY 10159.

Interstitial Cystitis, P. M. Hanno, D. R. Staskin, R. Crane, and A. J. Wein. New York: Springer-Verlag, 1990.

Interstitial Cystitis, Parts I & 2, P. M. Hanno and A. J. Wein. *AUA Update Series,* Vol. 6, No. 9 & 10, 1987. This concise synthesis of current medical information on interstitial cystitis offers an excellent overview of the topic.

"Interstitial Cystitis: Pathophysiology, Clinical Evaluation, and Treatment," Grannum R. Sant. *Urology Annual* 3, 1989.

"Summary of the National Institute of Arthritis, Diabetes and Digestive and Kidney Diseases Workshop on Interstitial Cystitis, National Institutes of Health, Bethesda, Maryland, August 28–29, 1987," Jay Y. Gillenwater and Alan J. Wein. *The Journal of Urology,* Vol. 140, July 1988, pp. 203–205.

Supplement to Urology, G. R. Sant, ed. Vol. 29, No. 4, April 1987. This state-of-the-art medical review covers interstitial cystitis from every angle. The articles are fairly technical, but brief and, in general, comprehensible. Required reading for all physicians and medical personnel who have an interest in or might be called upon to deal with interstitial cystitis.

CHAPTER 7

Prostate Problems

AT FORTY-EIGHT, TERENCE HAD AN ACTIVE SOCIAL life and had just been appointed head of the accounting department in a growing movie production company. He jogged almost every day and played racquetball once a week at his health club. For several months, he had been urinating more frequently, and recently started waking up at night to urinate. He had also noticed low back pain, but did not associate it with the changes in his urinary habits. One day after his racquetball game, he noticed that he was having difficulty in urinating. "I was really embarrassed because my racquetball partner called me from the shower and asked why it was taking so long." Terence didn't think too much about any of these changes until the next time he had sex with his girlfriend. "When I ejaculated, I had a very sharp pain. Afterwards, I felt like I needed to pee all the time." Terence hadn't been to a doctor since he broke his leg playing basketball in college, and didn't know what to do. He called an internist who belonged to his Sunday morning jogging group and asked for advice. From listening to his symptoms, the internist thought that Terence could either have an infection in his prostate or his prostate was beginning to enlarge, and suggested that he see a urologist. Terence was shocked when the internist mentioned the prostate. He thought only older men had prostate trouble.

The *prostate* is a complex and somewhat secretive gland. It plays a minor but essential role in male reproduction, adding an alkaline sperm-preserving ingredient to the seminal fluid containing the sperm and increasing its bulk by about 15 percent. Unless it becomes infected, the prostate remains conveniently out of sight, out of mind until men are between forty and fifty years old, when it begins to enlarge. From then on, although prostate enlargement is not generally life-threatening, for many men the prostate can become an Achilles' heel. In all, prostate problems constitute the bulk of the urologist's practice, amounting to more than 3 million visits annually. If you have noticed a change in your urinary habits, the Self-Evaluation Checklist below can help you to determine if you have a prostate problem.

SELF-EVALUATION CHECKLIST

____ Are you experiencing painful, urgent, frequent, or hesitant urination?

____ Do you sense that urination is often incomplete or that your bladder does not empty completely?

____ Do you regularly wake up at night more than once to urinate?

____ Have you had a bladder infection recently?

____ Have you experienced intense cystitis-like symptoms, but have gotten a negative urine culture?

____ Is your urine flow much slower than it used to be?

____ Is ejaculation painful?

____ Have you been told that you have an enlarged prostate?

____ Has the frequency of sexual activity increased or decreased lately?

____ Are you contemplating surgery for an enlarged prostate?

____ Do you suffer from incontinence or the inability to have an erection as a result of prostate surgery?

____ Have you been diagnosed with prostate cancer and are confused about the treatment options?

WHAT THIS CHAPTER CAN DO FOR YOU

In spite of a significant amount of research, the prostate is still somewhat of a mystery. Numerous theories about its structure, function, and malfunction have been proposed, but none of them has completely elucidated its essence. After a great deal of research, it is still not entirely clear how bacteria get into the prostate, why it becomes inflamed, or exactly what stimulates it to enlarge.

This chapter describes the different types of prostatic disorders, explains the tests that are normally done to diagnose them, and provides information on treatments. As you read it, you may want to refer to Chapter 3, pages 38–41, for details on the structure and function of the prostate.

Each year, more than 1 million men develop prostate disorders, in three broad categories:

- *prostatitis,* which includes infections, inflammation, and non-bacterial conditions;
- *benign prostatic hyperplasia (BPH),* the non-malignant enlargement of the prostate gland; and
- *prostate cancer.*

The symptoms of all these conditions may be so similar that it is frequently difficult to distinguish them. When something is amiss in the normally silent prostate, you can experience two types of prostatic symptoms: *irritative* symptoms, caused by infection or inflammation of the prostate, and *obstructive* symptoms, caused by prostatic inflammation or growth which causes narrowing of the urethra. The Symptom Chart on pages 28–29 graphically delineates the symptoms of these conditions, showing how similar their outward signs are to each other, and how similar they are to other disorders of the bladder. The following information should help you distinguish between the prostatic disorders and provide you with information that will help you obtain appropriate diagnosis and treatment.

PROSTATITIS

Prostatitis literally means "inflammation of the prostate" and accounts for more than 3 million urologist's visits every year. Urologists are the first to admit that prostatitis is an ill-defined term that covers several difficult-to-treat, sometimes confounding disorders. Dr. T. A. Stamey, one of the most respected urologists in this field, has gone so far as to term prostatitis "a wastebasket of clinical ignorance,"[1] referring to our poor understanding of why the prostate gets infected or irritated, the difficulties in diagnosing what exactly is wrong with it, and the lack of reliable treatments.

Nevertheless, after years of controversy and uncertainty in diagnosis, a group of leading urologists brought some order to the chaos by developing a classification system for prostatitis that helps doctors differentiate between genuine prostatic disorders and other conditions with similar symptoms such as prostate enlargement, urethritis, and prostate cancer.[2] This system divides infection or irritation of the prostate into four categories:

- *chronic bacterial* prostatitis, in which vague irritative voiding symptoms may exist for a long time before they become genuinely bothersome, and bacteria can be found in your urine or prostatic secretions;
- *acute bacterial* prostatitis, in which irritative and obstructive voiding symptoms flare up suddenly and bacteria can be found in your urine or prostatic secretions;
- *non-bacterial* prostatitis, in which irritative symptoms are present, but no bacteria can be found in spite of other signs of inflammation (pus cells) in the prostatic secretions;
- *prostatodynia,* in which prostatic discomfort or pain and/or irritative voiding symptoms are present, but no signs of prostatic infection or inflammation can be found in the urine or prostate secretions.

Classification under this system depends upon your symptoms, the results of your urine tests, and the findings from examination of prostatic secretions collected through prostate massage. (See page 284 for a description of how a prostatic massage is done.) Separating prostatic conditions into these categories takes some of the uncertainty out of diagnosis and offers more realistic guidelines to treatment.

Like the female bladder, the male bladder and prostate have some natural defenses that protect them against bacterial invasion. The prostate's most significant natural defenses appear to be *prostatic antibacterial factor (PAF)* and *spermine,* two substances composed of amino acids and high levels of zinc, which are known to have antibacterial properties.[3] Several researchers have also found what appears to be a strong immune response to bacterial invasion within the prostate itself.[4]

Chronic Bacterial Prostatitis (CBP)

Larry, a forty-two-year-old truck driver, has had one or two episodes of prostatitis over the past ten years. One day, he had another flare-up. "When I got back from a long trip, I noticed that my lower back hurt and I was having difficulty in urinating," he says. He came to see Kristene, who found he had bacteria in his urine and some stones in his prostate. Because of several recurrences, Kristene gave Larry a three-month course of antibiotics in the hope of controlling the infection. "Dr. Whitmore said that sitting for so long in the truck was probably contributing to my recurrences," he says. "She suggested that I consider changing jobs, but I'm not trained to do anything else." Larry still had symptoms after several long-term courses of antibiotics, so Kristene finally removed the affected tissue surgically, using a transurethral procedure (see page 194), and he had no more problems.

Although CBP does not present much of a threat to life or overall health, a badly infected prostate can occasionally cause urinary obstruction, kidney or testicular infections, and can sometimes result in infertility.

Symptoms of Chronic Bacterial Prostatitis

You may hardly notice the onset of CBP at first, and when symptoms do arise, they may endure for several weeks before you are bothered enough to seek treatment. Symptoms may wax and wane, even be episodic, separated by periods that are relatively normal. In fact, many men with CBP can be completely asymptomatic. And *all* of the symptoms are signs of a host of other prostatic conditions and can be extremely misleading to both you and your doctor.

Like the symptoms for other prostatic and bladder disorders, the symptoms for CBP are divided into three distinct categories, with the irritative symptoms being the most prominent.

Irritative symptoms
- urgency
- frequency of urination
- waking to urinate *(nocturia)*
- painful urination *(dysuria)*
- low back or perineal pain
- painful ejaculation

Obstructive symptoms
- hesitant urination
- weak or interrupted urinary stream
- feeling of incomplete bladder emptying
- post-void dribble

Signs (things that can be observed)
- recurrent urinary tract infections
- low-grade fever, fatigue
- painful or bloody ejaculation

The Causes of Chronic Bacterial Prostatitis

The precise means by which bacteria enter the prostate are still somewhat murky. It is assumed, however, that bacteria can either colonize the urethra and sneak through the prostatic ducts, or they can infect the urine and then enter the prostate ducts as the urine passes through the urethra. In spite of the blood-prostate barrier, bacteria may reach the prostate by way of either the bloodstream or the lymphatic system. (See illustration on page 41.)

As with urinary tract infections, the bowel bacteria *E. coli* is by far the leading offender in prostatic infections. Other types of bacteria account for a small percentage of infections, and more than one type may be present. There are numerous means by which these organisms can find their way into the bladder and/or prostate:

- prior urinary tract infections;
- intercourse (spreading bacteria [*E. coli*] through anal intercourse, or through vaginal intercourse if there is an *E. coli* infection in the vagina);
- catheters and instruments such as a cystoscope being inserted into the urethra and bladder;
- obstruction of the urinary tract by stones, tumors, or prostatic enlargement;
- nervous or structural dysfunction of the bladder caused by diseases such as diabetes or an enlarged prostate.

Diagnosis

A detailed medical history is essential to the accurate diagnosis of chronic bacterial prostatitis. Your doctor especially needs to know if you have had other prostate infections, prior urinary tract infections, what treatments you have received, and what your response to them was. He or she will also want to know your pattern of sexual activity, i.e., do you have a regular partner or more than one sexual partner, if you engage in anal intercourse, and if so, whether or not you use condoms, if you masturbate regularly, and if any of these patterns have changed recently. (See Preparing for Your Doctor's Visit on page 24.)

THE TESTS NOTED HERE ARE DESCRIBED IN DETAIL IN THE INDEX OF DIAGNOSTIC TESTS, BEGINNING ON PAGE 278.

During your physical examination, the doctor will try to determine if your prostate is tender and soft or "boggy," or normal in size and consistency. To determine this, he or she will insert a gloved, well-lubricated finger about 4 inches into your rectum.

Clearly the causes of prostatic infections are numerous, often not very specific, and in some cases it is not possible to definitively pin down a cause. It is therefore difficult to know what things or types of activities to avoid to reduce your risk of another attack. However, if you have chronic bacterial prostatitis, it would be very useful to determine the cause if you can, so that you could try to avoid any known precipitating factors in the future.

A urine culture is an indispensable tool in identifying an infection in the prostate, but the one used to diagnose prostatic conditions is more complicated than the normal "clean-catch" specimen used for bladder infections. This test, called a *segmented urine culture*, helps your doctor identify and differentiate between urinary tract infections and genuine prostatic infections (acute and chronic bacterial prostatitis) and inflammation (non-bacterial prostatitis and prostatodynia). The urine is taken in three "segments," and between the second and third, your doctor will perform a prostatic massage, to feel the size and consistency of your prostate gland and to obtain a sample of your prostatic secretions. (This test is described in detail on page 284.)

If your doctor thinks that it is necessary, he or she may order a kidney X-ray (*intravenous pyelogram* or *IVP*) or a kidney ultrasound exam to exclude the possibility of kidney problems such as malformations, obstruction, or stones. He or she may also do a cystoscopy to make sure that your symptoms are not being caused by bladder stones, tumors, or other anatomic malformations. For difficult or complicated cases, a *prostatic ultrasound* may be helpful in determining the presence of an abscess (a collection of pus), tumors, or stones in the prostate, which are present in up to 75 percent of men with CBP and may act as a source of repeat infections.

Biopsies are a routine and definitive way to identify many cancers and other diseases, but are not generally done to diagnose prostatitis.

Treatment for Chronic Bacterial Prostatitis

Only a few types of antibiotics have been found to be effective against chronic bacterial prostatitis, and unfortunately their effectiveness is not spectacular. The cure rate in urological studies using different drugs over different periods of time has varied widely. At best, about 80 percent of men in some studies have been cured, and at worst, only about 40 percent have had successful treatment. Because of the blood-prostate barrier (see page 313), and the potential presence of infected stones in the prostate, chronic bacterial prostatitis is notoriously difficult—and sometimes impossible—to reach with effective levels of drugs.

Based on your medical history and the result of the culture and sensitivity test, you and your doctor can decide whether to attempt a therapy that is potentially curative or to opt for suppressive therapy, which will sterilize your urine and likely relieve your symptoms, but will probably not prevent reinfection once therapy is stopped. Curative therapy consists of short- or long-term high-dose antibiotic treatment, which may have significant side effects and may not cure the infection. Suppressive therapy consists of long-term low-dose antibiotic therapy. This treatment may or may not cure the infection and has the added disadvantage of being quite expensive.

The most frequently used drugs in the treatment of CBP are carbenacillin (Geocillin), trimethoprim-sulfamethoxazole (TMP-SMX), cephalexin, the tetracycline family, or erythromycin. There are also two new drugs in the potent fluoroquinolone family, ciprofloxacin and norfloxacin, which may prove helpful in treating prostatitis. (See Drug Glossary for information on these drugs and their side effects.) The duration of treatment ranges from two weeks to three months or more, depending on your medical history, previous therapies, and your doctor's preference.

If the goal of your therapy is to cure, as opposed to suppress, CBP, *it is essential* that you have repeat urine and prostate secretion cultures after your therapy is completed and a follow-up culture in three to six months to rule out recurrence. You could be asymptomatic for some time after the course ends and yet still have infection in the prostate. If your infection is not cured at the end of the designated treatment period, and you still have infection with the same type of bacteria, a second round with the same antibiotic, or courses with a different antibiotic, may be prescribed. If this doesn't work, you may want to try a course of low-dose suppressive antibiotic therapy lasting up to six months or more, with a follow-up culture after completion. The drug most frequently used in suppressive therapy is trimethoprim-sulfamethoxazole.

Since prolonged therapy may be required, the potential side effects from taking longer regimens of antibiotics can be significant —diarrhea being the most common. If you do experience diarrhea or other common antibiotic side effects such as nausea, vomiting, fluid retention, tiredness, rash, or difficulty in breathing, report it to your doctor. He or she will probably decide to lower your dosage or change your prescription.

One alternative treatment for difficult cases of CBP that has been used in the past and has attracted new interest is the injection of antibiotics directly into the prostate. A group of Belgian doctors reported that up to 60 percent of men who had antibiotics injected directly into the prostate responded to this form of therapy for at least six months. While the treatment can be fairly uncomfortable, the benefits might outweigh the discomfort or risk of long-term antibiotic therapy, and because the stomach and bowel are bypassed, typical antibiotic-related side effects such as nausea and diarrhea may be eliminated.[5]

Non-Medical Remedies

If you do not want to take antibiotics, they do not work for you, or you have undesirable side effects from them, you may want to try self-help remedies and lifestyle alterations. Even if you do take antibiotics, changes in lifestyle or adjunctive self-help measures may maximize your chances of success with them.

Over the years some men have found that certain dietary substances (coincidentally, the classic bladder irritants) often cause
their prostatic symptoms to flare up. The most frequently mentioned substances are alcohol, caffeine, and acidic or spicy foods.
It also seems that certain activities promote a flare-up in prostatic
symptoms, including prolonged driving, heavy lifting, and vigorous exercise. Additionally, periods of stress or anxiety have been
associated with increased symptoms. Possible solutions to these irritative symptoms include dietary modifications, changes in daily
work-related or recreational activities, and stress management.
(See page 163 for information on stress management.)

If you have significant hesitancy, decreased urinary flow, or
post-void dribbling (the classic obstructive symptoms), you may
benefit from medications that will help relax the prostatic portion
of the urethra. The most commonly used drug is prazosin (Minipress, also used for treating high blood pressure), which may cause
the urethra to open enough to restore near-normal urination and
help you empty your bladder completely. Prazosin may have significant side effects, so its use, especially for an extended period of
time, must be carefully evaluated by both you and your doctor
before you begin therapy. (See page 297 for information on the
use of prazosin to treat prostatic enlargement.)

Non-steroidal anti-inflammatory drugs such as ibuprofen or naproxen definitely have a place in the treatment of chronic bacterial
prostatitis by reducing perineal and low back pain. Warm baths,
heating pads, and rest may also be of some help. If you have
urinary urgency and frequency resulting from prostatitis, your
doctor may decide to give you Pyridium or Urised, two of the
widely used bladder analgesics that deaden irritated nerves. These
drugs will do nothing for your infection, but they can ease your
symptoms a great deal.

Now, you may wonder: "If the prostate is such a pesky little devil
and is so difficult to reach with drugs, why not just remove it?" As
you will discover in the section on benign prostate hypertrophy,
the surgery for benign prostate enlargement is intricate, and for a
significant number of men has undesirable physical effects (see
page 205). In some cases, where the symptoms are long-standing
and there are other compelling circumstances, surgery may be a
pragmatic solution; but because the entire prostate is not removed,
some infected tissue or stones may remain and cause symptoms to
recur.

Acute Bacterial Prostatitis (ABP)

Paul is a twenty-eight-year-old computer analyst who has been sexually active with men since he was seventeen. He thought he had the flu and stayed home from work, but he also developed severe low back pain, fever, and painful, difficult urination. The night after he came down with these symptoms, he had to get up several times to urinate and had severe pain when he ejaculated. "I felt so bad the next day that I went to see Dr. Whitmore," he recalls. Kristene suspected an attack of acute bacterial prostatitis and hospitalized him immediately. In the hospital, Paul was given intravenous (IV) antibiotics, and two days later, his urine culture revealed that *E. coli* was the cause of the prostate infection. Paul was sent home after three days of IV antibiotics, and when his symptoms subsided, he returned to his urologist for a complete examination. Aside from the infection, nothing unusual was found. Paul's doctor discouraged him from having anal intercourse because of the significant risk of getting AIDS, and reminded him that if he did engage in this type of risky behavior, he should use condoms.

Symptoms of Acute Bacterial Prostatitis

Some of the symptoms of acute bacterial prostatitis are similar to those for chronic bacterial prostatitis (see Symptom Chart for Bladder Disorders on pages 28–29 and Symptoms of Chronic Bacterial Prostatitis on pages 184–85), but the onset is usually sudden and painful and often accompanied by fever, shaking chills, and flulike symptoms. Unlike chronic bacterial prostatitis, with its gradual onset, the symptoms of acute bacterial prostatitis usually declare themselves like a banshee and, like Paul, you may end up in your doctor's office or the emergency room.

Because of the intensity of the symptoms, acute prostate infections can be frightening, and since you often have to be hospitalized to receive IV antibiotics, can be very disruptive to your life. They can also cause severe systemic illness and even life-threatening infection if not treated appropriately. But with immediate treatment, your chances of a complete cure are very good.

According to several studies, the incidence of the recurrence of acute bacterial prostatitis is up to 40 percent, and men who have had this type of infection appear to be at higher risk for developing chronic prostatic infections.[6] Therefore, even after you have received a clean bill of health from your doctor, it's important to keep a watchful eye for a recurrence of symptoms.

Diagnosis

If you experience symptoms that appear to suggest ABP as described above, call your doctor, but do not take any antibiotics before getting a firm diagnosis. The antibiotics may invalidate the blood tests and urine cultures that are necessary to confirm your diagnosis and the type of antibiotic you will be given. Your doctor will carefully examine your prostate to determine if it is tender, "boggy," and swollen, and a midstream urine specimen will be sent for culture. Prostatic massage should not be done when ABP is suspected, since the manipulation of the prostate can cause the bacteria to spread or move into the bloodstream and cause a more severe, generalized, systemic infection. Otherwise, the diagnosis of acute bacterial prostatitis is very similar to the diagnosis of chronic bacterial prostatitis (see page 186).

Treatment for Acute Bacterial Prostatitis

Because of the danger that the infection may spread to the bloodstream, hospitalization and the administration of intravenous antibiotics are often necessary. If you respond well to the IV antibiotics after a few days, you can be discharged and switched to oral antibiotics for up to six weeks. If your symptoms are not very severe, you will probably be given carbenicillin or trimethroprim-sulfamethoxazole, the drugs of choice. Norfloxacin and ciprofloxacin, two drugs which achieve high concentrations in the prostate tissue, have been found to be very effective and are now being used more frequently. Whether or not the drug you are given is effective will be shown by a culture and sensitivity test.

If during your treatment you develop a fever, be sure to report it to your doctor right away. It could be indicative of a relapse, or it could mean that an abscess (collection of pus) has developed in the prostate. It could also mean that the infection may have spread to the testicles or, rarely, to the kidneys. If you do have a relapse, it is essential to look for an underlying problem within the genital or urinary tract. Your doctor may also do an intravenous pyelogram or renal ultrasound to rule out infection or abnormalities in the kidneys.

Non-Bacterial Prostatitis (NBP)

Steven is a highly successful lawyer in a very busy law practice. He discovered that he had a prostate the day after he celebrated being made a partner in his firm. What was more distressing than his hangover was the fact that he couldn't pass any urine. Since it was Saturday, he went to the emergency room, very embarrassed and very upset. A catheter was placed in his bladder. Much to his surprise, the impact of the pain that the catheter created was much less than the relief he experienced when nearly a half-gallon of urine was drained from his bladder. "In the past, there were a few times when a week would go by when urination would be painful and it wouldn't all come out at once," Steven recalls. "I would also have pain in my lower back and would have to get up at night to urinate. These spells usually occurred during examinations or at times when I was under a lot of pressure." Steven left the emergency room with a catheter in his bladder and a prescription for antibiotics, and was referred to Kristene for further evaluation. Three days later, at her office, Steven had the catheter removed. Kristene found that he had non-bacterial prostatitis and gave him an anti-inflammatory drug. She suggested that he take warm baths and that he investigate some type of stress management program to help prevent future recurrences.

Non-bacterial prostatitis is the most common condition in the prostatitis category. Men who have the irritative voiding symptoms characteristic of prostatitis, with no identifiable infection, but who have evidence of an inflamed prostate, are classified as having *non-bacterial prostatitis (NBP)*. This prostatic condition tends to be recurrent and episodic and is often associated with jobs that entail heavy lifting, sitting for long periods of time, or excessive intake of the classic bladder irritants: alcohol, caffeine, or acidic foods. (See pages 62–64 and 158–60 for more information on the role of diet in bladder disorders.) Men who are sexually active and have no evidence of infection in the urine or prostatic secretions may have a sexually transmitted Chlamydia infection. (See page 127 for information on Chlamydia.)

A complete medical work-up should be done to rule out neurologic problems, immune deficiency disorders, or malignancy.

Diagnosis of and Treatment for Non-Bacterial Prostatitis

The diagnosis of non-bacterial prostatitis is essentially the same as for chronic bacterial prostatitis (see pages 184–85). In general, heat, rest, dietary restrictions, stress management, and prazosin, a drug frequently used in the treatment of prostate enlargement, may be helpful. Non-steroidal anti-inflammatory drugs, such as aspirin, ibuprofen, naproxen, or Feldene, have also been found to be effective.

Prostatodynia

Men who have none of the above but have prostatic discomfort —real or perhaps referred pain—are said to have *prostatodynia.* This term literally means pain in the prostate, and is used when no cause for the pain can be found. Some skeptics have maintained that prostatodynia is one of those meaningless urological terms like "trigonitis" and "urethral syndrome," and suggest that men who have pain in their prostate glands but no identifiable cause for it might more appropriately be placed in the *painful bladder* category of disorders (see Chapter 6). Nonetheless, a significant number of men who have perineal, testicular, or low back pain without evidence of infection, inflammation, or enlargement of the prostate continue to be told that they have "prostatodynia."

The treatment for prostatodynia often includes heat, rest, dietary restrictions, stress management, and non-steroidal anti-inflammatory drugs, such as aspirin, ibuprofen, naproxen, or Feldene. Bladder stretching, described on page 283, might also be useful. If your doctor suggests that you might have prostatodynia and you don't get better with the recommended treatment, you might want to investigate the treatments recommended for interstitial cystitis and urethral syndrome and consider trying some of them.

BENIGN PROSTATIC HYPERPLASIA (BPH)

In 1987, when former President Reagan's surgery for an enlarged prostate was scrutinized by the unblinking eye of the media, many men found out for the first time that they had a prostate gland. Others, who had already encountered prostate trouble, found, much to their relief, that they were not suffering alone. Stretching over a period of more than twenty years, Reagan's prostate troubles provide a classic case study of the benign (i.e., non-cancerous) prostate enlargement many men experience between their middle years and old age.

When Reagan was in his fifties, while he was the governor of California, he experienced irritative voiding symptoms caused by a series of urinary tract infections. In 1967 he had surgery, a *transurethral resection of the prostate (TURP),* to remove (or "resect," in medical lingo) about thirty tiny calcified stones in the bladder and prostate as well as some prostatic tissue. At the time of this surgery he was told that he would probably need a second prostatectomy in the future. In 1982, Reagan again experienced irritative voiding symptoms, but a round of antibiotics cleared them up. It is not clear when the former president again began to have uncomfortable prostatic symptoms, but news of it was made public after a routine medical examination in August 1986 that was done in conjunction with his colon surgery. At this time, it was determined that

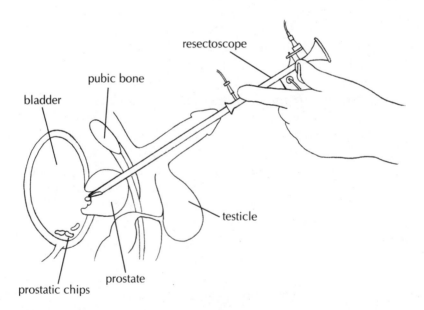

12. **Surgery for prostate enlargement (TURP).** The doctor inserts an instrument with either a sharp tip or a tip heated by electric current through the resectoscope and chips or burns away the affected prostatic tissue.

the president's prostate gland had enlarged to such a point that much of it would have to be removed.

In January 1987, Reagan entered Bethesda Naval Hospital for his second TURP. Before the surgery, he had an *intravenous pyelogram,* an X-ray procedure in which an opaque dye is injected into the veins, making the inner structure of the kidneys and bladder visible. His doctors also performed a *cystoscopy,* looking into the bladder with the aid of a tiny light on the end of a telescope-like device. These tests revealed no urological abnormalities other than an enlarged prostate, and the surgery proceeded uneventfully. There is no direct information about the former president's recovery, but it appears that he was able to carry on a full schedule during his last two years in office without any obvious urological disability.

How the Prostate Enlarges

Between the ages of forty and fifty, the prostate begins to enlarge, as glandular structures begin slowly to proliferate. Autopsy studies have revealed that this normal process of growth actually begins for most men in their early thirties. A few men will begin to experience noticeable symptoms of prostatic enlargement by the age of forty, and by fifty, benign growth (hyperplasia) occurs in at least half of all men. Almost all men who survive into their eighties will have significant enlargement.

The stimulus to this harmless prostatic enlargement has been one of the great urological enigmas. But it is now assumed that this normal proliferation of glandular tissue is the result of increased levels of *androgens,* the hormone responsible for the growth and development of a man's testicles and typical male characteristics such as body hair and deepening of the voice. (Women have androgens too, but in much less quantity.) One early clue to the androgenic cause of BPH was the fact that eunuchs (men who have had their testicles removed to prevent reproduction) and men castrated before puberty do not develop the symptoms of BPH (prostatism). It is also clear that BPH has *nothing* to do with previous prostate infections or with sexual activity—or the lack of it.

Prostatic growth generally begins near the urethra, in the so-called central zone, with proliferation of the glandular tissue, and proceeds inward, outward, or both. When the growth proceeds

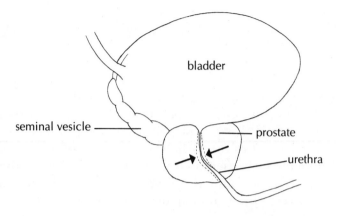

13. a. prostate enlargement with inward growth

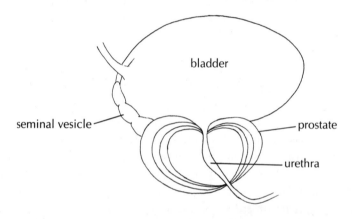

b. prostate enlargement with outward growth

13. **Benign prostate enlargement.** Benign prostate growth usually begins in the central zone and can progress both inward and outward. If growth is primarily inward, it can pinch the urethra and may eventually block it. If growth is primarily outward, there may be no symptoms at all.

inward, it impinges on the urethra, causing it to narrow. As this process occurs, urination is impeded, and in some men, it is eventually blocked. As the bladder muscle has to work harder to completely empty the bladder, it thickens like any muscle that is stressed and worked out. But unlike healthy muscle growth, bands of scar tissue (called *trabeculations*) eventually begin to form in the bladder wall. Trabeculations can be seen with a cystoscope and are one of the indicators of the severity of damage to the bladder from urethral obstruction. In the more advanced cases of BPH, weaker areas of the bladder wall between the areas of trabeculation begin to bulge outward, creating little sacs or pouches called *cellules* (an earlier, less pronounced stage) and then *diverticula,* where the cellules balloon and form little pouches. Occasionally, long-standing bladder outlet obstruction results in a poorly functioning bladder muscle, causing urinary retention, and this condition may not improve after prostatectomy. Untreated bladder outlet obstruction may also result in the formation of stones, or in reflux pressure (back-up of urine into the kidneys), causing kidney damage and perhaps, ultimately, kidney failure.

Trabeculations and diverticula are indicators that you may have more difficulty than usual urinating after prostate surgery, so if your doctor mentions that you have developed one of these conditions, be sure to ask him or her to explain your condition fully to you.

Unless the enlarging prostate begins to narrow the urethra and significantly hinder urination or is associated with urinary tract infections, or the enlargement is a result of cancer, prostate growth is not considered a health problem. Whether or not you experience urethral obstruction and hence difficult urination often depends on whether the growth proceeds inward toward the urethra or outward away from it. In other words, your prostate can be the size of a tennis ball (greatly enlarged), but if you have no symptoms or the symptoms are not disruptive, then you have nothing to worry about.

Symptoms

The symptoms of benign prostate growth begin gradually and can remain stable for some time, or they can progress fairly rapidly over a period of months to a point where they are uncomfortable for you. When symptoms endure over a long period of time, you may simply adapt to the gradual changes in your urinary habits, so that by the time you see a doctor, this adaptive pattern may seem quite normal for you.

Certain events, such as chronic illness, surgery, or injuries that require prolonged bed rest, or certain medications may precipitate a sudden worsening or acute onset of symptoms that can send you straight to your urologist or to the emergency room. In about one third of cases, the cause is temporary, such as too much alcohol or taking a certain medication, and when the underlying problem is resolved, the symptoms subside or disappear spontaneously.[7]

Like prostatitis, the symptoms of prostate enlargement can be divided into two categories: obstructive and irritative, with the obstructive symptoms being most prominent.[8]

Obstructive symptoms
• hesitant urination, or having to strain or "push" to urinate
• weak or interrupted urinary stream
• dribbling after finishing urination *(terminal dribbling)*
• feeling of incomplete emptying
Irritative symptoms
• frequent urination
• waking at night to urinate *(nocturia)*
• urgency
• urge incontinence (see page 52)

When acute symptoms develop, the most alarming are usually the inability to urinate and visible blood in the urine. (There are other causes of blood in the urine, such as bladder cancer, but this is uncommon in men under sixty.) Many men who experience these particular symptoms arrive at their doctor's office or emergency room distraught and anxiety-ridden—usually without a clue as to what could be causing them. In general, obstructive symptoms are indicative of prostate enlargement, but the irritative symptoms can also be due to several other conditions such as cystitis, interstitial cystitis, or bladder cancer (see Symptom Chart on pages 28–29). If you have only irritative symptoms, these conditions need to be ruled out before treatment of BPH is carried out. On their own, none of the symptoms of BPH provides a good indication of how much prostatic enlargement has occurred. The severity of the symptoms usually indicates, however, how much the enlargement has *narrowed the urethra.*

The symptoms of prostatitis and BPH are often similar and can be confused. In prostatitis, irritative voiding symptoms predominate, and often include burning during urination and pain in the low back or perineum. In BPH, on the other hand, obstructive symptoms are most common. Urinary retention can be precipitated by alcohol consumption, an accident, or illness that requires confinement to the bed or wheelchair, or by taking certain over-the-counter cold or allergy medications. Some of the chemical constituents of these medications can block the nerve signals that make the bladder contract or cause the urethral muscles to contract, making it more difficult to urinate.

HOW PROSTATE PROBLEMS CAN BE PRECIPITATED IN ELDERLY MEN

Dr. Neil Resnick, director of the Harvard Continence Clinic, who has done some pioneering work on incontinence in the elderly, has a fictional but realistic vignette that aptly illustrates how acute symptoms of prostate enlargement can be unwittingly brought on in older men, and inadvertently lead, in many cases, to unnecessary surgery.

George and Martha are a paradigmatic Beacon Hill couple who have been living happily in their townhouse for years. One Friday, George, who is sixty-seven, gets a cold, which keeps him up all night. Martha, lamenting George's plight but not wanting to call the doctor, wanders down the hill to the pharmacy. She enters and marvels at the wondrous medicinal advances that have occurred. She notes that we now have an array of cold pills, time-release capsules, nose drops that will last for twelve hours, and medications to help you sleep. She makes her purchases.

Martha comes back to a grateful George. Combined, these pills actually consist of more than just two or three ingredients. The time-release capsules have at least one, and probably more than one, *antihistamine* (which, among other things, blocks nerve impulses), and at least one *decongestant*—and frequently more—which tightens the bladder neck and makes it more difficult to urinate. The nose drops contain another decongestant, and the over-the-counter sleep medication includes another antihistamine. In one fell swoop, Martha brings home several drugs that cause the bladder neck to close and several more that ensure the bladder can't contract sufficiently to overcome this closure.

Not knowing all of this, George takes all of the pills and has a pleasant day. But Sunday night, he is in the emergency room with abdominal discomfort. In fact, he cannot urinate. The urologist on call, having kept abreast of developments in the field, knows that drugs can be a problem and asks George if he takes any. George says that he takes two drugs prescribed for heart problems, but he fails to mention the other medications because, like many of his peers, he believes that *medications* are prescribed by the doctor and *nostrums* are what you pick up at the drugstore. The urologist calls George's internist to tell him that he is going to

(continued)

do a prostatectomy in the morning. The internist racks his brain to see if there is anything else that might be causing George's problem. But George never called him about his cold or difficulty in sleeping. In truth, what George needs is someone to take his medical history and put a catheter in to drain the bladder, and once the medications have been identified and stopped, George will likely escape the need for a prostatectomy.

Every year, up to one third of men who have moderate prostate enlargement like George have unnecessary prostatectomies because they have urinary retention brought on by drugs or sometimes by constipation. The story vividly illustrates how easy it is for misdiagnosis of prostate enlargement to occur.

Diagnosis of Benign Prostatic Hyperplasia

Because the symptoms of benign prostate enlargement are not initially acute, and probably also because of the difficulties of discussing them with their family and peers, men usually do not seek medical help until their symptoms become fairly severe. On your first visit to the doctor, it is not possible to tell how fast your prostate is growing. But the results of your tests should provide an overall picture of the present state of enlargement. Before you go to your doctor, you might want to review the section in Chapter 2 on Preparing for Your Doctor's Visit.

THE TESTS NOTED HERE ARE DESCRIBED IN DETAIL IN THE INDEX OF DIAGNOSTIC TESTS, BEGINNING ON PAGE 278.

Diagnosis of prostate enlargement consists of a thorough medical history, a physical examination, several laboratory tests, and X-rays. When taking your medical history, your doctor will want to find out when your symptoms started, how they have progressed, how severe they are, what other medical problems you may have that could cause abnormal voiding, what surgeries you have had, and what medications you are taking. He or she may also ask you about your pattern of sexual activity.

During the physical examination, your doctor will feel your lower abdomen, looking for bladder distention—a sign of urinary retention. He or she will also insert a gloved and well-lubricated finger into your rectum to feel your prostate. Although the doctor cannot feel the core of the prostate—where enlargement most often occurs—on a rectal exam, he or she can get a general idea about the size of the prostate and feel its consistency (normal, soft or "boggy," which might indicate infection or inflammation), or detect hard spots that may be indicative of stones or prostatic cancer. In addition to the medical history and physical exam, the following tests may be done.

- A *urinalysis* and *urine culture* will rule out the presence of a urinary tract infection. The urinalysis will also reveal the presence of red blood cells, which might be due to BPH or indicate a separate problem in either the bladder or kidneys, in addition to the prostate.
- *Blood tests* can show an increase in creatinine, acid phosphatase, or prostate specific antigen. Elevated levels of creatinine suggest possible kidney damage due to urethral obstruction. Increased levels of acid phosphatase or prostate specific antigen may indicate the presence of prostate cancer, but they can also suggest prostate enlargement.
- Since BPH has the potential to cause kidney problems, visualization of the kidneys is still routinely done by most urologists prior to treating BPH. This can be done with a *kidney X-ray* or *IVP*, an ultrasound scan of the kidneys. These tests will show if prostate enlargement has resulted in obstruction of the ureters, blocking the kidney, or if there are any other conditions that may be contributing to your symptoms, such as kidney stones or tumors. An ultrasound is sufficient for this purpose if there is no blood in the urine. If the kidney is already damaged, the IVP may be harmful, especially for people who have diabetes or have an allergy to shellfish or iodine, the dye that is used.
- A test of your *urine flow rate* and *residual urine* after voiding will help to confirm the extent of urethral obstruction. These tests provide information that may be helpful in evaluating whether or not surgery is necessary.
- A *cystoscopy* is done by looking into the prostatic urethra and bladder with a cystoscope, so your doctor can assess whether the prostate is causing obstruction. The cystoscope exam can also reveal other changes in the bladder, such as trabeculation and diverticuli caused by BPH, as well as the presence of stones or tumors.

201

The symptoms that are characteristic of BPH can also be caused by inflammation, infection, bladder problems, or other conditions such as diabetes or neurological disorders, or by taking certain medications that interfere with bladder function. Therefore, if there is a possibility that you may have any of these conditions or you are less than fifty-five years old and have significant symptoms, you should have a *urodynamic evaluation,* especially a *uroflow study* and a *residual urine test* to determine the function of the bladder before undergoing surgery for BPH. These studies are vitally important in clarifying if, in fact, your symptoms are being caused by prostate enlargement or some other condition. According to several studies, about one third of men who are told that their incontinence is due to prostate enlargement actually have another cause when urodynamic studies are performed.[9]

Treatment

At the present time, there are two basic approaches to the treatment of prostatic enlargement. The first, and generally the most reasonable, is the wait-and-see approach. Unless you have severe symptoms, urinary retention, recurrent urinary tract infections, a lot of blood in your urine, or obstruction of the kidneys, there is no need to rush into surgery. As it is, *about 75 percent of men with enlarged prostates never have any treatment at all.* If your doctor recommends prostate surgery, be sure to ask him or her about alternatives and ask why each one is not appropriate in your case.

Some urologists believe that the overall results of prostatectomy are not that great, all things considered, and that men with mild to moderate symptoms might be helped by looking for other causes and more conservative therapy, or what doctors have come to call "watchful waiting."

Alternatives to Prostate Surgery

Even though the symptoms of prostatic enlargement are usually not acute, they can become disruptive for some men. Frequency of urination, urgency and urge incontinence, getting up several times at night to urinate, an inability to empty the bladder completely, and terminal dribbling can affect the quality of one's life considerably. If your symptoms are troublesome but you don't want to have surgery, there are a few possible alternatives that can make living with prostate enlargement easier:

Alpha Blockers. These relax the smooth-muscle tissue of the bladder neck, urethra, and prostate, resulting in decreased obstruction of the prostatic urethra. (See Drug Glossary on page 295.)

Prostatic Balloon Dilation. In this relatively new procedure, a catheter with a balloon at its tip is inserted into the urethra and blown up under pressure in the area of the prostate. After 10 to 20 minutes, it is deflated and removed, resulting in enlargment of the prostatic urethra, which allows the urine to pass more freely. Doctors at the University of Minnesota, where this procedure was popularized, report that obstructive symptoms disappeared or were significantly lessened in nearly 74 percent of cases for up to two years in certain patients who had minimal obstruction, no previous surgery, no evidence of cancer, or who had enlargement of only a certain portion of the prostate. This procedure is an attractive form of therapy because it can be done as an outpatient procedure in many cases. In addition, local anesthesia with intravenous sedation may be used instead of general or spinal anesthesia, which may allow patients with other significant medical illnesses (stroke, heart disease, neurological diseases, lung disease) to safely have non-surgical treatment of their BPH. At this time, the long-term effectiveness of this procedure remains to be determined.

Hormonal Therapy. Testosterone, the hormone produced in the testicles that is responsible for sexual development and function, appears to be a stimulus for prostatic enlargement. Several centers have been participating in the investigation of an experimental drug developed by Merck Sharp & Dome, called MK 906 or Prostim. This drug prevents testosterone from getting into the prostate cells and further stimulating growth, and may also decrease the size of the prostate. Up to 70 percent of men who have taken this drug have experienced good results, and minimal side effects have been encountered thus far.

Catheterization. If you have urinary retention and are too ill to undergo other forms of therapy, your doctor may insert a catheter to alleviate your symptoms until you are able to undergo surgery. If at all possible intermittent catheterization should be used instead of an indwelling catheter (see page 87).

Zinc. It is a dietary element that is found in fairly high concentration in the prostate. Although its role in prostate function is not well understood, the prostates of many men with BPH have been found to have lower concentrations of zinc than normal. While no scientific studies have shown zinc to be effective in inhibiting prostate growth, some men report that taking zinc helps keep prostate symptoms under control.

Surgery

Today, about 450,000 prostatectomies are performed in the United States each year, and 80 percent of these procedures are on men aged sixty-five and older.[10] In the past, the prostate was notoriously difficult to reach, so a surgeon had to cut through many layers of tissue. Consequently, the complication rate for surgical procedures was quite high. The development and use of the *resectoscope* in the 1930s allowed surgeons to approach the prostate through the urethra and thus avoid the problems that are often created by a deep incision in the pelvic area.

Traditionally, two approaches have been used to reach the prostate surgically, either through the abdomen or through the perineum—the short bridge between the anus and the scrotum. Both of these types are "open" prostatectomies, which require an incision. In recent years, approaching the prostate through the urethra has been favored because it is thought to be technically more efficient and to have a lower complication rate. This operation, called a *transurethral resection of the prostate* and commonly referred to as a *TURP*, literally means reaching the prostate through the urethra, "transurethrally," to cut or "resect" it. This type of operation is classified as a "closed" procedure because no incision is made. The primary indications for the use of the *open* procedures (in which an incision is made) are (1) if the prostate has grown extremely large, (2) if the shape of your prostate is such that your doctor believes that a TURP would be less effective or more risky, or (3) if there is another urologic abnormality that requires an incision through the abdomen for treatment.

A safe and successful prostatectomy requires a highly skilled surgeon, so if you are contemplating surgery, make sure the one you have chosen has had a lot of experience in performing the procedure. (See Choosing a Surgeon on page 22 for suggestions for how to find a doctor who is experienced in the type of surgery that you need.)

The decision to have prostate surgery rests upon three factors:

• your own perception of your symptoms and how disruptive they are to your life;

- your doctor's assessment of your physical condition; and
- the objective results of laboratory, radiology, and urodynamic tests.

If you are working and the symptoms are interfering with your ability to function, you might consider surgery sooner than a man who is retired or is in frail health. Indications for surgery may include the inability to urinate (acute urinary retention), a significant residual urine, decreased urine flow rate, evidence of urethral obstruction revealed by urodynamic studies, repeated urinary tract infections, or evidence of kidney damage because of prostatic enlargement.

Ninety percent of prostate surgeries performed today are by *transurethral resection.* In this procedure, the surgeon reaches the prostate by inserting a resectoscope through the urethra (see illustration 12). The prostatic tissue is carved away with an instrument tipped with an electric current. The bits of tissue removed, known as prostate "chips," are washed out of the bladder and urethra and sent to the pathology lab to check for malignancy. After the surgery, you will have a catheter in place that allows the bladder to be continuously irrigated for one to three days until the urine clears of blood.

Because of modern technology and experience, the rate of complications following a TURP is quite low and the chance of dying as a result of the procedure is less than 1 percent. Men can expect to be infertile after a TURP because the ejaculate usually travels backward into the bladder, called *retrograde ejaculation.* The sensations of orgasm are basically unchanged. The difference is that the ejaculate goes into the bladder instead of emerging from the tip of the penis. This occurs because the internal sphincter muscle is damaged during surgery, so it can no longer close reflexively to prevent the seminal fluid from entering the bladder. You should be carefully counseled about this condition before surgery. Most men adjust to the difference, but some find it disconcerting.

There are some serious complications associated with the TURP procedure—the major one being the transurethral resection (TUR) syndrome. When this occurs, dilution of your blood and body fluids can take place when some of the fluid used to irrigate the bladder during the procedure leaks out of the prostate area and into your veins. This disrupts the normal concentrations of the essential chemical constituents of the body fluids, known as *electrolytes,* and can result in convulsions, seizures, coma, and even death if an imbalance is not recognized and treated. You can also expect some post-operative bleeding that may occasionally necessitate getting a blood transfusion or another surgical procedure. Up to 65 percent of men suffer from irritative voiding symptoms —urgency, frequency, and urge incontinence—after the surgery. These symptoms usually disappear or improve within a few weeks or a few months, but very rarely they can be permanent. The most bothersome long-term complications following a TURP are urinary retention, urinary incontinence, and erectile dysfunction.

Urinary retention occurs in 5 or 6 percent of the men who have surgery for prostate enlargement. In one recent study, half of these men regained the ability to void comfortably, and the other half had to use a catheter intermittently for some period of time or had to rely on a permanent indwelling catheter.[11]

Incontinence following a TURP for benign prostate enlargement occurs in less than 1 percent of men, and resolves within six months in about half of these. The remainder have permanent incontinence, which may be dealt with by pelvic-floor exercises, biofeedback, medications, or further surgery. In the more radical surgery for prostate cancer, the rate of incontinence is higher, perhaps as much as 5 to 15 percent.

Erectile dysfunction occurs in up to 8 percent of men who have TURPs or open prostatectomies. The loss of the ability to achieve an erection has a varying impact on different men. Some men are able to take it in stride, while others feel very keenly that they have not only lost the ability to achieve erections but are missing a treasured part of their identity. However, *the loss of the ability to have an erection does not necessarily diminish the ability to achieve an orgasm.* Nor does it necessarily decrease the quality of sex. Although it may be a small comfort to many men who lose the ability to have erections, some find that sex can still be intensely pleasurable and that it actually improves when the focus of activity is no longer exclusively on intercourse. (See page 252 for information on coping with erectile dysfunction.) If the loss of erection is an important issue for you, you should talk about it with your doctor and explore the various treatment options if this problem does occur.

There is a significant difference between the surgery done for benign prostate enlargement and a radical prostatectomy, the type of procedure done for prostate cancer. Both TURPs and to some extent open prostatectomy for BPH leave some prostate tissue and its skin, known as the *prostatic capsule* (somewhat like coring an apple and leaving the rim of pulp and skin). This tissue is subject to the same diseases as the normal prostate—regrowth, inflammation, or cancer. The radical prostatectomy removes the entire apple—pits, pulp, and skin.

PROSTATE CANCER

While Lloyd and his wife were traveling in Europe, he came down with a bad cold, and the antihistamines that he took seemed to cause urinary frequency, which was unusual. "When I got back, I decided to get a check-up and my doctor discovered prostate cancer." Since most prostate cancers, like Lloyd's, are slow-growing, his doctor told him that he had some time to make a decision about treatment. He chose his surgeon carefully and had a radical prostatectomy. His doctor used a new surgical technique that preserved his ability to have an erection, but the surgery left him incontinent. "I was very fit for seventy and my doctors assured me that I had a 90 to 95 percent chance of not being incontinent," says Lloyd. "I never thought it would happen to me."

Prostate cancer is the most prevalent cancer in men, but it is relatively uncommon in men under the age of fifty. Since there is no way to reduce the risk factors for prostate cancer (short of removing the testicles to eliminate testosterone, the hormone responsible for prostate growth), this might seem like very bad news. The good news, however, is that prostate cancer is far from the leading killer. Far more men die of lung cancer each year than of cancer of the prostate. The reason for this is that most prostate tumors are slow-growing, so you may be far more likely to die of some other condition before succumbing to prostate cancer.

Survival Rates

Because symptoms of prostate cancer tend to occur late in the disease, only about 30 percent are caught before they spread beyond the prostatic capsule. In cases where the cancer is contained within the prostate, the cancer is usually cured when the prostate is removed. If cancerous cells have spread to lymph nodes but not to other organs, the survival rate is about 50 to 60 percent at five years, 30 to 40 percent at ten years, and 10 to 20 percent at fifteen years after surgery. If the cancer has *metastasized,* that is, spread to other organs, the average survival is two to three years, although about 10 percent of these men may live ten years or longer.

What causes cancerous changes to begin in the prostate is still unknown. As with prostate enlargement, castrati, men who have their testicles removed before they start puberty, almost never get prostate cancer, suggesting that a hormonal factor may stimulate cancerous changes in the prostate. There is also a possible genetic predisposition, since men whose older male relatives develop prostate cancer are more likely to develop the disease themselves.[12] Black men seem to develop prostate cancer earlier and tend to have more aggressive forms of it, suggesting an ethnic predisposition as well. In addition, black men are twice as likely to die from prostate cancer as white men, but this figure may be inflated due to minorities' traditional lack of access to health care in the United States.

Epidemiological data has identified some other groups of men as having a higher likelihood of developing prostate cancer: men who live in urban areas, and those who work with industrial chemicals that are commonly used in manufacturing rubber or textiles or who work as printers, painters, mechanics, loggers, ship fitters, porters, janitors, farmers, and shipping clerks.[13,14] If you work in any of these occupations, it's extremely important to have a yearly urological examination to check for early signs of prostate cancer.

Symptoms of Prostate Cancer

Lloyd was unlucky to have landed in the 5 to 10 percent or so of men who develop permanent incontinence as a result of radical prostate surgery, but he was exceedingly lucky that the antihistamines he took affected his voiding function and reminded him to have a urological check-up. Prostate cancer can grow silently for a long time before noticeable symptoms develop. A symptom that can bring men with prostate cancer to the doctor's office is lower back or pelvic pain—a symptom that men do not normally associate with a prostate problem. If there is not another cause of this pain, then it probably indicates that cancer has broken through the prostatic capsule and spread through the bloodstream to the bones of the pelvis and spine.

When symptoms of prostate cancer do occur, they can include the following:

Irritative symptoms
- urgent need to urinate
- frequency of urination
- waking to urinate *(nocturia)*
- painful urination *(dysuria)*

Obstructive symptoms
- hesitant urination
- weak or interrupted urinary stream
- feeling of incomplete bladder emptying

Other symptoms
- pain or infection in the kidneys due to obstruction *(hydrone-phrosis)*
- lower back or pelvic pain or other "bone" pain that lasts more than two weeks
- weight loss, loss of appetite, fatigue, loss of vitality
- weakness in legs, urinary or fecal incontinence, numbness or decreased sensation in the legs or perineum (the area between the scrotum and anus)
- blood in the urine

The irritative or obstructive symptoms are similar to those of benign prostate enlargement, but may not become noticeable or bothersome early in the development of the disease. This is because BPH usually begins near the core of the gland, and if it proceeds inward, it will press on the urethra, causing obstructive, and possibly irritative, urinary symptoms. Ninety percent of cancerous growths, on the other hand, begin near the outer (peripheral) part of the gland, and may not cause irritative or obstructive symptoms until they are quite large.

Diagnosis

If every man above the age of fifty had a yearly prostate exam, many more cancers would be discovered earlier, allowing treatment to begin before the cancer has spread to the lymph nodes, bones, and other parts of the body. Less than half of men take advantage of this routine, live-saving examination.

Whether you are having a routine exam, have made an appointment because you have symptoms, or have been referred by your family physician or internist, your urologist will take a thorough medical history and do a physical examination. He or she will be particularly interested in how long you have had symptoms (if you have any), if you have any immediate family members who have developed prostate cancer, and what type of work you do.

THE TESTS NOTED HERE ARE DESCRIBED IN DETAIL IN THE INDEX OF DIAGNOSTIC TESTS, BEGINNING ON PAGE 278.

The most important part of your physical examination will consist of a *digital rectal examination (DRE),* in which your doctor will insert a finger into your rectum and feel the size and consistency of the prostate, looking particularly for any hard or irregular areas. In addition, screening and diagnostic tests will be done.

Screening tests to rule out other problems
- A *urinalysis* and *culture and sensitivity test* of the urine will determine if you have infection or if there is any blood in the urine.
- A kidney X-ray or *intravenous pyelogram (IVP)* will routinely be done to rule out obstruction of the kidneys by enlarged pelvic lymph nodes or from a large prostate tumor. If you are allergic to the iodine dye used in this test, an *ultrasound* and *renal scan* can be substituted. If a CT scan is done and no blood is found, then an IVP is not always necessary.
- A *chest X-ray (CXR)* will be done to make sure that the cancer has not spread to the lungs, and to make sure you don't have any condition in the chest area that might preclude or postpone surgery.

Diagnostic tests to determine if cancer is present
- A *biopsy* of the prostate, performed with a very thin needle, will be done. A positive biopsy is a clear sign of prostate cancer.
- A *prostatic ultrasound* may aid in identifying prostatic nodules and help your doctor easily locate them to do biopsies if cancer spread is suspected.
- A *blood test* will check for an elevated prostate specific antigen (PSA), a substance normally manufactured by the prostate. PSA levels may be mildly elevated in cases of prostate enlargement, but if they remain or become elevated after surgery, this is a strong indication that there is persistent cancer, or that it has spread.

Staging to see how far cancer has spread
- Your doctor will look into your urethra and bladder with a *cysto-scope* to see if the tumor is pressing on your urethra and if the cancer has invaded the bladder.
- A *bone scan* (an X-ray of the bones) will be done to make sure that the cancer has not spread to the bones.
- A *CT scan* will make sure that there are not any enlarged pelvic lymph nodes or evidence of spread to nearby organs.
- A *blood test for acid phosphatase:* elevated levels of acid phosphatase, a substance normally manufactured by the prostate, can indicate that cancer has spread to the lymph nodes or to other sites in the body.
- Other *blood tests* will evaluate your blood chemistry to check your liver function, since prostate cancer can spread to the liver. A *complete blood count (CBC),* showing a decrease in normal red blood cells, white blood cells, and platelets (important in immune defense mechanisms), can be another indication that the cancer has spread to the bones.

The results of the staging tests will indicate the stage of your cancer. See the box on page 212 for information on the classification of prostate cancer.

About 10 to 12 percent of the men who have a TURP for suspected benign prostate enlargement and have no obvious signs of cancer will have cancerous cells found in the prostate "chips" that are cut away during the surgery. In this case, the TURP is considered to be a diagnostic procedure for prostate cancer. If your doctor thinks there is a possibility that prostate cancer may have spread to the lymph nodes, but cannot be certain any other way, he or she may want to do a *pelvic lymph node dissection.* Most urologists feel that it is necessary to know whether the lymph nodes contain cancer in order to choose the most appropriate treatment.

211

THE CLASSIFICATION OF PROSTATE CANCER

Cancerous tumors vary widely in terms of size at the time of discovery, what they look like under the microscope, i.e., how different (or "differentiated") the cells are from normal cells, how fast they grow (how "aggressive" they are), and how much they have spread (how "invasive" they are), so all these factors affect the choice of treatment. In order to choose the (potentially) most effective treatment, each tumor is graded, or *staged*, depending upon various factors:

Stage A constitutes about 10 to 15 percent of all prostate cancers. There are no symptoms, and the prostate feels normal during a rectal examination. Cancer cells are found in the chips removed during surgery for benign prostate enlargement. *A1* indicates a few areas of cancerous growth, while *A2* indicates more widespread disease within the prostate.

Stage B comprises roughly 20 to 30 percent of prostate tumors and can usually be felt by a digital rectal exam, but has no noticeable symptoms. *B1* tumors are less than 1.5 centimeters wide and are growing in only one lobe of the prostate. Stage *B2* tumors are larger and have invaded more than one area of the prostate.

Stage C tumors make up about 25 to 30 percent of prostatic cancers. These tumors have grown through the capsule, but they are still considered contained and "locally invasive." Symptoms of obstruction may be present and virtually the entire prostate may be cancerous, but no cancer is found in the lymph nodes.

The remaining 35 to 45 percent of prostate cancers are classified as *stage D*. If the cancer has spread beyond the prostatic capsule and has invaded the lymph nodes, it is classified as *D1*. If the cancer has spread further to other organs, such as bones or lungs, it is classified as *D2*. Symptoms may or may not manifest themselves at the *D2* stage.

In addition to staging your cancer based upon physical examination and the results of laboratory tests, your doctor may also make use of the *Gleason score,* a system that evaluates the differentiation of cancerous cells that make up the tumor and the pattern of their growth.[15] A score of from 1 to 5 is given for each of the two largest clusters of cancer cells, with the lower scores indicating more well differentiated, and therefore (presumably) less aggressive, types of cancer cells. Then the two numbers are added together, yielding a result of from 1 to 9. The lower the number, the less aggressive the tumor, indicating to your doctor how quickly the cancer is likely to spread.

Depending upon a number of variables, stage A, B, and C cancers are considered potentially curable, and in general, the lower the stage, the higher the chances for cure.

Treatment for Prostate Cancer

Treatment for prostate cancer varies *considerably* among urologists and cancer specialists across the country, so what you read here may not coincide exactly with the way your urologist decides to treat your disease. In deciding which treatment to pursue, you will probably want to know the advantages and disadvantages of each treatment, the side effects, and the survival rates. If your cancer is in the range of A to B, probably the biggest decision you will have to make is whether to use surgery or radiation therapy as your primary form of treatment. Both treatments have advantages and disadvantages that must be carefully evaluated in terms of your personal situation and physical condition. Some doctors may prefer one type of treatment over the other and will have a well-supported rationale for their preference. However, it is important, and very appropriate, for you to have full information about each treatment option, and to express your preferences as well.

Based on the stage of your cancer, the following treatments are most frequently used:

If the tumor is truly A1, many doctors will adopt a wait-and-see approach, and this seems to be a very reasonable option, especially with an older man. Some urologists, however, believe that up to 15 percent of people with A1 tumors will show progression within five to ten years, and opt for treatment of the localized disease—either radiation or surgery—especially in younger men. Other doctors choose to adopt a moderate approach, doing repeat biopsies of the prostate two to three months after the initial exam, to make sure that the cancer has not grown significantly. If you have a strong preference on this score, you should talk it over with your doctor.

For stages A2 and B, when the cancer is confined to the prostate gland, there are three options: a radical prostatectomy, in which the entire prostate is removed; external radiation treatment; or the implantation of radioactive "seeds" or pellets into the prostate. Each has certain advantages and disadvantages.

Radical Prostatectomy. If the cancer is confined to the prostate gland, as it is in stages A2 and B, the treatment preferred by many urologists is a radical prostatectomy, in which the entire prostate gland, including part of the urethra and the seminal vesicles, is removed. The prostate is usually reached through an abdominal incision, approaching the gland behind the pubic bone (the retropubic approach). Your surgeon will remove nearby lymph nodes to confirm that the cancer is really confined to the prostate. If the cancer has spread, further treatment will be needed. A perineal approach (through the skin between the scrotum and rectum) is favored by a minority of urologists, but has produced equally good results.

Until recently, both incontinence and erectile dysfunction (commonly referred to as *impotence*) were the frequently expected after-effects of prostate surgery. In the last decade, Dr. Patrick Walsh and his associates at Johns Hopkins University have pioneered a nerve-sparing technique in the retropubic approach that preserves the ability to have an erection in many cases, depending on the patient's age and the degree of erectile function prior to surgery. Incontinence results in 5 to 6 percent of cases for stage B disease and is slightly higher for stage A disease. If you are having a radical prostatectomy, ask your doctor if he or she is familiar with the Walsh procedure. If your doctor is not, you might want to call some of the organizations listed on page 21 to ask for a referral to a surgeon who can do this operation.

Even though your surgeon is only removing a gland that is the approximate size of a walnut, a radical prostatectomy takes from three to four hours to perform. Since it is a relatively long operation, and because of the extensive network of veins encountered near the pubic bone, there is the potential for considerable blood loss. If you are healthy and have time between the dates of your diagnosis and surgery, you might want to consider storing 2 to 4 pints of your own blood, or having a family member or friend with compatible blood donate for you, to further reduce the small risk of complications that sometimes can occur when using blood from a commercial blood bank.

External Radiation Treatment. In delivering radiation to the prostate, there are two options: radiation from an external source (*external beam radiation*) or the implantation of radioactive "seeds" directly into the prostate. Of the two, external beam radiation is by far the most frequently employed. The treatments, which take about 30 to 40 minutes, are usually done every working day for about six or seven weeks. In general, radiation has some advantages over surgery—you do not have to endure the physical pain and emotional stress or potential complications of major surgery. Although the complications of radiation therapy are lower than those of surgery, they are not inconsequential. They include skin rash, water retention (edema) in the legs and feet, diarrhea, and cystitis (called *radiation cystitis*) with symptoms of urinary urgency and frequency and erectile dysfunction in about 50 percent of men. Usually, these symptoms dissipate over a period of time, but in some men, they may take up to a year to resolve. In some cases, they can become permanent and have a negative impact on the quality of your life. For some unknown reason, erectile dysfunction may not appear until one to two years after treatment.

Implantation of Radioactive Seeds. The implantation of "seeds" into the prostate has some potential advantages over the use of external beam radiation, but has been used on far fewer patients. Urologists and radiologists are still learning about the effectiveness of radiation in curing or controlling cancer. In this procedure, tiny pellets of radioactive iodine, gold, or palladium (a metal similar to platinum), or irradiated metal are implanted in the prostate, using a long needle inserted through the abdomen. The advantage of implanting radioactive pellets directly into the prostate is that it affords the ability to deliver a higher dose of radiation to the tumor, but with minimal effects on the adjacent tissue and nearby organs. However, this type of radiation treatment seems to work only on smaller tumors and it will not work if the cancer has spread to the lymph nodes or bones. In addition, there are many unanswered questions about its long-term effectiveness.

In a newer method of delivery, a few doctors are currently implanting palladium seeds into the prostate through the perineum while the patient is under local anesthesia and intravenous sedation. This procedure can be done as an outpatient procedure, which would appear to be a less traumatic and less expensive option. However, since a pelvic lymph node dissection is not done prior to implanting the seeds, potential cancer in the lymph nodes may go unnoticed and untreated. This procedure is very new, and long-term follow-up regarding tumor recurrence and complications is not yet available. Because most prostate cancer is slow-growing, accurate information about the effectiveness and curative potential will not be available for eight to fifteen years.

215

Many cancer specialists now prefer surgery over radiation therapy because the cancer seems to recur sooner with radiation—in about seven years instead of ten.

Hormonal Treatment

Stage D tumors, in which the cancer has spread (or metastasized) to the lymph nodes and bones and perhaps the liver or lungs, are *not* considered curable, and treatment is aimed at arresting the spread of the disease. Since about 85 percent of prostate cancers are androgen-dependent, that is, they need the hormone testosterone (a type of androgen) to grow, removal of the testicles, the source of testosterone, is the most direct way to deprive the cancer of its main source of sustenance. There are also other means of depriving the tumor of its testosterone supply. One is *the administration of estrogen,* which suppresses the production of testosterone quickly and efficiently. While this treatment is known to be effective, it may have significant side effects in those who have heart disease or a history of blood clots. Many men find taking estrogen undesirable because it decreases sex drive, causes erectile dysfunction, and stimulates breast growth (as it does in some women). Breast growth stimulated by estrogen is irreversible, so it can be suppressed by radiation treatment before starting therapy.

Another treatment that will reduce the production of testosterone to near zero is the administration of synthetic *LH-RH (luteinizing hormone–releasing hormone),* a drug that suppresses pituitary function. (The pituitary stimulates the production of testosterone in the testicles in men and in the adrenal glands of both men and women.) LH-RH does not have most of the side effects of estrogen, but it does cause erectile dysfunction. All of these treatments can cause "hot flashes," similiar to those women have when passing through menopause. In the past, the LH-RH preparation was given in daily injections, but a long-acting form (a once-a-month injection) is now available. Although such treatment certainly improves symptoms and the quality of life, it is unclear whether the use of any of these drugs actually increases the chances of survival.

Flutamide is a recently FDA-approved drug which is an oral anti-androgen agent, that is, it interferes with the production of androgen (the hormone that stimulates prostate growth and sexual functioning) within the prostate cells. When used in combination with a drug like LH-RH, or after removal of the testicles (orchiectomy), Flutamide suppresses androgen that is produced in other parts of the body as well. Since androgen stimulates the growth of prostate tissue—and prostate tissue that is cancerous as well—the elimination of this stimulus would be desirable to slow the growth of prostate cancer.

If the cancer fails to respond to hormonal therapy, as a last resort *chemotherapy* is sometimes used to slow the spread of the cancer and relieve symptoms.

Diagnosing and treating prostate problems can be challenging to both you and your doctor. Because so little is known about the prostate's function, overcoming the various disorders that can arise often requires diagnostic skill on the part of your doctor and, on your part, patience and perseverance, as well as diligence in adhering to prescribed treatment regimens.

PROSTATE PROBLEM REMINDERS

- Prostate infections are often difficult to diagnose, and may require long-term treatment.
- Prostate enlargement is generally not life-threatening, so there is no rush for surgery.
- A yearly rectal examination is your best defense against prostate cancer.
- Most prostate cancers are slow-growing, and are not likely to be fatal.

RESOURCES

The Prostate Book, Stephen N. Rous. New York: W. W. Norton & Co., 1988. This superbly illustrated book by a sympathetic male urologist describes how the prostate works, diagnostic tests, and treatment options. Its one shortcoming is that it provides no information on alternative remedies or coping mechanisms.

CHAPTER 8

Confronting Bladder Cancer

"YOU HAVE CANCER" IS SURELY ONE OF THE MOST dreaded phrases in any language. To the average person, who doesn't know lymphoma from sarcoma and doesn't particularly care to, cancer is the great unknown, a cruel game of cards in which the rules are written in an abstruse code and somebody else is holding all the aces. But after the initial shock of diagnosis has worn off, fear can be replaced by knowledge, and knowledge can give you the power to work with your doctor to fight a formidable and sagacious enemy. Sometimes, in spite of the best efforts, cancer prevails. But until it does, you need to make many decisions about your care and treatment.

Thus far, we do not have much concrete knowledge about the specific mechanisms that trigger cancerous growth at the cellular level. In the case of bladder cancer, it does seem clear that these changes can be precipitated by external environmental factors or by internal metabolic factors.

When compared to cancer in many other parts of the body, bladder cancer has a generally good prognosis. The vast majority of cancers found in the bladder are *superficial tumors* that arise and stay confined to the surface of the bladder and can be treated without disfiguring surgery.[1] Because of its tendency to unpredictable recurrence, the issue of "cure" in cancer is very controversial. Cancer specialists now think not only in terms of "cure," but also in terms of five-year survival rates. The key determinants of survival are the type of cancer you have, the "grade" (how similar it looks under the miscroscope to normal bladder tissue), and the "stage" (the degree of advancement), that is, if it is confined to the bladder's surface, if it has invaded into the deeper layers, if it has grown through the entire bladder wall, or, worst of all, if it has spread to lymph nodes or distant organs. Other important factors in survival are how long it was growing before it was diagnosed and how well you respond to treatment.

WHAT IS BLADDER CANCER?

Cancer is the chaotic, uncontrolled proliferation of cells called *neoplastic* (new growth) in an organ or area of the body that crowds out normal growth and ultimately destroys or replaces much of the structure it inhabits. Cells with cancerous characteristics can break away from the main tumor and spread to other parts of the body through the lymphatic system or bloodstream.

As scientists probe deeper into the inner workings of the cell, they are beginning to learn more about how normal cells function and, using the concepts of a science called molecular genetics. They are beginning to get some understanding of why cellular structures sometimes grow out of control. With the aid of the electron microscope, neoplastic changes have been observed almost as they happen, and a number of metabolic, viral, and environmental factors that appear to stimulate such growth have been identified.

The innermost surface layer of the bladder—the part that is in contact with the urine—is composed of several layers of *transitional cells.* These layers together comprise the *epithelium.* Below these "superficial" layers lies the *lamina propria,* a layer of fibrous connective tissue that is the division between the epithelium and the deeper muscular layer of the bladder wall. In terms of bladder cancer, the lamina propria represents the frontier beneath which cancer is classified as "invasive." Approximately 70 to 80 percent of all bladder cancers are classified as *superficial tumors,* meaning that they begin and remain in the epithelial, or superficial, layer of the bladder (see illustration).

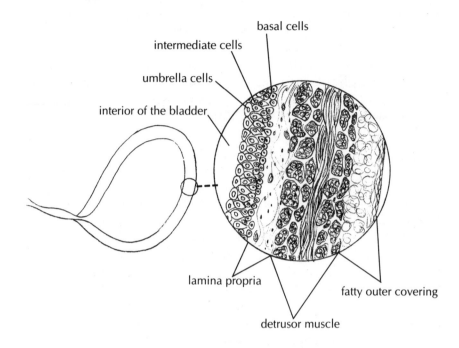

14. Bladder lining. The bladder lining is composed of several layers of cells. The innermost (epithelial) layer has three types of cells: umbrella cells, so called because they are rather large and flat, intermediate cells, and basal or base cells. The *lamina propria* is a thin, membranous tissue that divides the epithelial layer from the bladder muscle (the detrusor). Covering the detrusor muscle is a layer of fatty tissue.

CHANGES THAT LEAD TO BLADDER CANCER

The metamorphosis from normal cells to a cancerous tumor consists of four phases. The first is *hyperplasia,* which merely means an increase in the number of cells, without any change in their basic architecture. In the second phase, *metaplasia,* certain characteristic changes in the amount and arrangement of cells occur, but these are not yet characterized as cancerous. Some metaplastic changes are certainly pre-cancerous, but others, especially *squamous metaplasia,* occurring in the epithelial layers of the bladder, are probably not. In the third stage, *dysplasia,* the cells will have enlarged centers or nuclei and their arrangement is somewhat abnormal. In almost all cases, the dysplasia is usually classified as mild, moderate, or severe. Of these conditions, only severe dysplasia is considered pre-cancerous, although some researchers prefer to classify this condition as cancerous. In the final stage, *carcinoma*, the cell centers or nuclei are frankly abnormal and their usual arrangement is disrupted. This classification encompasses *carcinoma-in-situ, transitional cell carcinoma, adenocarcinoma*, and *squamous cell carcinoma*. There are other types of cancer as well, but they are rare.

TYPES OF CANCEROUS CHANGES

Carcinoma-in-situ, which is frequently referred to as CIS, is a self-contained, localized area of cancerous cells that has not spread beyond the innermost layer of the bladder lining, the epithelium. While CIS does not spread itself, it often co-exists with other types of bladder cancer, and if it does, the chances of progression to invasive cancer are quite high—perhaps even as high as 80 percent. The development of CIS does not follow a set pattern. Some people have it for a long time without symptoms, while others may experience severe irritative voiding symptoms early on. One study done several years ago found that 20 percent of people who had CIS also had other types of bladder tumors in various stages of development. Even under the microscope, benign growths are often difficult to differentiate from cancerous ones, and experts are sometimes divided on where to draw the line between non-cancerous and cancerous tumors.

Transitional cell carcinomas are the most common type of cancer in the bladder. They can be *papillary*, meaning that they project into the bladder on a stalk; these are not usually invasive. The less common *flat* tumors usually are invasive, often growing into the deeper layers of the bladder wall.

Cancers of the *squamous cell* variety account for about 7 percent of bladder cancers in the United States. These cancers are most often associated with bladder irritants such as long-term indwelling catheters, infection, and bladder stones.

Adenocarcinomas are not very common, accounting for only about 2 percent of all bladder cancers. This type of cancer is also thought by some to be associated with chronic inflammation and infection. A thorough evaluation should be done to make sure that the adenocarcinoma did not originate in another organ like the colon or prostate gland.

WHO HAS BLADDER CANCER?

Bladder cancer rarely affects people below the age of fifty, but it is the fifth leading cause of death in American men over the age of sixty-five. In 1989, an estimated 47,000 new cases of bladder cancer occurred (34,500 in men and 12,500 in women), and approximately 10,200 died. Men are at least three times as likely to develop bladder cancer as women are, and white men are more than twice as likely to develop it as are black men. White women are about twice as prone to this particular kind of cancer as black women, and they are about twice as likely to develop it. Bladder cancers occur much more often in urban areas than in rural ones and 40 percent more often in the North than in the South of the United States.

In recent years, bladder cancer has decreased significantly among women, and slightly among men.[2]

RISK FACTORS

Over the last two decades, exhaustive studies have been done to try to discern and document patterns in the incidence of cancer. In the case of bladder cancer, several clear-cut risk factors have been established and others are strongly suspected.

Cigarette Smoking. Studies on smoking and cancer of the bladder differ about how much risk is involved, but most have found it to be substantial—even as much as seven to ten times higher than for non-smokers, depending on the duration of smoking and the degree of inhalation. About 40 percent of bladder cancers have been said to be related to cigarette smoking. Cigarette smoke contains known carcinogens, predominantly nitrosamines, a breakdown product of nicotine.

Occupational Risks. Occupational hazards contribute to more than a quarter of all bladder cancers in the United States. Unusually high risks of developing bladder cancer exist in the dye, rubber, textile, cable, and printing industries. People who work in these sectors of manufacturing should without question have a urinalysis and urine cytology every year to check for blood or abnormal cells in the urine—telltale signs of bladder cancer. The incidence of bladder cancer is also significant in the following occupations, and routine screening could save your life:[3]

plastics industry	petroleum workers
leather workers	shoe-repair workers
metalworkers	plumbers
painters	hairdressers
tailors	sailors
engineers	photographers
carpenters	stoneworkers
food processors	

These industries make heavy use of chemicals containing *aromatic amines,* used in many manufacturing and chemical processes, which contain a chemical structure called a benzene ring and have been identified as carcinogenic. Chemicals used in the manufacture of plastics as well as petroleum and crude oil derivatives are suspected of causing bladder cancer as well.

Pelvic Radiation Therapy. Higher incidences of bladder cancer have been reported in people who have had radiation therapy for pelvic cancers such as colon, prostate, and cervix. Definitive studies, however, have not been done.

Bladder Infections Associated with Indwelling Catheters or Urinary Stones. It is thought that inflammation in the bladder from the long-standing presence of bacteria, especially *E. coli* and *Proteus mirabilis,* caused by long-term catheter use or bladder stones, may serve as a catalyst or *co-promoter* for bladder cancer.

Certain Drugs. Long-term exposure to large doses of *phenacetin* (a painkiller) or exposure to *cyclophosphamide* (a drug used for chemotherapy in many cancers) has been associated with the development of *transitional cell* carcinoma.

Caffeine Consumption in Coffee, Tea, and Sodas. The association between caffeine ingestion and bladder cancer has not been firmly established, but some studies have suggested a higher incidence of bladder cancer in heavy consumers of these beverages.

Consumption of Artificial Sweeteners. The statistical association between artificial sweeteners and bladder cancer in people is not very strong, but high doses are known to cause cancer in laboratory animals.

Bladder cancer is usually not seen for up to twenty years or more after exposure to one or more of the above substances.

SYMPTOMS

Bladder cancer is most often a silent intruder. It can remain asymptomatic for a long time without causing the physical signs, such as fatigue and weight loss, that often accompany other kinds of cancer. The first sign of bladder cancer is often accidentally discovered when your doctor finds blood in your urine *(hematuria)* on a routine urinalysis, when there is no infection or other obvious explanation such as cystitis or prostatitis. This blood, which is invisible to the naked eye, can be detected in up to 60 percent of cases. Visible blood is present in the urine in an additional 20 percent of people who have bladder cancer. If blood is discovered in your urine, it does *not* necessarily mean that you have cancer. Check the Symptom Chart on pages 28–29 to see the other conditions in which blood appears in the urine. There does not appear to be a direct correlation between the appearance of blood in the urine and the severity of the cancer.

The next most frequently occurring symptoms of bladder cancer are the classic irritative voiding symptoms—urgency, frequency, and painful urination. These symptoms, which occur in up to 25 percent of those with bladder cancer, are usually associated with extensive carcinoma-in-situ or invasive cancer. As the Symptom Chart indicates, these symptoms may also occur in many other bladder disorders.

DIAGNOSIS

Michael, a fifty-nine-year-old engineer at a large plastics manufacturing company in southern New Jersey, came to see Kristene after he noticed blood in his urine. His kidney X-ray was normal, and his urinalysis found no bacteria, but the cytology test, in which cells are examined under a microscope, revealed abnormal cells in his urine. When Kristene looked at Michael's bladder through the cystoscope, it did not appear normal. A biopsy revealed grade 1 transitional cell carcinoma in one area of the bladder. Kristene removed the tumor and told Michael that he needed to be monitored closely. "I went back every three months for a cystoscope exam, and my bladder was normal for nine months, when two new tumors appeared," Michael remembers. Biopsies from each of the two tumors showed grade 2 transitional cell carcinoma. A biopsy from an area of the bladder that appeared normal also revealed carcinoma-in-situ. "The appearance of the CIS tumor made my case more complicated, and meant that I had to have drugs put into my bladder every week for six weeks," Michael says.

Michael's experience is typical of that of many people who develop bladder cancer. He had no symptoms, but went to a urologist when he discovered blood in his urine. The diagnosis of his cancer was not difficult, and his treatment with chemotherapy appears to have arrested the growth of the cancer. He continues to be monitored every three months and after every visit when no more cancer is discovered, he and his wife have a special dinner to celebrate.

THE TESTS NOTED HERE ARE DESCRIBED IN DETAIL IN THE INDEX OF DIAGNOSTIC TESTS, BEGINNING ON PAGE 278.

If you come to your doctor and say that you have found blood in your urine or it is found on routine examination, the doctor will be looking for certain risk factors for bladder cancer in your medical history. He or she may ask you whether or not you smoke, and what your occupation is, to see if you may have been exposed to any of the occupational hazards mentioned on pages 222–23. He or she may also inquire about your past use of drugs, especially pain relievers, and whether you have had any other kinds of cancer and what kinds of therapy you received.

If blood is found in your urine but no bacteria are present, your urine will be sent for a *cytology test* to detect the presence of cancer cells. Cytology screening is highly accurate in confirming the presence of cancer cells in the bladder, but it is not foolproof. Up to 30 percent of cancers can be missed, especially if they are low-grade and less invasive cancers.

Since about 10 to 15 percent of people who develop bladder cancer will also get it in the kidneys or ureters, an X-ray of the entire urinary tract (an *intravenous pyelogram* or *IVP*) will be taken. This test will also show if the bleeding is being caused by a kidney stone or other abnormality. Your doctor will look into your bladder with a cystoscope to see if any abnormal growths are visible. This procedure is usually done right in the doctor's office, and can be uncomfortable, but it doesn't last long, and it provides a great deal of useful information about the number, size, and location of tumors and whether they are *papillary* or *flat*. Based on the results of the cystoscopy, your doctor will decide what other tests are needed to make the diagnosis and assess the extent, or *stage*, of the cancer.

If abnormal cells are seen on your bladder cytology test, or a suspicious growth is seen in the bladder, your doctor will schedule you for removal of the tumor, a procedure both *diagnostic* and *curative*. Once removed, the tumor can then be examined to see if it is benign or malignant, and if it is malignant, the type, grade, and stage will be determined. If the cancer is found to be non-invasive, the removal of the tumor may constitute a cure. This procedure is done in the operating room under anesthesia. While you are under anesthesia, a pelvic examination will be done to try to feel if the tumor has grown through the bladder wall or if there is evidence of spread to adjacent pelvic organs. If several tumors are found in your bladder, the likelihood of recurrence is thought to be higher, *and* recurrent tumors tend to be more aggressive.[4] Based on this assumption, your doctor may decide to take biopsies from several sites that appear normal to see if this process is already under way elsewhere. This information can be of great value in determining the best treatment options.

STAGING BLADDER TUMORS

After a positive diagnosis of bladder cancer has been made, you will want to know two very important things: what treatment is best, and what the *prognosis*, or chance for cure, is. Both of these questions are answered by *staging*, or evaluating, your tumor by looking at the type of cancer you have, the degree of abnormality of the cancer cells *(grade)*, how deeply it has invaded into the bladder wall, and if it has spread to adjacent pelvic organs, lymph nodes, or to distant organs. This will help you and your doctor choose the best available treatment. As Kristene explained to Michael, the staging of bladder cancer is very important. But because of the limitations of present technology, errors commonly occur. One study found that 10 percent of tumors were overstaged and 33 percent were understaged.[5] Because of the high possibility of errors in staging bladder tumors, you might consider getting a second opinion before undertaking radical therapy. The adjacent box explains staging of bladder tumors.

STAGING BLADDER CANCER

The primary staging system for **transitional cell carcinoma** of the bladder in the United States is the *Jewett-Strong-Marshall* system, which has been in use for several decades. A newer system called *TNM (Tumor Node Metastasis)*, developed by the Union Internationale Contre le Cancer, is gradually coming into use. This system takes into account depth of tumor growth (T), lymph node involvement (N), and the degree of spread, or *metastasis* (M). By comparing the categories of tumors described here with the accompanying illustration, you can get a good idea of how tumors are graded. The Jewett-Strong-Marshall system is printed in italics and the TNM system given in parentheses:

Stage O (Ta or Tis) includes *non-invasive* papillary tumors and carcinoma-in-situ.

Stage A (T1) indicates invasion into the lamina propria, the layer between the bladder surface (epithelium) and the deeper muscles of the bladder wall.

Stage B (T2 or T3) indicates depth of invasion, superficial or deep, into the muscle layers of the bladder.

Stage C (T3) signifies tumor growth into the fat that surrounds the bladder.

Stage D (T4, N1-3, M1) includes invasion of adjacent pelvic organs, spread to lymph nodes, as well as spread (metastasis) to other parts of the body.

If the cancer is invasive, your doctor will order a *CT scan (Computed Tomograph scan)*, popularly known as a "cat scan." This three-dimensional X-ray can provide information about the dimensions of the tumor, the depth of invasion into the bladder wall, involvement of the lymph nodes, and whether or not the cancer has spread to other organs.

A newer technique, called *magnetic resonance imaging* or *MRI*, also provides a computerized three-dimensional view of the skeleton, soft tissues, and organs much in the way that the CT scan does, but it remains unclear whether one is really better than the other. Even though both the CT scan and the MRI provide a lot of information, they are not definitive tests. The CT scan has been found to be inaccurate about one fourth of the time.[6] The MRI may be no more accurate. However, these tests are useful in determining lymph node involvement if the nodes are significantly enlarged

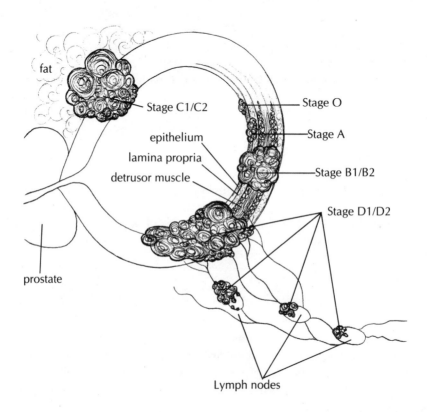

Labels in figure:
fat
Stage C1/C2
epithelium
lamina propria
detrusor muscle
prostate
Stage O
Stage A
Stage B1/B2
Stage D1/D2
Lymph nodes

15. Stages of cancer growth. In Stage 0, the cancer is non-invasive, self-contained, and has not spread beyond the bottom, or basal, layer of cells of the bladder lining. In Stage A, the tumor has spread into the *lamina propria,* the thin membranous barrier between the bladder lining and the bladder muscle. In Stage B, the tumor has spread into the bladder muscle. In Stage C, the cancer has broken through the bladder muscle and has invaded some of the tissue that surrounds it. In Stage D, cancer cells have traveled to nearby lymph nodes and pelvic organs and may have metastasized (spread) to distant organs.

and there is advanced spread to other areas such as the liver, lungs, or bones.

The early spread of cancer to the lymph nodes may readily be missed. Since bladder cancers often spread to the lungs and bones, several other tests will be ordered to complete the *staging* process. A chest X-ray or CT scan of the chest will detect spread to the lungs, and a bone scan will evaluate possible spread to the bones by injecting a radioactive substance into a vein that is selectively absorbed.

The degree of abnormality of the cancer cells, or *grade* of the tumor, is the most important factor in predicting prognosis or the likelihood of tumor recurrence and *invasion*. Transitional cell carcinoma is graded from 1 to 4: grade 1 tumors contain the least abnormal-looking cells and grade 4 contain the most. Low-grade (grades 1 and 2) tumors tend to be less aggressive than high-grade (grades 3 and 4) tumors, which progress in one third of cases.

Your doctor may order a test called *flow cytometry*, in which the amount and type of the protein substance *DNA* (found in all human cells) is determined to aid in predicting the potential aggressiveness of the cancer. Non-aggressive tumors, which tend not to recur, have an amount and type of DNA similar to normal benign cells. More aggresssive tumors, however, tend to have an abnormal amount and type of DNA. As knowledge about cancer grows, researchers are discovering new tests, called "markers," that can be used to predict tumor behavior.

TREATMENT FOR BLADDER CANCER

In any kind of cancer, the goal of treatment is usually to deliver a knock-out punch to the disease without knocking you out in the process. Unfortunately, people sometimes succumb to the physical effects of the remedy before they do to the disease. Enduring painful aftereffects and functional difficulties when the prospects of a cure are good may be worth it to some people. But on the other hand, living with a devastating illness and massive damage to the system from treatment, when the prognosis is not very promising, may not be worth it to others. You and your doctor will have to carefully evaluate all of these factors before proceeding with treatment. Faced with the prospect of major cancer therapy, it is your right to know all of the possible ill effects you may experience from the treatment and what your prognosis or outcome might be. Some types of therapy can cause severe side effects. If you don't think you can face enormous physical suffering, especially when the chance of a cure is not so good, then you should have the option to choose a less invasive treatment or to have treatment that is simply designed to make you as comfortable as possible.

Treatment for Non-Invasive Bladder Cancer

Transurethral resection of bladder tumor (TURBT) is the treatment most widely employed in the treatment of superficial bladder cancer. In this procedure, a *resectoscope,* an instrument with both a light source and a long electrified cutting loop, is inserted through the urethra *(transurethral)* and visible growths are cut away (or *resected*).

Laser therapy has been widely employed in medicine, especially in the treatment of cancer. A laser is a small, intensely focused beam of energy that produces heat and vaporizes tissue protein. Among the several types of lasers that have been used in the treatment of cancer, the neodymium-YAG laser is used to treat bladder cancer since it is effective in fluid environments such as urine and other solutions that pass in and out of the bladder during a cystoscopic procedure. Small or moderately sized tumors are vaporized by laser energy, which passes through a thin laser fiber placed through the cystoscope. The larger blood vessels found in large tumors prevent safe utilization of the laser for tumors greater than 1.5 inches in diameter, since the laser can only stop bleeding in small blood vessels. Larger tumors must be removed for a TURBT. The main advantage of using laser therapy as opposed to the TURBT procedure is that it can often be done under local anesthesia, often on an outpatient basis. With any laser treatment, too much laser energy can cause severe damage to surrounding healthy tissues if it is not properly controlled. Therefore, you should choose a urologist who is certified in the use of the neodymium-YAG laser and who has had abundant experience in treating bladder tumors with this form of therapy.

Intravesical chemotherapy involves drugs being instilled directly into the bladder and held there up to two hours once a week for six to eight weeks, after which the response rate or effectiveness of the treatment is checked by cystoscopy done at regular intervals. A biopsy is taken of any new tumors to make sure they are non-invasive, since recurrent tumors have a habit of becoming invasive, necessitating a new treatment plan. Monthly bladder instillations for up to a year or more are often given after the initial weekly treatments to help prevent cancer recurrence in people who have high-grade tumors, multiple tumors, or carcinoma-in-situ (CIS) in areas of the bladder that appeared normal.

BCG (bacillus Calmetté-Guérin) immunotherapy uses BCG, a naturally occurring bacteria similar to those that cause tuberculosis. When instilled directly into the bladder, it works like a vaccine, stimulating an immune response. One study found complete remission in nearly 60 percent of patients who had tumors and nearly 80 percent in those who had carcinoma-in-situ, making BCG the most effective of the agents used in intravesical instillation.[7] Almost all people who have BCG treatments experience irritative voiding symptoms that may last several days after therapy, and some people have flulike symptoms. If these symptoms last for more than 48 hours, a course of therapy with *isoniazid (INH)*, a drug used to control the symptoms of tuberculosis, can be given to lessen them.[8]

Thiotepa appears to work best for people with grade 1 tumors and is effective in about 50 percent of cases. The primary complication of this drug is its effect on bone marrow function. In 15 to 20 percent of cases, thiotepa is absorbed into the bloodstream, where it can affect the production of blood components, especially white blood cells, leaving you prone to infection. If this occurs, therapy will have to be discontinued until the bone marrow function returns to normal. If your bone marrow function remains suppressed, you may have to switch to another form of therapy. One study found that about 35 percent of the people who undergo thiotepa therapy experience complete remission and an additional 25 percent have a partial remission.[9] Thiotepa may also cause cystitis-like symptoms which almost always disappear over time.

Mitomycin C is an antibiotic that inhibits the synthesis of DNA, the genetic material of cells. Ten to 15 percent of those who take mitomycin develop chemical cystitis or a rash in the genital area or on the hands. In one study, approximately 40 percent of the people with superficial bladder cancer who had mitomycin C instilled in their bladders had complete remission, and an additional 40 percent had a partial remission.[10] Mitomycin C tends to be rather expensive at $450 a treatment, compared to thiotepa and BCG, which are about $100 per treatment.

Doxorubicin (Adriamycin) is also an anti-tumor antibiotic that is instilled directly into the bladder. It has been shown to have a complete response in up to 50 percent of patients and a partial remission in up to 35 percent. One of the main disadvantages of Adriamycin is that it is very caustic and may cause permanent scarring of the bladder lining resulting in chemical cystitis. And like mitomycin, Adriamycin is very expensive, but it has been shown to be especially effective in treating recurrent tumors.[11]

The treatment of superficial bladder cancer by instilling any of the above listed agents has similar effectiveness. Kristene chose to treat Michael, whose story appears on page 224, with BCG because she has found it to be the most effective agent available for his type of tumor. Based on the size, location, and number of tumors in your bladder, as well as the number of recurrences you have had and most importantly the grade of the tumor, your doctor may have a preference for one type of instillation over another. Other considerations might include the severity of the side effects and the cost of treatment.

Michael had two courses of six-weekly BCG treatments for non-invasive transitional cell carcinoma of the bladder. "Instilling the BCG solution into the bladder with a catheter just takes a couple of minutes, and isn't particularly uncomfortable," he says. "The hard part was holding it in for two hours. That part was pretty uncomfortable for me because my bladder was already irritated. Sometimes I couldn't keep it in for the whole time. The worst part is when you let it out. I had a terrible burning that would last for three or four days afterwards."

Treatment for Invasive Bladder Cancer

Surgery, radiation therapy, and chemotherapy are the treatment options available for people suffering from widespread carcinoma-in-situ, superficial bladder cancer that has not responded to the above therapies, or cancer that has invaded the muscle layers of the bladder wall or that has spread to areas outside of the bladder.

When Michael came back for his fifteen-month follow-up after his BCG treatments, he reported that he had again seen blood in his urine. Kristene did a cystoscopy exam, which showed that he had recurrent tumors in his bladder. A biopsy now revealed that one of the tumors was grade 3, had invaded the lamina propria, and was seen in the muscle layer of the bladder wall as well. Michael is very healthy and active for his age, but his cancer appeared to have progressed in terms of both grade and stage, so

Kristene ordered a "staging work-up." Michael's CT scan showed no evidence of spread outside of the bladder, and his bone scan was normal. Kristene explained that he could have radiation therapy or intravenous chemotherapy, but that his chances of long-term survival might be best with cystectomy, removal of the bladder. After careful consideration, Michael decided to have his bladder removed. Kristene explained that his pelvic lymph nodes would be examined for cancer while he was under anesthesia, and if they did not show positive evidence of cancer, his bladder would be removed. If many nodes showed signs of cancer, it would mean that his disease was too far advanced to be cured by removal of the bladder. Kristene further explained that if no cancer was found in his lymph nodes, there was at least a 50 percent chance that he would be cancer-free five years after the operation. She also asked him if he wished to donate some of his own blood before the procedure in case he needed any during surgery. He agreed, since the risks of using his own blood would be less than of using some-one else's. He could also have a family member or friend with compatible blood make a donation for him.

Cystectomy, the partial or total removal of the bladder, is normally reserved for treating Stage B and C (T2 and T3) invasive bladder cancer such as Michael's. If the tumor is confined to one region of the bladder and it is possible to remove a 1-inch margin of normal bladder around the cancer, only part of the bladder, a partial cystectomy, can be done. Unfortunately, only one in twenty people with invasive bladder tumors is a candidate for this form of therapy. The remainder are confronted with undergoing radical surgery, with the total removal of the bladder and prostate in men and uterus, cervix, and urethra in women.

After bladder removal, provision must be made to *divert* the urine from its usual path, since the bladder isn't there anymore. There are two ways that this can be done. In one, called an ileal conduit or ileal loop, the urine drains continuously through a conduit made from a small piece of bowel, to which the ureters are attached. The open end of the bowel segment is brought out through a hole in the skin of the abdomen, called a *stoma*. The urine then drains into a plastic bag. In the other, the Koch or Indiana pouch, a reservoir is created from a large piece of bowel, which somewhat resembles a bladder and stores urine inside the abdominal cavity. The reservoir is attached by a one-way valve to a stoma on the skin of the abdomen. It can also be attached to the urethra in men. The pouch is drained with a catheter every three to six hours without needing to use a bag. (See page 167 for more information on these two surgical techniques.)

Michael decided to have a conduit because it is a simpler operation and there was less chance of having to have a second operation to correct any problems with the pouch. His surgery went uneventfully and all of the cancer was removed.

Radiation therapy is one of the major techniques that have been employed in efforts to stop the growth of cancer. In the past, external beam radiation, in which a machine focuses a beam of radiation on a targeted area or organ, was given before radical cystectomy. But now it has been found that the survival rate for surgery is no better when it is preceded by radiation.[12]

Radiation therapy *alone* for the treatment of invasive bladder cancer is not very popular because the rate of tumor recurrence has been as high as 50 percent.[13] However, if you have already had your bladder out and you have a recurrence of cancer in the pelvis, radiation therapy is one of the options for treatment.

Radiation therapy does kill cancer in many cases, but radiation oncologists constantly walk a fine line between what is enough to kill the cancer but will not devastate the patient as well. As it is, about 70 percent of bladder cancer patients who have radiation treatments experience the acute irritative voiding symptoms of *radiation cystitis*, as well as diarrhea for a limited amount of time after the treatments are finished. About 10 percent of people who develop radiation cystitis continue to experience these symptoms for the rest of their lives. Ten to 20 percent of people who have radiation treatments may develop permanent swelling of the legs. The advantages of radiation therapy are that the body and the bladder remain essentially intact.

Systemic chemotherapy, as opposed to *intravesical chemotherapy*, in which chemotherapeutic drugs are placed directly in the bladder, is the injection into the veins of very toxic substances that are designed to kill cancer cells. Unfortunately, many normal cells are also killed, especially those of the hair follicles and lining of the intestines. Thus hair loss and severe nausea and vomiting frequently accompany the injection of chemotherapeutic agents. Chemotherapy is used in two ways to treat bladder cancer. Most commonly, it is given for patients who have evidence of spread outside of the bladder—metastatic cancer. The second way is as an option to possibly save the bladder. In this effort to *salvage* the bladder but cure the cancer, candidates include those who refuse surgery, those who may not be healthy enough to undergo major surgery, and those who want to try to save the bladder but are prepared to undergo surgery should chemotherapy fail. With this form of therapy, some studies reveal that from 20 to 30 percent of patients have been spared radical surgery, but the long-term results remain to be determined. This type of chemotherapy may also be coupled with radiation in an attempt to save the bladder. If you have invasive bladder cancer and are interested in this approach, you should ask your doctor about it.

Currently, the most effective form of chemotherapy has been to use a combination of drugs; the most popular combination at present is methotrexate, vinblastine, Adriamycin, and cisplatin (MVAC).

TREATMENT BY STAGE

- *Stage O* (Tis,Ta): laser, TURBT, BCG, intravesical chemotherapy.
- *Stage A* (T1): TURBT, laser, intravesical chemotherapy, BCG, partial cystectomy (for larger tumors). A radical cystectomy may be indicated if there are multiple recurrences in a short period of time, recurrence with increasing grade, or persistent CIS in the bladder.
- *Stages B and C* (T2/T3): radical cystectomy with urinary diversion (a conduit or a pouch). Radiation, chemotherapy, or bladder removal and radiation therapy may also be given in selected cases.
- *Stage D* (T3 and T4 N, M): radiation, chemotherapy, or bladder salvage plus radiation.

If you have widespread bladder cancer and the potential for cure is not great, and you have severe persistent bleeding, it may be necessary to instill agents such as *alum* or *formalin* (formaldehyde with methanol) into the bladder. These agents may help you to be more comfortable and may control the bleeding for a variable period of time.

SURVIVAL RATES

As we mentioned in the introduction to this chapter, in the case of cancer, it may be less useful to talk in terms of "cure" than to

235

look at *survival rates.* And these rates are both disease-dependent, i.e., dependent upon how far the cancer has spread when treatment was started, and treatment-dependent, i.e., how well the treatment worked. Unfortunately, when one begins to look at survival rates, they are confusing. The survival rates for any specific study are dependent upon many factors: who was included in the study, what their ages were, what part of the country they were from, what their occupations were, how advanced their disease was when it was discovered, what kinds of other treatments they may have had previously, and how long the patients were followed up after the treatments ended—and who was *excluded* from the study for various reasons. Because there are so many variables involved, the survival rates for any individual study are accurate *only* for that particular study. If there is more than one study on a particular facet of a subject, a range of rates will be given, usually the highest and the lowest. Frequently, this range will be enormous and thus, in a sense, meaningless to the average person. In this case, you have to look at the individual studies and see what the criteria for inclusion and study standards were. It is also important to know if certain study results, especially ones that seem very attractive, have been duplicated by other researchers using similar criteria and standards.

The most useful way to look at survival is to look at five-year survival rates—that is, how long a person has lived after treatment. The chart below summarizes the accepted survival rates for bladder cancer by stage.

BLADDER CANCER SURVIVAL	
Stage	Survival five years after treatment
O/A (Tis, T1)	60–83%
B1 (T2, T3)	41–70%
B2/C (T3)	17–53%
D1 (T4)	0–35%
D2	0–5%

SELF-HELP FOR BLADDER CANCER

Vitamins are essential for health and normal bodily function. Their primary task, which is similar to that of enzymes, is to regulate metabolic processes. Unlike some of the amino acids, vitamins are not formed in the body, with the notable exceptions of A and D, and must be derived from food intake or supplements.

Although mainstream medicine has not embraced vitamin therapy in large part, some investigation has been done suggesting that vitamins may play a therapeutic role in prevention or recovery. Urological researchers have carried out a few studies on the role of vitamins A *(retinoids)*, B_6 *(pyridoxine)*,[14] and C in preventing recurrences of bladder cancer. Although these studies are not definitive, they do offer encouragement to anyone who wants to do all that they can to prevent the recurrence of bladder tumors.

PREVENTION

If preventing cancer were a realistic possibility, millions would no doubt be following the recommended regimen. Unfortunately, no one has come up with a surefire panacea yet. At this point, the best thing you can do is to assess the known risk factors, especially cigarette smoking and the occupational hazards noted on pages 222–23. You may not be able to change your job, but you can quit smoking, and you can get a urine test every year to help with early detection.

BLADDER CANCER REMINDERS

- Most bladder cancers are superficial tumors that can be easily treated if they are detected early enough.
- If you work with industrial chemicals in a high-risk industry, you should have a yearly urinalysis, and if blood is found in the urine, a cancer cytology test.
- If you have irritative voiding symptoms and no bacteria in your urine, you should be tested for bladder cancer.
- If you have a long-term indwelling catheter, you should have periodic urine tests to rule out bladder cancer.
- Stopping smoking may reduce your risk of bladder cancer.

RESOURCES

BOOKS

Cancer as a Turning Point, Lawrence LeShan. New York: E. P. Dutton, 1989. The author, a pioneer in mind-cancer research, gathers information on self-healing from a wide variety of sources.

Our Bodies, Ourselves, The Boston Women's Health Book Collective. New York: Simon & Schuster, 1984. The section on cancer (pp. 522–539) is an excellent primer for anyone who has been diagnosed with cancer.

Ourselves, Growing Older: Women Aging with Knowledge and Power. Paula Brown Doress and Diana Laskin Siegal and the Midlife and Older Women Book Project. New York: Simon & Schuster, 1987. The section on cancer contains helpful resources and a useful discussion of various issues people with cancer must face.

MEDICAL SERVICES

Cancer Information Service (1-800-4-CANCER), funded by the National Cancer Institute. Provides information on diagnosis, treatment, and prevention of cancer, including bladder cancer, and will send pamphlets on various aspects of the disease free of charge. Also provides referral to centers that specialize in different types of treatment.

Physician's Data Query (PDQ) is a free computer listing of physicians and treatment programs throughout the United States sponsored by the National Cancer Institute.

United Ostomy Association, 2001 West Beverly Boulevard, Los Angeles, CA 90057 (213-413-5510), provides information about how to live with a stoma. This organization also coordinates a nationwide network of support groups of people who have stomas.

CHAPTER 9

Staying Sexual: Strategies for Enhancing Sexuality

"Dear God, next time please don't put the sexual organs so close to the excretory organs. It makes for trouble later."
—Overheard on a bus

BLADDER DISORDERS CAN BE EXTREMELY INTRUSIVE in our lives, and nowhere are they more intrusive than in our sexuality. If you have a leaky or painful bladder, or can't achieve an erection spontaneously, sex, which should be one of our most dependable comforts, can become an unwelcome or painful obligation. To compound the problem, difficulties resulting from bladder dysfunction can affect our sexual partners as well. Not wanting to be demanding or afraid of causing pain or embarrassment, they may emotionally distance themselves, and the resulting tension can spill over into other parts of our lives. In this chapter we will explore some of the most frequently mentioned problems about sex and bladder disorders, and make some suggestions that may help you move toward positive, comfortable solutions.

Mimi, the mother of three in her early fifties, developed diabetes during her second pregnancy when she was thirty-one, and later began having episodes of urinary leakage. Her doctor always brushed aside her concern about incontinence, passing it off as "a side effect of childbirth." Now, she has frequent episodes of moderate urine loss, which get much worse when chronic bronchitis flares up, causing fits of coughing. "I just don't go to work then," she says, "and it's not because of my lungs. I'm just wet all day." Mimi adjusted to daytime leakage after a while—learned which pads worked best for her and always had a change of clothes in the car for emergencies. "The big adjustment was sex," she says. "I just couldn't face up to the idea that I was going to wet the bed before I could have an orgasm." For two or three years Mimi used every excuse she could invent not to have sex, claiming pulled muscles, the proverbial headaches, even feigning a case of mono for a while. Whenever she sensed that her husband, Bill, was just about at his limit, she would give in and be as passive as possible in the hope that she wouldn't leak. "I'll tell you," she says, "the womanly art of faking orgasms came in very handy in those years."

Eventually, tension began to develop between the two. Bill knew that the leakage distressed Mimi, but he began to get offended about being put off so often. He became reluctant to initiate sex, and when he did, he often could not sustain an erection. Mimi noticed that Bill was going out with his friends more often and coming home drunk, which he rarely did before. "I began to feel sorry for him," she recalls. "Then, one day, I was thinking about it and realized, I should feel sorry for *myself* too. Sex was a great part of our marriage, and now it's so difficult. I still feel like we're very stable, but in the back of my mind I sometimes wonder, 'Why would anyone put up with this?' "

Claire, a lab technician, is thirty-eight years old, has suffered from interstitial cystitis for about fifteen years, and has had numerous medical treatments but has not responded very positively to any of them. She experiences pressure and burning in her bladder day and night, and on a "good day" she has to urinate between twenty and thirty times. She is married to Rob, the swimming coach at a small college, and describes their sex life prior to the advent of IC as "active, aggressive, and satisfying." Like many people with IC, Claire finds intercourse painful, but, she says, "we indulge about once a week anyway. You can't deny those urges." Afterward, she usually has increased burning and frequency for one or two days, sometimes longer. Claire used to masturbate once or twice a week, but rarely does so now because the friction irritates her urethra. Contraception has also been a problem for her. "I could never use a diaphragm again, since I think that's what caused infections when I first became sexually active, and there's no way I am going to go on the Pill." Claire and Rob are resigned to diminished sexual activity. "We both regret the loss of the spontaneity we had. And since I am always worse afterward, we have to choose a night when I know I don't have to function well the next day."

These personal experiences illustrate some of the fears and frustrations that people with bladder disorders commonly face: difficulties in communication, fear of urinary leakage, fear of precipitating pain or a urinary tract infection, anxiety about sexual performance, as well as a lack of interest in sex and a poor self-image. These are all problems that people with normal bladders face at one time or another (yes, even fear of wetting the bed), and they all have solutions—if you are willing to think creatively. With more open communication, a broader definition of what good sex is, and a willingness to be more assertive about your own needs in sex, you can not only cope with bladder dysfunction, in the process you might make some significant improvements in your sex life.

COMMUNICATING ABOUT SEX

Sex is the most difficult issue for most of us to talk about—sometimes with our lovers, usually with our friends, especially with our families, and even with our doctors—and we have few positive role models to guide us to comfortable resolutions when problems arise. When communication breaks down completely, both partners can be deprived of the affection and nurturing that they need the most. Of course, difficulties in communicating about sex can occur in any relationship. "Having a bladder disorder just exaggerates the problems everybody has with sex—communication, relationships, how to please our partners," observes Ella, who has had interstitial cystitis for eight years.

"Communication is the critical element in solving problems posed by bladder disorders," says Geraldine Hirsch, a psychologist who has interstitial cystitis and has worked with a number of people who have the disease also. "I've found that if people are able to talk about what's bothering them, they can work out their difficulties."

In talking to many people with bladder disorders and their partners, we found that partners are often confused about how to confront a bladder disorder. Fear of causing embarrassment or pain often results in a reluctance to initiate sex, and sex itself is often less than optimal because of that fear. Many partners feel helpless in the face of difficult disorders, but are anxious to know how they could be supportive. Some people with partners choose not to have intercourse at all, while others, like Claire, are content to please their partners and suffer the consequences. Julia, a lesbian who has interstitial cystitis, hasn't been sexually active in a while, but worries that potential partners might be afraid that they could catch the disease, and wonders how to explain such a complex, mysterious illness without frightening them away.

Andrew, a thirty-year-old environmental consultant who has had severe incontinence since he was a child, recalls his last relationship three years ago. "I had been dating Danielle for about seven weeks, but I hadn't told her about my problem until we went to bed early on New Year's Day. When I told her, she was shocked and exclaimed, 'You wear diapers? Oh, my God!' She promptly turned her back to me and that was the end of our relationship."

Although it might have been difficult, one of the things that Andrew could have done to avoid such a traumatic ending was to explain his condition to Danielle ahead of time. If he had great difficulty in getting the words out, he might have given her some literature on incontinence from the educational organizations mentioned at the end of Chapter 4.

Lauren, a lesbian whose story appears on page 46, has moderate daily urinary leakage and always wears absorbent pads. She has a policy of explaining her urine loss to potential partners as soon as she gets involved with them. That way, if they are sympathetic, she sees them as having potential for a deeper relationship. If they do not respond positively, then their potential for a future relationship decreases.

Geraldine Hirsch says that she has seen people make significant breakthroughs by bringing their problems to a support group or therapist, then inviting their partners to attend as well. In a support group, you may encounter new ideas and get encouragement to break out of old patterns. Then, by inviting your partner to therapy or to a group session, you can expose him or her to new ideas as well.

If you are in a support group, you could talk to your coordinator about arranging a series of sessions on sexuality and invite one or two sex therapists to participate. At the first meeting, you might have a therapist facilitate a discussion for the regular members who are fairly comfortable in sharing their problems with the group. At this meeting, you might also ask participants to bring any books on sexuality that they have found helpful and share information from them. At a second meeting, you might invite partners to participate, arranging ahead of time for the therapist to address issues that came up at the last meeting. At a third meeting, you could do role playing, having partners exchange roles.

Mimi, whose story is told above, finally got so worried about her relationship that she decided to see a therapist. After a few sessions, she invited Bill to come to her session where they did some role playing. This time, *Mimi* initiated, or tried to initiate, sex. Bill said, "Gosh, honey, do you mind if we don't tonight? I'm just wiped out." (This was Mimi's most frequently used excuse.)

"I was really hurt," says Mimi. "I felt, 'Maybe he's not attracted to me anymore,' and almost wanted to cry." Bill learned something too. "Switching roles forced me to see what a dilemma Mimi is in. I saw how hard it is to protect yourself *and* please the other person." Sessions of this type can stir up the waters a great deal, and set the stage for positive change.

One of the primary aspects of good communication is learning how to assert your own needs without being too pushy or demanding. First of all, you need to pinpoint what your needs are in terms of sexual activity, including frequency, what types of activity are comfortable for you and what types aren't, and changes you would like to make. Then you might want to prioritize them and work on the ones that are the most important first. If you, like millions of others, find being assertive about your sexual needs difficult, you might want to review the information on being assertive in Chapter 2, and perhaps read one of the books on assertiveness recommended in the Resources on page 30. Naturally, talking is the most direct way to communicate your needs, but some people find it very difficult to talk about sex. So, if you find that you can't make any headway on your own, you might consider seeing a therapist for advice and support, or if you have not already done so, find a support group. You don't have to do it all by yourself!

LOSS OF INTEREST IN SEX

One of the questions that people with bladder problems frequently ask is, "How can I maintain an interest in sex when I don't feel very sexy?" *Libido,* or the desire for sex, is an elusive force that is controlled by our hormones but is also influenced considerably by our conscious minds. The loss of libido is sometimes as mysterious as its presence, but factors such as low self-esteem or depression, as well as anxiety or fear, can play a part.

People with bladder disorders frequently suffer from a poor self-image that can contribute to a lack of desire for sex. As noted in the epigraph to this chapter, having the sexual apparatus so close to the plumbing (or in the case of men, having them be one and the same) causes lots of trouble. For example, an episode of incontinence can make a person feel unclean, and therefore unattractive and unlovable. And people who need to wear diapers say that they feel less attractive. People who use an indwelling catheter, or have had bladder surgery that requires them to wear a urine collection bag, may think that having an appliance makes them undesirable and may experience intense inadequacy and shame.

If you suffer a genuine loss of interest in sex, it's important to reassure your partner that it's not because he or she is no longer attractive. Dr. Naomi McCormick, another psychotherapist who also happens to have IC, suggests telling your partner directly, or at least communicating the message that your lack of interest in sex is the result of illness or disability rather than indifference to your partner.[1] At the same time, it is important to remind yourself that you have a medical condition that prevents the full range of sexual activities. In her excellent book *Living with Chronic Illness*, Cherie Register articulately addresses this issue: "Self-love is a prerequisite for healthy sexuality, but it is difficult to achieve when your body is not working properly. Hatred of your own body is certainly not conducive to good health, sexual or otherwise, but it is a common consequence of chronic illness."[2] Register suggests that people with chronic illness accept some degree of disability, stop measuring themselves against impossible "Hollywood myths," and then enjoy what measure of sexuality they can. One way to improve your self-image is to focus on things that you do very well, and accept the fact that no one gets gold stars in every area of life.

Depression goes hand in hand with low self-esteem, but it is more difficult to treat. The loss of libido is often a clue that something serious is going on. If you have a bladder condition and sense that it is contributing to depression, it is essential that you get appropriate treatment; when your condition has improved, your interest in sex may return as well.

VARIATIONS IN SEXUAL ACTIVITY

Many of the sex therapists Rebecca interviewed indicated that, in addition to good communication about sex, employing alternatives to intercourse, on either a regular or a part-time basis, is probably the most useful concept for people with bladder problems to explore. Getting sexual pleasure and orgasms by means other than having the penis in the vagina not only takes the focus and pressure off the urethra (and hence the bladder), it can greatly enhance the quality of sexual enjoyment for both partners. For women who have incontinence or urethral tenderness, non-intercourse sex usually provides quicker, more reliable, and more intense orgasms. For men with erectile dysfunction, it means that you can still have great sex even though you don't have an erection.

In the post-Freudian world, intercourse and sex have become synonymous and many, if not most, heterosexual men and women still firmly believe that sex without intercourse just isn't "real" sex. Somehow, when we were getting our sex education in high school locker rooms and the back seats of cars, we all learned that intercourse was *the* way to have sex, and that other forms of sexual activity were definitely second-rate. And there is probably a good reason for this. Men learn very early that intercourse is a convenient and sure route to an orgasm. Unfortunately, this knowledge generally puts an end to their exploration of other forms of sexual pleasure. The problem (for women, anyway) is that once intercourse is initiated, it must be done in a certain way, usually with a certain intensity, and a great many other sensual possibilities are lost. Polls and surveys have repeatedly shown that for women, intercourse is *not* the bonanza it is for men. In fact, many women say that they get better and more reliable orgasms through masturbation, but they rarely venture to incorporate self-stimulation into sexual activity with their partners. Gay men and lesbians have always known that there was more to sex than intercourse, but because of social prejudices against homosexuality, their experiences haven't been taken very seriously.

Of course, intercourse can provide a very dynamic sexual experience, but there are some variations that can be beneficial to people with bladder problems. Allowing the woman to choose the position and control the angle of penetration and pace of the thrusting can offer both partners opportunities for orgasm. Some

245

women who have interstitial cystitis say that both partners lying on their sides is a more comfortable position and others say that they prefer rear entry, since both of these positions take pressure off the vaginal opening. Some couples find that one or both partners can achieve orgasm through a sort of "false" intercourse, in which the woman lies on her back and crosses her legs, forming a small triangular space between the upper thighs and the vulva. This affords stimulation to both the penis and the glans of the clitoris. If both partners are aroused enough before beginning, this technique provides an acceptable substitute for the "real thing."

Another widely held assumption about sexuality is that orgasm is the only goal of sexual activity. Even though they may feel relaxed and revitalized after a session of cuddling or heavy petting, many people still feel cheated, or feel as if they failed if orgasm didn't occur for one or both of the partners. While orgasm is usually the goal in sexual activity, it certainly does not have to be in order for the experience to be enjoyable and rewarding. Some of the alternatives to intercourse that don't necessarily have orgasm as their goal are sensual massage (if you find that your imagination is not enough, there are a number of excellent books on this subject), bathing or taking showers together, cuddling and kissing, petting with clothes on or off, sharing sexual fantasies, looking at erotic pictures or videos, and dancing. These sexually stimulating activities take the focus off the urethra, which can be exquisitely tender in severe cases of interstitial cystitis, or off sexual performance in the case of erectile dysfunction.

Many people who answered Rebecca's survey on interstitial cystitis said that they rely on oral sex when intercourse is impossible. "If they held championships in oral sex, I should get a prize," says Melanie, a New York City IC sufferer who has apparently perfected her technique to a fine art. "I could show those girls down on 42nd Street a thing or two."

Many people have found that vibrators provide more rapid, intense, and reliable orgasms, and these devices are often recommended by sex therapists for people who have problems in achieving orgasm for various reasons. A vibrator could be very helpful to women with incontinence who, like Mimi, have anxiety about leaking before they come to orgasm. Many women with interstitial cystitis say that they are reluctant to try vibrators because vibrations of any kind cause pain. If intercourse is too painful, it may be that a vibrator may be too painful as well. If you have intercourse regardless of how bad your symptoms are, a vibrator might help you come to orgasm quicker and thus minimize friction around the vagina and urethra. Like transcutaneous nerve stimulation (described on page 153), the vibrations from a hand-held vibrator might distract you from the pain, at least as long as you are using it. Experimenting alone is a good way to see if a vibrator might be effective for you. After you are comfortable with the device, you can share it with your partner.

BREAKING OLD PATTERNS: SENSATE FOCUS EXERCISES

Sensate focus exercises are often recommended by sex therapists to cure a variety of conditions, especially the failure of women to have an orgasm and the inability of men to get or sustain an erection or to prevent premature ejaculation. They can also be very helpful in exploring non-intercourse ways of having sex and incorporating them into your sexual routines.

Although there is some variation in how these exercises are taught, the framework is essentially the same. Over a period of about two months, intercourse as the goal of sexual fulfillment is put aside, and other ways to have sexual pleasure are explored. These exercises are typically done in sets of several similar sessions, to give you a chance to become very familiar with the concept and perfect new techniques before moving on to another set of exercises. Therapists usually recommend that you do the exercises several times a week.

- The first set of sessions is devoted to sensual touching, but specifically avoiding the breasts and genitals. One partner lies face down while the other caresses every part of the body from head to toe, then turns over and the touching is repeated. Then the partners change places. Both partners are often surprised to discover areas that are particularly sensitive to touch.
- The next series expands the types of stimulation to include the breasts and genitals, but is limited to gentle caressing, without having orgasms.
- Sexual fantasies or looking at erotic pictures or videos might be added to touching. You could also add kissing and other activities that you find stimulating, still avoiding orgasm.

247

- The final series puts all of the techniques together and includes orgasm, in this case without having the penis in the vagina, for one or both partners.

If orgasm is not comfortable for one partner, then the other should now have a good idea about what is comfortable and exciting and be able to have enjoyable sex in new ways.

FEAR THAT SEX WILL PRECIPITATE LEAKAGE

Like Mimi, fear that you are going to lose urine during sex can kill your desire as quickly as anything. Luckily, Mimi's urine loss was moderate. After seeing Kristene, she undertook a course of biofeedback coupled with electrical stimulation and her urine loss improved dramatically, but was not cured entirely. In her support group, she picked up a few tips that helped her minimize the loss she did experience during sex. Since she and Bill only had sex at night, Mimi stopped drinking sodas in the afternoon and usually had only one glass of iced tea with dinner. She routinely emptied her bladder before sex. "I would still lose a little urine with orgasm," she says. Because of this, she also ordered some special washable sheets that are plastic on one side and flannel on the other.* "I keep one on top of the regular sheet. Then I can just remove it after sex and sleep in a dry bed."

Mimi's attitude toward losing a little urine has changed a great deal. "After talking about it a lot in the support group, I was less embarrassed," she says. "Besides, there are people who have no control at all. Compared to that, I'm pretty lucky."

Bernadette is one of the people in Mimi's group who is not so lucky. While she is not normally incontinent, until she got treatment she regularly lost urine—all of it—at the moment of orgasm. "I even had trouble in movies sometimes if a scene was very arousing," she recalls. She saw a doctor, but he told her that there was nothing physically wrong. "I was so devastated in so many ways that I stopped being sexually active," she recalls. Finally, a sympathetic woman gynecologist referred Bernadette to Dr. Suzanne Frye, a urologist in New York, who assured her that the condition

---

* Distributed by Bryam, Inc. For other special bed coverings, see the *Resource Guide for Continence Aids and Services,* 3rd edition, HIP, Inc., P.O. Box 544, Union, SC 29739.

was not psychological. "When I finally realized that it wasn't my fault, I broke down and cried," she confesses. "It took so long for somebody to understand." Bernadette was referred to a urody-namics lab, and went through a series of tests, which included reproducing the urine loss during orgasm. "It was the hardest thing I did in my life—harder than giving up smoking," she admits. "But the doctors and technicians in the lab were super." The tests showed that Bernadette's bladder nerves were not sending the proper signals—a dysfunction caused by spina bifida, a common birth defect. When the bladder got full, it would become paralyzed, and Bernadette was unable to urinate. That's why an orgasm would trigger a flood—it relaxed everything. Dr. Frye gave Bernadette a prescription for oxybutynin chloride (Ditropan) which helped her bladder to relax, so that she could release urine voluntarily. "It was an incredible ordeal," says Bernadette, "but now it's over. Finally I was able to recover my sense of dignity and have normal sex again."

It's not clear how many people have problems as severe as Bernadette's, but it is fairly certain that people who do have sexually related bladder dysfunction of any sort experience a great deal of difficulty in talking about their problem and in finding help. Bernadette's story clearly shows that with the right doctor or therapist, and determination not to be deprived of your right to satisfying sex, help is available, even for seemingly hopeless problems.

One way women can minimize the effects of urinary leakage is to wear a pair of sexy underpants and a Serenity pad through part of a session of sex play. Because the pad is infused with a powder that turns to gel when it becomes wet, when you remove it, you should be relatively dry.

In spite of the logistical difficulties, some people with intractable incontinence manage to have satisfactory sex with the cooperation of their partners. Most people and even some doctors may be unaware that you can have intercourse with an indwelling catheter in place. In a chapter on sexuality in *Managing Incontinence,* Rosemarie King, a rehabilitative nurse who has a special interest in sexuality, explains that an indwelling catheter does not necessarily prevent enjoying intercourse. She points out that the catheter can be left in place during the early stages of sexual play and then removed, or it can be folded back along the penis and held in place by a condom.[3] Men with minimal or moderate leakage can empty their bladders just before sex and use a condom to collect any urinary leakage. If you have a bladder disorder and are in a relatively stable relationship, there can be immediate experimentation with the suggestions in this chapter.

Fear of leakage can present enormous stumbling blocks to finding a relationship. Single people with incontinence seem to have quite a bit of difficulty in establishing new relationships and may be celibate for long periods, choosing to masturbate as frequently as is comfortable, or not at all (see page 252).

PAIN RELATED TO SEXUAL ACTIVITY

If you have interstitial cystitis and pain is a major component of your symptoms, there are some things that you can try which might minimize discomfort when you do have intercourse or other types of sexual activity.

During sexual response, an enormous amount of blood rushes to the pelvic region, playing a major role in the dynamic changes of sexual arousal: erection in both women and men, vaginal lubrication, and, ultimately, orgasm. Stimulation of the genital area is one of the primary ways to effect this process. But if you find the friction from thrusts of the penis or fingers too intense, there may be alternative ways to help stimulate the increased blood flow that is necessary to have an orgasm. A heating pad or warm gel pack on the genital area for five or ten mintues before sex will bring more blood to the pelvic region and may help facilitate orgasm with less friction.

Once sexual activity is finished, it takes several hours for the pelvic area and genitals to return to normal. In the meantime, tissues that are already sore and inflamed may be even more puffy and sensitive. In this case, you might try using a *cold* gel pack (available at pharmacies and most athletic stores) on your genital area to reduce swelling and temporary inflammation of irritated tissues. If you find that you really like cold packs, use them the way athletes do: 20 minutes on and 20 minutes off. Then 20 minutes on again (this prevents frostbite). On the other hand, some IC patients have found that taking a hot bath afterward helps to reduce swelling and tenderness. You could try experimenting with both heat and cold and see which works best.

Interestingly, Masters and Johnson learned that "it is not unusual . . . to find many older women having to contend with a sense of urinary urgency shortly after coital connection [intercourse] and being forced frequently to urinate immediately after coition. Some of these individuals even may complain of urinary burning and frequency for as long as two or three days after an episode of extended coital connection."[4] Here they are referring to post-menopausal women, but it is possible that IC patients, especially those who are not very sexually active, experience similar irritation in the bladder, urethra, and vagina.

If friction is a problem with intercourse, use of a lubricant can help to reduce it. If you find that the water-based lubricants that you can buy at the drugstore don't really do the job, you might consider trying Astroglide,* an industrial-strength lubricant that has been designed especially for use in sexual activity and is heavier and smoother than the normal household or drugstore lubricants.

SEXUAL SECRETIONS

Several kinds of secretions are involved in sexual response and orgasm, and these are often confused with urine. A woman's major secretion is vaginal "sweat," which is squeezed through the walls of the vagina as sexual tension increases, lubricating the vaginal opening and the entire interior of the vagina. Often, this mucouslike secretion is enough to make a small wet spot on the bed.

Some women may also ejaculate a small amount of fluid from the paraurethral, or Skene's, glands on each side of the urethra (see illustration on page 32). These glands, which some sex researchers regard as the female equivalent of the male prostate gland, can produce a significant amount of alkaline fluid, somewhat like the male prostatic secretion.[5] Many women mistakenly believe that this dampness is caused by urinary leakage. But if you check carefully, you will not find the characteristic acrid smell of urine that you would if you had "wet the bed." In addition, the vulvovaginal, or Bartholin's, glands, located on either side of the base of the inner lips (labia minora), near the perineum, also produce a mucous secretion during sexual arousal that is often mistaken for urine.

---

* Astroglide and other special lubricants can be ordered by mail from Eve's Garden (see Resources at the end of this chapter).

MASTURBATION

Aside from the myth that there is only one way to have inter-course, another unfortunate myth perpetuated by marriage man-uals of the past is the idea that each partner is responsible for "giving" the other partner pleasure and an orgasm, and you weren't supposed to help yourself—if you didn't get an orgasm from your partner, you just didn't get it. This unstated rule has discouraged many people (especially women) from exploring their own sexuality through masturbation.

The Victorians thought masturbation caused everything from rotten teeth to mental illness, but today we know it's not true. In fact, it is now generally accepted that masturbation is a healthy and eminently rewarding form of sexual activity. Indeed, it has signifi-cant advantages—especially for people with leaky or painful blad-ders. Masturbation allows you to control the amount and type of direct stimulation to the vaginal/urethral area in women and the penis or urethra in men. For women who are having difficulty in achieving orgasm, solitary masturbation can help you find out how much and what type of stimulation works best for you.

Discovering what pleases you is the easy part. Integrating mas-turbation (which by definition means "self-stimulation") into sexual activity with a partner may be more difficult. It is usually easier for men, who are used to initiating and determining the format of sexual activity. Some women, even fairly "liberated" ones, find in-corporating masturbation into sex play very difficult indeed. If you find it too hard, you might try some of the suggestions in the section Communicating about Sex on page 241.

ERECTILE DYSFUNCTION

Every man suffers from the inability to have an erection some-times, and past the age of forty, the failure to achieve an erection on command is extremely common. Causes of this problem include stress, anxiety, alcohol, illness or diseases such as diabetes or mul-tiple sclerosis, prescription medications, recreational drugs, and surgery.

The term *impotence*, meaning "weak, powerless, and ineffec-tual," is widely used to describe this problem, but it is both incor-rect and unnecessarily judgmental. *Erectile dysfunction* is correct and more appropriate, taking the blame off the victim and placing it on the physical and psychological causes.

Urologists specialize in male sexual dysfunction and can usually pinpoint the cause, even if it is not an obvious one such as drugs or surgery. If stress, psychological factors, medications, or alcoholism appears to be a significant factor, your urologist will refer you to a specialist for further treatment. If no physical reason for your problem can be found and a psychological cause is suspected, a psychologist can prescribe a program of sensate focus exercises (see page 247), which nearly always solves the problem or improves it significantly.

Men who have transurethral resections (TURPs) for benign prostate enlargement usually recover from surgery with the ability to have an erection intact, although it may take up to a year for function to return to normal. Most men who have TURPs or prostatectomies (removal of the prostate) experience retrograde ejaculation, also known as "dry ejaculation," in which the bladder neck can no longer close automatically during orgasm to prevent the semen from entering it. The ejaculate simply flows backward into the bladder, and flows out with the next urination. There is absolutely no health risk attached to this phenomenon, but men who have retrograde ejaculation will be infertile. Since most men who develop infertility as a result of prostate surgery are older, infertility may not be a significant issue for them. If you are younger and feel you would still like to have children, you might want to investigate the possibility of storing sperm at a sperm bank. The sperm can be stored indefinitely at a cost of about two hundred dollars a year.

In large part, the ability to achieve erections after a TURP is dependent upon two factors: what your ability was prior to surgery, and the type of surgical procedure you have. A relatively new procedure, devised by Dr. Patrick Walsh of Johns Hopkins University, cuts fewer nerves than old procedures did, thereby preserving nerve function in many more cases.

TAKING ACTION

Because of the bladder's close proximity to our sexual organs, their functions are intimately related, and their dysfunction can cause fear of sex and may prompt some people to abandon it altogether. The sexual problems created by bladder disorders are sometimes thorny and frustrating, but they can usually be improved or even solved with some thoughtful work on your part and, if that isn't enough, with a proper medical evaluation and the help of a sympathetic doctor or therapist. Finding a doctor who is willing and able to help you may not be easy, and you may have to go to several before you find someone who has a special sensitivity to sexual issues. You might want to review Finding the Right Doctor on page 18, to get some ideas about the kinds of questions to ask. A careful medical exam should determine whether there is a physical cause for your problem, and appropriate treatment can be undertaken. Then, with determination and perseverance, you should be able to make changes in your sexual habits and routines that can make sex better for both yourself and your partner.

SEXUALITY REMINDERS

- Communication is the first step toward improving sexual relations.
- A healthy self-image—one that acknowledges disabilities as a normal part of life—is an important component of the desire to have sex.
- Intercourse is not the only way to have satisfying sex.
- If your bladder is ruining sex, there may be something that can be done about it, so get a competent urological evaluation.
- Many people who have bladder problems still have very satisfactory sex lives.
- Since erectile dysfunction is a possible outcome of surgery for prostate cancer, and occasionally for benign enlargement, it is important that you be aware of this before you have surgery.

RESOURCES

Eve's Garden, 119 West 57th Street, Suite 1406, New York, NY 10019 (212-757-8651). This feminist sex boutique for women sells items to enhance sexuality such as vibrators, body oils, lubricants, condoms, and positive, informative books on sexuality for women. Write or call for a complete catalog of books and products.

For Yourself: The Fulfillment of Female Sexuality, Lonnie Garfield Barbach. New York: Doubleday/Anchor Books, 1976. This classic sexual primer teaches women how to have orgasms through masturbation and offers advice on how to integrate self-stimulation into sexual activity.

The G-Spot and Other Recent Discoveries About Human Sexuality, Alice Kahn Ladas, Beverly Whipple, and John D. Perry. New York: Holt, Rinehart & Winston, 1982. The existence of the elusive "G-Spot" has been hotly debated and generally dismissed as insubstantial. The real value of this book is its discussion of female ejaculation.

Healing Love Through the Tao: Cultivating Female Sexual Energy, Mantak Chia and Maneewan Chia. Santa Fe: The Healing Tao Press, 1985.

Male Sexuality, Bernie Zilbergeld. New York: Bantam Books, 1978. Written by a widely respected psychologist, this classic work on male sexuality exposes myths and covers such issues as masturbation and sexual dysfunction. The book also includes exercises designed to increase understanding and pleasure for both sexes.

A New View of a Woman's Body, The Federation of Feminist Women's Health Centers. New York: Simon & Schuster, 1981. This book contains "The Redefinition of the Clitoris," the Federation's groundbreaking examination of women's sexual anatomy. Available from the FFWHCs, 6221 Wilshire Blvd., Suite 419 A, Los Angeles, CA 90048.

Sex for One: The Joy of Self-Loving, Betty Dodson. Available from Eve's Garden (see above).

MEDICAL RESOURCES

Sexuality and Chronic Illness: A Comprehensive Approach, Leslie R. Schover and Søren Buus Jensen. New York: The Guilford Press, 1988. Although this book does not deal specifically with bladder disorders, it contains helpful information for therapists, physicians, and other medical personnel who treat and counsel people suffering from sexual dysfunction as a result of chronic illnesses.

CHAPTER 10

Strategies for Daily Survival

BLADDER DISORDERS, LIKE MANY OTHER SERIOUS DIS-eases, have a way of insinuating themselves into almost every aspect of life. They can make parenting and family responsibilities difficult, disrupt school or work, make a disaster out of social occasions, inhibit your ability to travel, make sports and recreational activities impossible, and disrupt countless other miscellaneous pursuits that make our lives rich and worthwhile. With appropriate diagnosis and treatment, many bladder problems can be cured completely. But even with proper treatment, you may still be left with some dysfunction, and have to cope with a certain amount of discomfort and inconvenience.

Many people have learned how to cope with bladder disorders quite well, but because of a reticence to discuss such problems openly, their secrets for leading near-normal lives usually remain just that—secrets. With few role models to follow, each person with a bladder problem ends up having to invent the wheel again. And very little has been written on the subject, so you can't just sneak off to your local library and bone up on the latest coping strategies for balky bladders. To help remedy this situation, we have put together a collection of coping mechanisms devised by veteran bladder sufferers who have been living with bladder dysfunction on a daily basis. In order to carry on with their lives, they have been forced to find new, inventive ways of doing perfectly ordinary things. As you will see, many have risen to the challenge.

GAINING ACCESS TO RESTROOMS

For people with all types of bladder disorders, there is surely nothing so dear—and sometimes so rare—as a clean, well-lighted restroom, stocked with toilet paper and without a line. It's understandable if people are reluctant to let strangers into their houses to "use the restroom," but almost every business has a restroom, yet people are routinely denied access on the grounds that they are not paying customers. Even when you pay, it is sometimes difficult. Estelle told us that in spite of spending hundreds of dollars on clothes and accessories, when she begged the manager to let her use the toilet, she was rudely ushered from the store.

This rigid attitude about public access to restrooms is virtually universal in the United States. The denial of bodily functions is so deeply ingrained in our culture that it is actually possible for people to be cruelly unsympathetic about the need to use a toilet, even though they have probably been in similar situations themselves on occasion. Many people, however, have found ways to gain access to even the most well-defended restrooms.

If just asking for a restroom appears nearly hopeless, here are some ingenious ploys. "If I have my son with me, I use him as an excuse," Rhonda says. "It's hard for anybody to refuse a child." Jean says that she claims to be pregnant and about to throw up. Elsie reports that once or twice, in a desperate situation, she has approached a police officer and asked him or her to intercede. "That definitely works," she says. Barbara has had some success masquerading as a health inspector. If all else fails, says Diane, "I just tell them I have a bladder disease and if I can't use the restroom *now,* they will have a mess."

In addition to these strategies, a number of people have found that carrying a letter from a doctor stating that they have a bladder disorder is very useful in difficult situations. Sometimes, a handicapped parking permit will work miracles. Getting such a permit is very simple. Call your state motor vehicle department and ask for the handicapped licensing bureau. When you reach the bureau, someone will inform you of the kind of documentation you need. Normally, a letter from your doctor is sufficient. Rosalind, who has had life-long incontinence as the result of a serious birth defect, found that a Medic-Alert bracelet has been very useful. "People take the Medic-Alert bracelet very seriously," she says. "It has helped me gain access to bathrooms even in restaurants." The official Medic-Alert bracelets are for people with serious health problems, but if you have severe incontinence because of surgery or interstitial cystitis, you should be able to get one. The phone number is 1-800-432-5378. You can also buy an unofficial bracelet at many pharmacies to carry in your purse or pocket to show to a restaurant or shop manager in case of emergencies. Many, many people say that they have given up going to theaters or sports events because the lines for the restroom are always so long. Instead of giving up events that you enjoy, you might try showing your doctor's note, handicapped permit, or bracelet to the first few people in line and ask them if you can go ahead. Some people find this intimidating at first; after a few successes, you may be encouraged as to the value of this particular strategy.

Gaining access to restrooms is one thing. But you have to find them first. On your own turf, you may be like Edith, who "knows every restroom between here and anywhere and can tell you the rating." But when you have to deviate from your normal route, or are in a strange town, you may have to ferret out new facilities. Places where you can reliably find a restroom include department stores, libraries, hospitals, museums, schools, restaurants, bars, parks (not always so clean), and hotels (in larger hotels, there is often a restroom adjacent to the lobby for the use of hotel patrons and their guests). Some experienced restroom sleuths have found that just looking as though you belong there, especially in bars and restaurants, often works. Sometimes, a smile and a request will get you what you want.

Restrooms of the World

For people with moderate to severe incontinence or interstitial cystitis, longer trips, whether for pleasure or for business, require a good deal of forethought, scheming, and for anyone who experiences urinary frequency and urgency, downright guts. Travel on the interstate highway system seems to offer predictable—if too infrequent—rest stops. But if you get off the beaten path, you may need to make some provisions of your own. Traveling in Arizona, Patsy and Frank found this especially true. "There were no restrooms or roadside accommodations of any kind anywhere we went," Patsy says. "We became convinced that the people of Arizona never have to go to the bathroom." In the good old United States, this certainly isn't an isolated experience.

Refusing to be housebound because of lack of public facilities, some people have improvised quite effectively. "Wear loose clothing and keep a porta-potty in the car. It can be a real lifesaver on trips," advises Toni. Dorothy, who has interstitial cystitis, describes her initiation with a portable toilet. "My husband and I were traveling through rural Pennsylvania when I needed to try out the potty. I crawled in the back seat and threw a heavy bedspread over myself. The next thing I knew, we were speeding down some back road—there was a car behind us and my husband didn't want it to get too close. I was trying to balance on the wobbly potty without doing a back flip. It worked, but I emerged from my camouflage in disarray."

Carrie, who has interstitial cystitis, balked at the idea of giving up her freedom. "I purchased a mini-van with smoky windows, removed the middle seat, and installed a portable toilet I bought at Sears, Roebuck," she says proudly. "Now I go anywhere I like and don't even think about it." Other models of portable toilets can be found in stores that carry camping equipment. Estelle thinks that attitude overcomes all obstacles. "I've given up this ridiculous modesty," she says. "When I have to go, I will go *anywhere*, including behind bushes, buildings, or cars, and I *always* carry tissues." Leah says that she also carries toilet-seat covers. Katrina has made effective use of a device, designed for campers, that allows women to urinate standing up. "Now I don't have to sit on dirty toilet seats or cactus spines when camping," she says. "And if you live in a cold place, you can avoid squatting in two feet of snow in winter."

Asking to be let ahead in line in a theater or boisterous stadium restroom may not present much of a threat after you get used to doing it, but some people find that asking to go ahead in the more intimate environment of a crowded airplane is just too difficult. On long flights, this can present a serious problem to someone with interstitial cystitis, who may have to go several times an hour.

Even though air travel may be difficult, there are a few simple, common-sense things you can do to make your trips less difficult.

- Arrange ahead of time for an aisle seat near the toilets.
- Sit on a couple of pillows to minimize vibration.
- Restrict fluids, especially coffee and alcohol, before and during the flight.
- Wear loose clothing for comfort.
- Women can wear absorbent pads and men might consider using

259

a condom catheter (see page 264) in case the flight is delayed on the ground or has to circle a while before landing (both very common occurrences these days).

• Tell the head flight attendant that you have a medical problem and perhaps show him or her a note from your doctor. You may be allowed to use the toilet in the first-class section, if the plane is large.*

The Need for Public Toilets

Even though you may not have to urinate twenty or more times a day, as people with interstitial cystitis do, you can probably relate to the desperate need to find a public bathroom. The famous psychoanalyst Sigmund Freud, who suffered from diarrhea, is said to have hated the United States because, among other things, it had few public toilets. Sadly, nothing much has changed since Freud's day. European travelers must be dismayed, to say nothing of inconvenienced, by the scarcity of public bathroom facilities in the United States. In Europe, a concerted effort has been made to have clean, attended public toilets on street corners, in parks, subway stations, and public transportation facilities. You generally leave the attendant a tip or pay a set fee—usually the equivalent of 25 to 50 cents. The primary complaint that Europeans seem to have about their own facilities is that they are often not wheelchair-accessible.

Now that it is possible to conduct some rational public discussion about bladder disorders, perhaps we can hope—and work—for much-needed changes in the way we respond to the normal need of people to empty their bladders in an appropriate and timely manner. The most desperately needed changes are in the provision of sufficient toilet facilities for both women and men in public settings and the installation of safe, clean public restrooms in many locations where they are not currently available.

The issue of sufficient toilet facilities in theaters, stadiums, and other places that serve large numbers of people at the same time is just now beginning to be addressed. These places almost universally have token numbers of toilets for the numbers of people that they serve—and are especially deficient in providing adequate fa-

* Thanks to Debra Slade, executive director of the Interstitial Cystitis Association, for these suggestions.

cilities for women. The owners seem oblivious to the long lines of women, standing, night after night, inching ever so slowly toward relief, all the while wondering if they will get back in time for the second act or the kick-off.

Recently, there has been a glimmer of hope that those agonizing waits in line will one day be a thing of the past. Several cities and states have made attempts to remedy this intolerable situation. As is frequently the case, New York City was in the vanguard. In 1984, the City Council passed a bill requiring all new theaters, restaurants, and other public places that hold more than seventy-five people to install equal numbers of toilet fixtures for women and men.[1] California, Virginia, and New York State also passed "potty parity acts" in 1989, requiring equal numbers of toilets for women and men.

These laws, likely to be copied by other states in the foreseeable future, are important steps in the right direction. But they fail, at the outset, to address the central issue. The point is not *equality* per se, but *sufficiency*. How much is enough? Women require from two to four times as long to initiate and complete urination as men do. Real equality, then, would be to provide enough toilets for men, based upon the average occupancy of the facility, then provide not an equal number, but at least *twice* as many toilets for women and perhaps more. And this requirement needs to be imposed on existing structures as well as new ones. If enough people write to their city councils and state legislators, demanding that sufficient restroom facilities be universally provided, perhaps this basic necessity, which some would argue is a right, would become a reality.

Spending Time in Your Own Bathroom

Many people say that having to use the toilet so often, or having to stay there for a long time, eventually becomes degrading. Others complain it's a big waste of time. These feelings may hark back to toilet training, which for many was a profoundly unpleasant experience, even though we may not remember it consciously. It may not be possible to overcome these deeply ingrained feelings all at once, but there are some concrete things you can do to make trips to the bathroom less of a negative experience.

Keeping a stock of magazines or newspapers in the bathroom has long been an American tradition. If this is one of your standard distractions, you might think about upgrading your library a bit.

Books of poetry or quotations are good because the individual items don't take as long to get through as, say, *War and Peace*. And you can quote them to your friends, who may wonder where you found the time to learn so much. Some people like a radio or tape player to keep them company. If you can rig it to go on when you turn on the light or shut the door, the bathroom can be filled with beautiful, soothing music, a symphony or a Broadway extravaganza every time you walk in. If your bathroom has a window, you could fill it with plants and create a minitropical forest. With a little daily sunlight, plants will thrive in the concentrated humidity of the bathroom. If there is no window, plants won't do very well, so you might consider having an ever-changing art show. You'll be surprised at how much you can see in a picture the longer you study it. Maggie solved her boredom factor by taking the Sunday crossword puzzle to the copy shop and having it enlarged. She tapes it to the wall and works on it all week.

The point of these rather whimsical suggestions is, if frequent bathroom sessions are a fact of your life, they don't necessarily have to be entirely negative experiences.

OTHER COPING MECHANISMS

Absorbent Products

Before Hillary came to see Kristene, she was trying to "make do" with super-absorbent menstrual pads. "One pad was never enough to get me through a long game. In tennis, you just can't say, 'I'll be back in ten minutes' and trot off to the clubhouse."

Fred, who developed incontinence as the result of a childhood accident, has some specific complaints about wearing diapers. "Disposable diapers rustle and the cloth ones are too bulky to wear under clothing, and pads have a tendency to slip unless they are taped to your underwear." Fred, who has tried everything, says that there are two myths about incontinence products: the "one size-fits-all myth" and the "size-range myth." "As for myth No. 1, bottoms come in a range of sizes, so one size can't possibly fit all," he observes. "And as for No. 2, extra large runs from 46 to 52 inches in the waist and large goes from 38 to 45 inches. How the hell can someone wear a garment with that large a range? If your waist is 41 inches, you are out of luck."

Although many excellent absorbent products are now available, 32 percent of all menstrual products and 28 percent of baby diapers sold are used for incontinence, even though they are not designed for this purpose.[2] Thanks to consumer demand and TV advertising, the variety and availability of absorbent products has increased quite a bit in the last five or six years. Knowing what types of products are available and where to find them can help you maintain or regain a sense of independence and precious personal freedom. An exhaustive and very up-to-date catalog of these products, including information on where to order them, has been put together by HIP, Inc. You can order the *Resource Guide for Continence Products and Services* from HIP, Inc., P. O. Box 544, Union, SC 29738, for $3.

There are quite a number of absorbent pads and fitted underpants designed to accommodate them that you could use instead of your basic diaper, a panty made of stretch mesh to help hold the pad in place. There are even several types of boxer shorts for men with a built-in absorbent pad that could make going to the gym more comfortable, as well as a specially designed jock strap that can hold an absorbent pad.

One excellent recent innovation is the development of pads and other absorbent products that are impregnated with a substance that turns to gel as it absorbs fluid. If you have moderate urine loss, you can wear one of these products for several hours without needing to change. Women who have interstitial cystitis have also found this type of product (Serenity is one brand) to be useful for riding in a car or getting through a meeting or movie.

For men, there are also absorbent dribble collectors, some of which have a thin lining that turns to gel when it becomes wet. Many people, especially older people, find that their incontinence is containable during the day but is worse at night. In this case, there are a host of disposable bed pads, some of which have gel linings, and even reusable rubber sheets, with lightweight rubber on one side and cotton fabric on the other.

Many people who have to wear incontinence products develop skin problems sooner or later. There are quite a number of moisturizers and barrier creams that are specifically formulated to deal with heavy-duty chafing. Skin infections can be uncomfortable and, because affected areas are constantly being reexposed to moisture, very difficult to heal. Therefore, using these products *before* a problem develops would be very prudent.

Many people who have moderate to severe incontinence find that odor is an even worse problem than wetness. Bernice, who developed incontinence after a hysterectomy, observes, "Wetness only affects *you*, but odor affects anyone you come in contact with." Odor can often be dealt with by taking frequent showers and changing pads and clothes often. However, if it is a severe problem for you, there are several over-the-counter medications you can take that act on urine to neutralize the odor. The HIP *Resource Guide* lists a number of these products. You can also find some of them locally at surgical supply houses, which are usually listed in the Yellow Pages under "Surgical Appliances and Supplies."

It's helpful to be aware of the various products that are available, but they are expensive if used on a regular basis and many retired people who live on fixed incomes simply can't afford them. The cost of diapers for someone who has to wear them around the clock can be around $1,200 a year.[3] This cost is clearly prohibitive for many people. Private insurance and Medicare will pay for external and indwelling catheters, and some "collection devices," but they won't pay for absorbent products. This is ludicrous, since incontinence is a medical problem. One solution to the ongoing expense of absorbent products is the use of reusable pads, which can be washed numerous times. After all, many of us can remember when all baby diapers were reusable. Larger towns may even have services that will pick up and deliver.

As helpful as absorbent products are, the exclusive use of diapers or devices for incontinence fosters dependence on these products and may contribute to the loss of independence and self-esteem. Therefore, before you begin using these products or devices regularly, be sure that you have gotten a full urological evaluation and a diagnosis and have tried all of the treatments that are available to you.

DEVICES

A special open-ended latex *condom catheter* with elastic or self-adhesive tape around the inner part of the top is placed over the penis and connected to a drainage bag. The leg bag needs to be emptied periodically, but the same condom can be left on day and night for a day or two. Each time you change it, you need to check carefully for signs of skin irritation or sores, and each time you replace the condom, you need to coat the skin with a special skin-care product to protect it from irritation. For men who have urge, reflex, or transient urinary incontinence, condom catheters may be used on a temporary basis. Long-term use of these devices is generally only appropriate for men who have spinal cord injuries or who are very frail or ill and cannot take advantage of other forms of therapy. Men who have urinary retention because of urethral obstruction from prostate enlargement or underactive bladder muscles should not use condom catheters.

Several attempts have been made to design a *female collection device*. The National Aeronautics and Space Administration (NASA) has made a concerted effort to design such devices for both men and women to be used when bulky space suits make using the toilet impossible. Millions of dollars have been spent on this endeavor, but so far, the design of a genuinely comfortable, efficient female collection device has eluded NASA engineers. Given the inadequate provision of public toilet facilities for women, the perfection of such a device could benefit not only women who have bladder problems but women with normal bladders as well.

For many years before better absorbent products were available, the Cunningham clamp was the standby for some men who had severe incontinence but wanted to remain active. *Penile clamps* are still prescribed today for short-term use after prostate surgery. The Cunningham clamp compresses the shaft of the penis to stop the flow of urine. It must be removed about every four hours so that you can urinate. If you use a clamp, you need to carefully inspect the penis at frequent intervals for evidence of injury or infection, and you should not use it at night, because prolonged clamping can cause injury to the penis. The HIP *Resource Guide* makes note of an inflatable cuff, which might provide a more comfortable alternative to the standard metal clamps.* In general, penile clamps are discouraged for long-term use, so if your doctor suggests that you use one, be sure to find out how long you will need to use it, and ask if there are any alternatives, such as timed toileting, bladder training, pelvic muscle exercises, or condom catheters.

* The cuff is manufactured by VPI, P.O. Box 266, Spencer, IN 47460.

COPING WITH OSTOMIES

People who have surgery for bladder cancer or interstitial cystitis, or incontinence from birth defects or accidents that cannot be treated any other way, often have stomas—surgically constructed outlets for urine—on the lower abdomen. For these conditions, the most commonly employed procedures are the Koch or Indiana pouch, in which the urine is stored in a bowel segment inside of the abdomen and emptied periodically, or the ileal conduit procedure, in which a bowel segment serves as a passageway for urine, which drips constantly into a waist or leg bag.

Some stomas protrude a tiny bit from the skin like a small nipple, while others may be flat, more like a tight buttonhole. In either case, they are not disfiguring, and with proper care you can lead a normal life.

After an initial adjustment period of several months, the primary issues that people with ostomies have to deal with on an ongoing basis are skin care, proper attachment of the urine collection bag to the body, and keeping the bag or "appliance" clean to reduce the chances of infection.

The United Ostomy Association (UOA), an educational organization that promotes the dissemination of information on the care of ostomies, points out that 99 percent of skin problems can be avoided if the appliance fits properly. Choosing the proper style from the array of available products is essential to a well-functioning device. There are one-piece and two-piece styles, with standard-size custom-fitted face plates (the part of the appliance that fits over the stoma and prevents leakage). If your stoma leaks, certain manufacturers will custom-make face plates for you. Several styles of collection bags are available. Normally a knowledgeable representative of the manufacturer will help you choose the appliance that will work best for you.

If you are faced with bladder surgery, investigating the various options for ostomy care is essential before you have your operation. That way, you won't get any unpleasant surprises after the fact. If you already have a stoma but are having problems, there may be remedies available for you. In either case, your best bet might be to contact the United Ostomy Association (36 Executive Park, Suite 120, Irvine, CA 92714; 714-660-8624) for aid in finding an experienced enterostomal therapist who can help you. This organization coordinates local support groups, holds annual conferences, publishes *The Ostomy Quarterly,* a professional journal, and provides free information booklets and pamphlets. By going to support group meetings, you can meet other people who have successfully adapted to living with ostomies.

EXERCISE

Exercise plays an important part in both physical and mental well-being, but for many people with bladder disorders—especially incontinence and interstitial cystitis—and those who have had extensive bladder surgery, vigorous exercise is difficult to do. If you have physical limitations that interfere with your ability to exercise normally, or you are older and have not exercised in many years, it is not easy to find some form of exercise that is comfortable for you, yet requires you to extend yourself physically. Regular exercise may help you cope better by improving your fitness, attitude, and self-image. Yet even low-impact aerobics may be too strenuous for people who have had extensive surgery, those who lose urine easily, or those who have interstitial cystitis in which bladder pain is a significant factor.

One alternative to aerobics is "Body Recall," a system of exercise that was developed especially for elderly people but could be extremely useful for people with a variety of disabilities, especially where jarring precipitates urinary leakage or is uncomfortable. This comprehensive program encompasses relaxation, flexibility, coordination, and the gradual building of strength. There are over 200 exercises, many of which can be done even if you are in a wheelchair or in bed. "Body Recall provides an opportunity to learn how to take charge of the physical equipment we have and bring it to full potential," says Dorothy Chrisman, developer of the Body Recall system, who teaches physical education at Berea College in Berea, Kentucky.

Kay, a regal woman in her early sixties who has severe interstitial cystitis, discovered the Body Recall program through word of mouth. Since there were no certified instructors in her area, she traveled to Berea to learn the technique. "Starting this program was the turning point in my illness," Kay says. "I found that it helped to take the focus off the pain and put it on myself." Kay became a certified instructor and has been teaching classes for four years. "Some people can barely walk around the block when they begin, but everybody sees results."

An illustrated guide to the Body Recall program and a list of certified instructors can be ordered from Body Recall, P.O. Box 412, Berea, KY 40403. If there is no certified instructor in your area, perhaps you could consider becoming one yourself. If you have a relative in a nursing home, perhaps you could try to get a program started, either by becoming an instructor and volunteering your own services or by encouraging the home to hire a part-time instructor.

People with the worst cases of interstitial cystitis often find that vibrations or jarring movement precipitate or intensify bladder pain. Yet many people who have moderate to severe cases report that regular exercise and even sports activities are an essential part of trying to maintain physical fitness, energy, and mental equilibrium. The people who answered our survey on interstitial cystitis appear to be quite active in spite of their pain, and engage in a wide variety of physical pursuits, especially walking and low-impact aerobics, but also swimming, jogging, bicycle riding, stationary bicycling, weight lifting, tennis, dancing, skating, bowling, stretching exercises, NordicTrack, rowing, racquetball, and skiing (both downhill and cross-country).

Many people, like Sheila, find that they must accommodate their exercises to the waxing and waning of symptoms. "On good days, I can do just about anything, and on bad days, just about nothing," she says. Although Sheila has severe urgency, moderate pain, and sometimes extreme frequency, she still manages to swim a mile four times a week. Gabrielle, who even had to give up walking because the motion exacerbated her symptoms, found that she could still do upper-body exercises on rowing or exercise machines. Sharon finds that when her symptoms are severe, she can't run, but when they lighten up, she runs three miles five times a week. "The first half mile is somewhat uncomfortable, but after that I feel great, and am much better for some time afterward." Samantha was an avid tennis player before coming down with IC. She noticed that playing on hard courts caused her symptoms to flare up, but that playing on a clay surface was much better. "Now I can play often without worrying too much," she says.

VISUALIZATION

Visualization, using mental images to control bodily processes, has probably been used since the beginning of time to help people cope with extraordinary circumstances in their lives. Athletes have used it to enhance performance, soldiers have used it to confront the terrors of war, prisoners have used it to endure the interminable boredom of incarceration, and so on. This technique has been adapted for use by people with chronic pain, devastating diseases, and depression. If you have incontinence, visualization can help you cope with an embarrassing accident. If you have interstitial cystitis, it would seem essential to have some safe, dependable mental strategies to be used on a routine basis to provide positive reinforcement against pain, frustration, and fatigue.

Many people practice visualization on their own, either consciously or unconsciously, and it is certainly a skill that you can learn without much outside help. However, if you want to utilize visualization to its maximum potential, you might want to get some help. Psychotherapists are usually versed in visualization techniques and can give you some useful pointers, and courses are frequently taught at YMCAs/YWCAs or at alternative learning centers. If you can't find a therapist or course, you can learn from reading one of the several excellent books on the subject, such as *Creative Visualization* by Shakti Gawain, or Bernie Siegel's popular bestseller, *Love, Medicine and Miracles*.

Leslie, who has a very severe case of interstitial cystitis, has successfully used visualization "to get through rough spells." Since she began using the technique several years ago, she has created a number of soothing, healing images that have helped control bladder pain. "At one period when I was having an especially rough time, I pictured a white chalky substance coating the inside of my bladder. It filled all the cracks and lesions and my bladder became calm and healthy." Because of the constant need to urinate, Leslie gave up going to the theater, but on a lark decided to treat a friend to a show. She was in a panic all the way there, worrying about how she would manage. "I knew I had to calm down, so I made up this jingle: Pink air, blue light, everything will be all right. I said it over and over. Amazingly enough, I was fine. I went to the bathroom during intermission just like everyone else."

PAIN CLINICS

For people with interstitial cystitis or bladder cancer who have unremitting bladder pain, a pain clinic might offer some as yet untried options in controlling pain when coping techniques and standard medical remedies have not been helpful. Such facilities generally provide comprehensive diagnostic services and offer both medical and psychological treatments, which may include biofeedback, electrical stimulation such as the TENS unit (see page 153), relaxation techniques, visualization, acupressure and acupuncture, hypnosis, massage, medications—both narcotic and non-narcotic pain relievers, as well as antidepressants—and medical treatments such as procedures that interrupt nerve pathways, including surgery and epidural blocks.

To find a certified pain clinic in your area, you can contact Oryx Press, 2214 N. Central at Encanto, Phoenix, AZ 85004-1483. You might also contact the American Pain Society, 1200 17th St. N.W., Suite 400, Washington, DC 20036 or the American Academy of Pain Medicine, 43 East Ohio Street, Chicago, IL 60611.

DISABILITY

Half of the people with interstitial cystitis say that they are unable to work, but very few have applied for Social Security or private insurance company disability benefits. Many people assume that they are ineligible, or will be arbitrarily turned down, and others believe that having to wade through the bureaucratic swamp to get qualified simply isn't worth the time and expense. Yet there are some surprising benefits to getting disability if you are eligible, and it is not prohibitively expensive for most people.

If you are eligible, there are a number of advantages to qualifying for benefits:

- you will have a minimum income, based upon the amount of time you have worked since you were eighteen and how much you earned in the last three years, until you are able to work again;
- after two years on disability, you will be eligible for Medicare;
- if you are judged eligible, any minor children will become eligible for Medicare benefits also;

• if you miss several years of work but receive disability payments, these can be counted toward your retirement.

In spite of the reported difficulties in getting processed for disability, 40 percent of those who apply are approved without having to retain a lawyer. If you are turned down on the first round, appealing with the help of a lawyer is definitely worth it. Seventy percent of the people who appeal are eventually qualified for benefits. You can find a lawyer who is experienced in representing Social Security claimants by calling the National Organization of Social Security Claimants' Representatives at 1-800-431-2804. Federal regulations prohibit lawyers from charging a fee in advance on a Social Security claim. Many lawyers take Social Security cases on a contingency fee basis, that is, they only get paid if you win the case, and the average fee is about $1,500—about 25 percent of the past due benefit.

It does take a while to get processed, so you must be prepared to be patient. It usually takes between two to three months to get an initial decision and another two to three months for the second hearing. If you are turned down and appeal again, you will go before an administrative judge, which may take up to five months. After that, you should get a decision in two to three months.

The key to getting your disability claim accepted is to word the claim very precisely. It's important to tie your physical disability to your symptoms. For example, explain that you have a hard time functioning during the day because of sleep interrupted by urinary frequency. Having a psychologist submit a written statement validating your emotional suffering can also be helpful.

Applying for disability is a complex issue. For some people, it is an admission of defeat, a signal that the disease is calling the shots. Others, however, find that they cannot function well enough on a day-in-day-out basis to hold a full-time, responsible job, and these may consider applying for disability. While disability may seem like an attractive option, many, many IC patients say unequivocally that idleness, or periods when they have too much time to focus on themselves, intensifies symptoms and allows the pain to take over. Each disability case is individual. Before you do decide to apply, be sure to weigh all of the pros and cons carefully. It may be that you could take a lesser job or try to make an arrangement with your employer so that it is still possible for you to keep working within the limits imposed by the disease.

271

The National Organization of Social Security Claimants' Representatives (19 East Central Avenue, Pearl River, NY 10965 (800-431-2804 or 914-735-8812) provides an informative free brochure called "Social Security Disability and SSI Claims: Your Need for Representation" that answers some of the most frequently asked questions about getting disability and notes the many things an attorney can do for you. If you are faced with filing an appeal, you might consider contacting the Interstitial Cystitis Association (see page 177). This group has supplied supportive documentation about the disease in a number of cases, and reports that appeals have been successful in many states.

DON'T TAKE IT SITTING DOWN

If a leaky bladder is making you feel powerless and depressed, or pain and urinary frequency are getting the best of you, doing something substantial and constructive to help yourself and others can take your mind off your troubles and if nothing else, provide a distraction. Some people have found this very powerful medicine indeed. Cheryle Gartley, who had severe incontinence and got no help from doctors, did her own research and started the Simon Foundation. Of course, most people with incontinence aren't likely to start a foundation, there are things you can do, such as joining a support group. If one doesn't exist in your community, you could start one. (See page 16 for information on where to find or how to start a support group.) You could also engage in some "anti-incontinence" activities, such as writing to your city council representative or state legislator, asking him or her to introduce legislation requiring adequate public restrooms. Many incontinence experts would like to see absorbent products labeled, similar to the labeling on all cigarette packs, to the effect that incontinence is a treatable condition and that these products should not be used in place of treatment. If you are looking for an "anti-incontinence" activity, you could write to the companies that manufacture any product you are using and ask if they have any plans to label their products in the near future and what the label will say. Letting each company know that you will only buy from a company that does label its product appropriately might also be helpful. A few thousand letters could make the difference! If you have interstitial cystitis, you could contact the Interstitial Cystitis Association and participate in their annual letter-writing campaign to Congress, asking for more funding to study the disease. You could, as Mary Louise does, visit new supermarkets in your area and encourage them to have well-marked, accessible restrooms.

People with interstitial cystitis have been especially motivated to take action. Arta Chastain, the Arkansas state coordinator of the Interstitial Cystitis Association who has had severe IC for eighteen years, got tired of having a condition that no one knew about and decided to try to raise the visibility of the disease. She conducted a PR campaign and succeeded in getting articles into thirty newspapers in Arkansas. She also got a notice in her church bulletin. The response to that was so encouraging, she decided to reach out to religious organizations and initiated "Operation Clergy," writing letters to 400 bishops and rabbis. She received more than 100 replies from bishops, rabbis, chaplains, and nuns, as well as from one archbishop and a cardinal. Information about the condition was included in church bulletins and newspapers; a special Catholic mass was said for IC sufferers; one chaplain invited a urologist to give a seminar for other chaplains on how to recognize the condition when counseling patients; and information about it was disseminated at a church conference. "I decided ahead of time that the number of responses didn't make any difference," Arta says. "Just having reached out made me feel so much better. The fact that many people reached back was also gratifying."

MIND OVER BLADDER

Humor has traditionally been one of the mechanisms people have used to help them maintain perspective or gain some much-needed psychic distance from the pain, discomfort, and humiliation of bladder problems. And since you can't take your bladder out at night and put it in the cupboard along with your contacts or dentures, there are probably times when you need all of the psychic distance you can get.

Most people would deny that there is anything funny about having bladder problems. Some, in fact, became irate when Rebecca asked them if they had any humorous anecdotes they would like to share with others. Yet, when presssed, even those who were the most adamant about the humorlessness of their situations seemed to be able to find a funny story to tell or remember a family joke that helped them make light of difficult situations. Here are some of the jokes and humorous stories, and even some humorous fiction, that have helped people cope with bladder disorders.

Anyone who has ever tried to do pelvic muscle exercises might appreciate this anecdote that Fran Wright, R. N., tells about her famous boss, Dr. Arnold Kegel.

Kegel was a dedicated advocate of the pelvic muscle exercises, not only for incontinence but to improve sexual satisfaction as well. He was also an avid researcher, looking far and wide for examples of their use in other cultures. Once he discovered an illustration of post-natal pelvic muscle exercises in a copy of an Egyptian papyrus. In the picture, a woman sits on a low stool placed over hot stones. Pomegranate seeds are placed on the stones and when they begin to pop (like popcorn), the woman reacts by sharply contracting her pelvic muscles. According to Fran Wright, Kegel tried to get his wife and daughter to try out this technique—certainly the first recorded biofeedback mechanism—but they declined. So Kegel himself tried it with apparent success. "Mrs. Wright," he reported, "when the pomegranates started scattering, I drew my testicles up to my tonsils!" Convinced that such mechanisms could work, Kegel invented the perineometer, the first modern biofeedback device. Perhaps researchers who are on the lookout for cures for stress incontinence will appreciate this anecdote as well.

Hilda developed overflow incontinence as a result of diabetes about twenty years ago. As a result, she often had no warning when she was going to urinate. "I wore pads, but in those days, they didn't work so well." One day, she was visiting some friends and drank a lot of iced tea for lunch, which she usually didn't do. "I was having a great time and sat on their Queen Anne couch with a gorgeous raw silk covering. Suddenly I realized that my bottom was wet." She waited nervously until both of her friends left the room, then threw their small Pekinese dog, Mei-Ling, on the couch and began yelling about how the dog had wet the couch, and started scolding it abusively. Years later, when the dog died, Hilda got up the nerve and admitted that it had not been the culprit. Her friends laughed and told her that they had known all along, since the dog *never* urinated inside the house. Hilda says that she felt very relieved to be able to confess, and they all had a good laugh over it in memory of Mei-Ling.

Fred, whose critique of absorbent products appears on page 262, found the adjustment to wearing diapers very difficult, but his two-year-old nephew, Benjie, saw it in an entirely different light. "I slept over at my sister's house one night and Benjie walked in on me after I had removed my pajamas," Fred recalls. "He saw me in my diapers and waterproof panties and beamed, saying, 'Oh, boy, Uncle Fred, you wear diapers, too! You and me are the only ones that do. How come Mommy and Daddy don't wear diapers?' By that time, I was laughing so hard, I couldn't think of an answer to his question."

Eileen has severe interstitial cystitis, but hates to be confined, so she usually carries a wide-mouth plastic jar in the car for those inevitable times when she won't be able to get to a toilet in time. "One day I missed my exit on the New Jersey Turnpike and the next exit was closed because of an accident. So I had to drive about twenty-five miles more than I normally would to get home. I had to go so bad, but I couldn't stop, so I decided the only thing to do was to drive faster." She finally reached an exit and pulled off the road at the first opportunity, only to notice to her chagrin that a patrol car had pulled up just behind her. "I didn't care," she says. "I really had to pee and figured it was their problem." When the officers came to the window, Eileen smiled serenely and explained what she was doing. "They were a little sheepish but very understanding," she says. "And thank goodness I didn't get a ticket. It would have been an expensive bathroom stop."

"I've always been a housewife," says Janice, who has had interstitial cystitis for many years. "Our family joke is that if I ever went to work, I would have to work as a bathroom attendant, since it's the thing I know best." Donna, who had her bladder removed and has to catheterize her internal reservoir, says she has finally achieved a rare kind of equality with men: "I can pee standing up!"

Betty Lynn Warren, the Alabama state coordinator for the Interstitial Cystitis Association, had such bad bladder pain that she didn't think she could live another day with it. Then she decided to name her bladder and give it its own identity. That made her feel so good that she made up a story about it. "I laughed so hard writing that story that I began to come out of my depression," she says. Here is the story of Betty Lynn and Elvira:

Elvira and I are constant companions. She goes everywhere I go and much to my dismay, I have to endure the places she takes me. Elvira is a witch. To look at her she is beautiful and healthy, but under the veneer she is deceptive, cunning, and totally unpredictable. She and I are in continuous battle. Some days I tell her, "Elvira, I don't care. You take charge." I give in to her, hoping it will pacify her, and possibly she will "let me be." Then some days I take charge. "Now, Elvira," I say, "I want to give you my plans for today. I choose to pay the consequences for these choices: (1) I'll be sitting for three hours. (2) I plan to drink eight ounces of real coffee. (3) I'm going to eat a pizza with lots of tomato sauce. (4) I'm going to cross my legs today. You'll be crowded but that's your problem. (5) I'll be playing tennis. Get ready to be bounced and jolted around. It's my way of paying you back for the misery you cause me."

One day Elvira and I took a trip. She didn't want to go, but I insisted. No, I demanded that she go. I told her we'd be going to some new bathrooms. Some she would like, but I would detest. Our first stop was a grocery store. I asked the clerk where the restrooms were and he said, "Through the double doors, behind the boxes, past the produce, and the next to the last door on the right." When we finally got there, I decided it should be condemned as unsafe and unclean for both employees and public use. But I had my individually wrapped tissues so it was okay. After taking care of Elvira, I worked my way back to the front, deciding to write a letter to the store manager.

From then on, I decided that if a particular restroom didn't meet my personal requirements, I'd leave a large note on the door, stating, "Bathroom unclean, use at your own risk," and sign it "Elvira." Maybe I should call my son who is almost through law school and find out if I can be held liable for claiming to be a health inspector wherever I go. I know he will quote me ten reasons that I will. But why should I worry? I won't implicate myself, only Elvira. I'd love to see her panic, just once!

RESOURCES

Creative Visualization, Shakti Gawain. New York: Bantam Books, 1982.

Living with Chronic Illness: Days of Patience and Passion, Cheri Register. New York: The Free Press/ Macmillan, 1987. Based on in-depth interviews with thirty people (including the author) who live on a day-by-day basis with chronic, often painful illnesses, this book shatters some myths about long-term illness and provides some penetrating insights into its impact on people's lives.

Love, Medicine and Miracles, Bernie S. Siegel, M.D. New York: Harper & Row, 1986. This bestselling book on coping with cancer contains an excellent section on visualization.

The Mind-Body Effect, Herbert Benson. New York: Simon & Schuster, 1980.

The Relaxation Response, Herbert Benson and Miriam Z. Klipper. New
York: Avon Books, 1976. A classic book on stress reduction.
Resource Guide for Continence Aids and Services, 3rd ed. To order, send $3
to HIP Resource Guide, P.O. Box 544, Union, SC 29739. This comprehensive guide covers the range of absorbent products and other
incontinence aids.

277

INDEX OF
DIAGNOSTIC TESTS

The following tests, listed in alphabetical order, are the ones you will normally encounter in a urologist's office. Many people find some of these tests very embarrassing, especially the urodynamic tests, which involve having to urinate while being watched by a doctor or other health professional. In addition to being embarrassing, some tests that involve inserting instruments into the bladder can also be uncomfortable. Knowing what is likely to happen and what will be expected of you can help lower your anxiety level and perhaps make the tests that require your active participation more accurate.

ACID PHOSPHATASE TEST (see BLOOD TESTS, opposite)

BIOPSY OF THE BLADDER

Used in the diagnosis of interstitial cystitis and bladder cancer
A cystoscope is inserted into the bladder and a cold cup biopsy forceps, a long tweezerlike instrument, is inserted into the bladder. Several samples of tissue are snipped from the bladder wall, both superficial and deep. In the case of interstitial cystitis, these tissue specimens may reveal evidence of inflammation and/or mast cells

in the bladder wall, and in the case of bladder cancer, they may reveal cancerous cells. A biopsy can be done on an outpatient basis, but occasionally an overnight stay is necessary.

BIOPSY OF THE PROSTATE

Used in the diagnosis of prostate cancer

A long needle with a hollow center is inserted into the prostate through the perineum or rectum, and some tissue is removed by vacuum. The procedure is mildly uncomfortable and usually takes about twenty minutes.

BLOOD TESTS

Acid Phosphatase

Used to help determine if prostate cancer has spread beyond the prostatic capsule

Acid phosphatase is an enzyme manufactured in the prostate gland. This enzyme continues to be manufactured by cancerous prostate cells; if these cells break through the prostatic capsule and migrate to other parts of the body, they will go on making the enzyme, so that eventually, elevated levels can be detected by a blood test. This test should not be done 48 to 72 hours after a rectal exam, since an exam may cause the release of acid phosphatase, causing a false positive result.

Blood Urea Nitrogen (BUN)

Used to evaluate kidney function

Urea nitrogen is one of the by-products of protein breakdown that takes place in the liver and is filtered out of the bloodstream by the kidneys. If the level of urea nitrogen in the bloodstream is higher than normal, kidney damage will be suspected. BUN levels may also be affected by dehydration or intestinal bleeding. Therefore the creatinine test (described below) is often more specific.

Creatinine

Used to evaluate kidney function and in the diagnosis of prostate enlargement

Creatinine, a normal by-product of muscle breakdown, is filtered from the blood by the kidneys and excreted in the urine. Elevated levels in the bloodstream usually indicate decreased kidney function, sometimes because the urethra is obstructed and urine is backing up to the kidneys.

Prostate Specific Antigen (PSA)

Used to detect or confirm benign prostate enlargement or prostate cancer

Prostate specific antigen is a substance normally manufactured in the prostate. Slightly elevated levels can indicate prostate enlargement, simply because there is more prostate to make the antigen. If cancer cells leave the prostate and migrate to the nearby lymph nodes or to other tissues or organs, they will continue to produce PSA, and higher levels may be found in the bloodstream. The higher the level, the more likely that the cancer has spread to other parts of the body. To avoid false positive results, this test should not be done 48 to 72 hours after a rectal exam.

COTTON SWAB TEST

Used in the diagnosis of stress incontinence

If you have stress incontinence, it is usually because your urethra slips out of its normal position during certain movements or activities. This simple test will provide a rough measurement of how much slippage has occurred. You will be asked to lie on your back and a long-handled cotton swab, well lubricated, will be gently inserted into the urethra. If the bladder is in its normal position, the swab handle will be parallel to the exam table. If the urethra has slipped from its normal position, the handle of the swab will rise. (The illustration opposite shows how slippage is measured.) If the handle rises more than 30 to 40 degrees, then your doctor can assume that the bladder neck has slipped significantly.

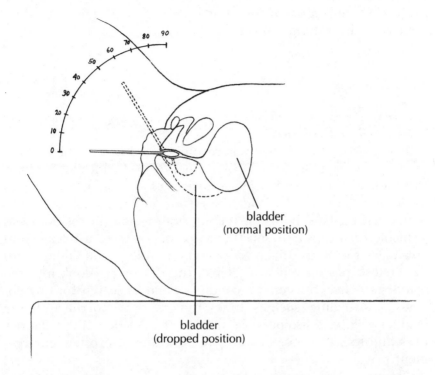

bladder
(normal position)

bladder
(dropped position)

16. **Cotton swab test.**

CT SCAN AND MAGNETIC RESONANCE IMAGING

Used in the staging of bladder or prostate cancer

Computed Tomography (CT or "cat scan") is a three-dimensional X-ray taken of a limited area of the body. A radioactive beam is rotated 360 degrees around the body and a computer translates the data into tiny dots of varying density. In order to get sharper detail on the X-ray, a dye or contrast medium is often given orally or intravenously. Magnetic resonance imaging (MRI) is a more recently developed technique that makes use of a magnetic field and radio-frequency signals instead of radiation to form three-dimensional pictures of organs and tissues. Even though both the CT scan and the MRI provide a lot of information, they are not definitive tests. The CT scan has been found to be inaccurate about one fourth of the time and the MRI may be no better. However,

281

each of these tests can be useful in determining lymph node involvement if the nodes are significantly enlarged and whether cancer has invaded tissues around the bladder or spread to other areas such as the liver, lungs, or bones.

CYSTOSCOPY

Used in the diagnosis of incontinence, interstitial cystitis, prostate problems, and bladder cancer

The practice of urology was revolutionized in the 1920s when urologists were able, for the first time, to see inside the bladder, although with the crude optical devices of the day it was only as through a glass darkly. With the advent of high-resolution fiber optics in the 1950s, however, the interior of the living bladder was available for inspection and the cystoscope became a reliable and invaluable tool in the diagnosis of certain urologic conditions. With the cystoscopes currently available, the doctor can look into the bladder to check its general condition, and to search for any obvious abnormalities such as stones, tumors, or hemorrhages in the bladder wall. It is also possible to check the position of the bladder neck and to see if obstruction is present due to prostate enlargement.

The cystoscope might be compared to a skinny periscope. It has two very thin channels—one through which fluid can be instilled into the bladder, and released again, and one fitted with a light and lenses that allow viewing of the interior of the bladder.

The typical cystoscope exam takes just one or two minutes. Because of the length of the male urethra, this procedure takes a little longer and may be slightly more uncomfortable for men than it is for women. You will be asked to empty your bladder before the procedure begins. Then the urologist gently inserts the lubricated shaft of the instrument through the urethra. While the cystoscope is being inserted, he or she can see the walls of the urethra and note if there are any obvious abnormalities or if the urethra has been narrowed by prostate enlargement. If there is any urine left in your bladder (residual urine), it will be allowed to drain and will be measured. Then the bladder will be filled with sterile water so that its interior walls can be examined. A sample of this fluid will be sent to the laboratory to be examined for cancer cells. This is called a urine cytology test, or bladder washing. This procedure has the advantage of picking up cells from the entire bladder surface if no tumors are seen in the bladder.

For people who have interstitial cystitis, a cystoscope examination can be somewhat more uncomfortable or even painful. If your symptoms suggest IC, the examination should be carried out under general anesthesia, not only because insertion of the cystoscope can be very uncomfortable, but also so that the bladder can be overdistended with water or gas to reveal tiny hemorrhages called *glomerulations* in the bladder wall.

HOME URINE TESTS (see URINE TESTS, page 286)

INTRAVENOUS PYELOGRAM (IVP)

In diagnosing bladder problems, the IVP is used to look for abnormalities in the urinary tract and to rule out kidney problems as the source of symptoms

The intravenous pyelogram is an X-ray of the kidneys and urinary tract done by injecting a dye into the veins which is concentrated by the kidneys and can be "seen" on the X-ray, outlining the kidneys, ureters, and bladder. If you are allergic to iodine, you should not have this test, but should have an ultrasound done instead.

Because of the risks of X-ray exposure and of injecting dye into the veins, this test is not done as frequently as it once was.

OVERDISTENSION OF THE BLADDER

Used in the diagnosis and treatment of interstitial cystitis

Bladder overdistension, or overstretching, is the most essential test for interstitial cystitis. Because this procedure is painful, it should be done while you are under general anesthesia. A cystoscope is inserted through the urethra into the bladder and the bladder is filled to its *true* capacity (as much as it will hold without bursting), as opposed to its *functional* capacity (the amount it holds under normal conditions), and the water is left in the bladder from two to seven minutes, depending on your doctor's preference.

After the water is drained from the bladder, your doctor will look again through the cystoscope to inspect the bladder wall carefully for ulcers, hemorrhages (called glomerulations), or scarring. This diagnostic procedure is also the first line of treatment for interstitial cystitis.

PHYSICAL EXAMINATION

Regardless of what your symptoms are, your doctor will do a thorough physical examination in the hopes of discovering clues as to the cause of them. He or she will focus on the pelvic and abdominal areas of the body, searching for tenderness and masses, and checking muscle tone, especially of your pelvic muscles. To do this for women, the doctor will put two gloved fingers into the vagina and ask you to contract the muscles that you would use to stop the flow of urine. With fingers still inserted in place, he or she will check for signs of protrusion of the bladder or urethra (or both) into the vagina. Removing the fingers from the vagina, your doctor will insert a speculum, a metal or plastic instrument that has two long bills somewhat like a duck's bill, into your vagina to look for signs of estrogen deficiency, including the lack of lubrication, easy bleeding, loss of elasticity, discoloration, and thinning of the vaginal walls. Sensation and nerve reflexes will also be checked. In men, a rectal examination will be performed to determine the size of the prostate and any hard spots on it that might suggest cancer. (See below for more information on this exam.) In both men and women, the genitals will be examined for any sign of inflammation, infection, or other abnormalities.

PROSTATE SPECIFIC ANTIGEN TEST (see BLOOD TESTS, page 279)

RECTAL EXAMINATION AND PROSTATIC MASSAGE

Used in the diagnosis of prostate cancer and prostatitis

The prostate lies adjacent to the rectum, about 1½ inches from the anal opening. It is thus fairly easy to reach with a finger or instrument. Most cancers occur in the back or posterior lobe of the prostate, and if they are large enough (about half an inch or larger; 1 to 1½ cm.), many of them can be felt. If infection or inflammation is suspected, the prostate can also be stroked or "massaged," through the rectum, to release prostatic secretions into the urethra. Since prostate enlargement most often occurs in the portion near the urethra, benign enlargement is not easy to detect through an anal prostate examination. To do a prostate exam or massage, the doctor inserts a gloved finger into the rectum and presses toward your pubic bone. He or she will be feeling for hard bumps or nodules that are raised or embedded within the prostate tissue, as well as for soft or "boggy" places that might indicate infection (see illustration). In prostatic massage, the doctor strokes the prostate six or seven times on each side, covering all of the gland that it is possible to feel. A few drops of the secretion produced may

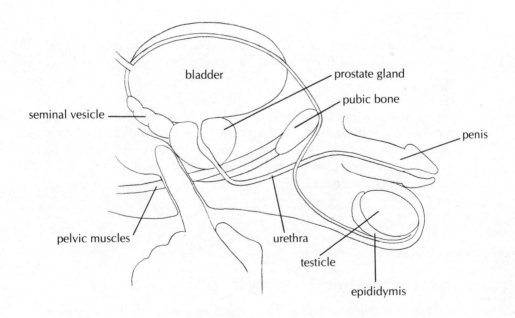

17. **Digital rectal examination of prostate.**

emerge from the tip of the penis. If nothing comes out, the secretions can be washed out by urinating a small amount into a cup. This test is frequently referred to as a "digital rectal exam" because the prostate is massaged with a physician's digit, or finger.

STRESS TEST

Used in the diagnosis of stress incontinence

This test is sometimes called the "full-bladder provocative stress test." It is designed to determine whether or not your bladder leaks when full when certain pressures are exerted on it.

While you are lying down, a catheter is inserted into the bladder, the bladder is filled with water, and the catheter is removed. Then you will be asked to cough. If you have leakage, this is considered a positive test. If you experience no leakage, you will be asked to stand, with legs slightly spread, and cough again. If no leakage occurs while you are standing and you have experienced incontinence at other times, further tests may be ordered.

ULTRASOUND

Used in the diagnosis of bladder stones and for establishing the size, shape, location, and function of the kidneys, ureters, bladder, and prostate

In ultrasound, very high frequency sound waves are aimed at certain parts of the body, and because the waves pass through tissues of different densities at different rates, the outline of organs or masses can be seen. In urology, an ultrasound test will aid in identifying the shape, size, and location of the kidneys, ureters, bladder, and prostate. If masses or other abnormalities are found, more extensive testing may be required.

URINE TESTS

Culture and Sensitivity Test (C&S)

Used in the diagnosis of cystitis, prostatitis, and to rule out bladder infections in interstitial cystitis

This test identifies the specific type of bacteria you have and which drugs will get rid of them. A few drops of your urine are placed on a dish with a special culture medium and incubated for about twenty-four hours. If infection is found, a sample of the same urine specimen is then placed on a blotter that is treated with different kinds of antibiotics and incubated for another twenty-four hours. If the bacteria are "sensitive," i.e., they can be killed by a certain drug, there will be bare spots on the blotter where these drugs are located. This test usually identifies a selection of several drugs that will kill a given bacteria. The results are normally available in about two days.

Until recently, the culture and sensitivity test had always been considered essential in diagnosing cystitis. But today, if your doctor is familiar with your case and you have had the necessary evaluation, he or she may decide to treat you without doing a culture and sensitivity test. The C&S test usually confirms the diagnosis, but does not often change the chosen course of treatment for uncomplicated infections. Urinalysis (see below) is important, however, in helping to determine the presence of bacteria that are causing repeated attacks, and it provides useful information in developing an effective treatment strategy.

Urinalysis

Used in the diagnosis of cystitis, interstitial cystitis, prostate problems, and bladder cancer

This test, done in a doctor's office or clinic, gives a general idea of whether infection is present. It is often done in two parts. First, a chemically treated plastic strip, called a *dip stick*, is dipped into the urine. Parts of the strip turn specific colors in response to various substances in the urine. The dip stick can reveal the presence of white blood cells, red blood cells, glucose (sugar), and show if the pH of the urine is acid or alkaline. White blood cells usually indicate that you have an infection. Based on this information, your doctor will probably treat you for an infection and order a culture and sensitivity test to confirm the diagnosis. The second part of the urinalysis (which may or may not be done) is spinning the urine in a centrifuge to separate substances, such as blood cells and bacteria (called *sediment*), from the urine itself. Then the sediment is examined under a microscope for bacteria. Although the *type* of bacteria cannot be identified, their presence can be seen and a general idea of their numbers can be obtained. Today, many doctors do a dip-stick test first, and if white blood cells are found, order a culture and sensitivity test, and if red blood cells are found, order a cancer cytology test.

Providing a midstream, clean-catch urine sample, i.e., one that is free of contaminants, is of vital importance in arriving at a correct diagnosis. Many urine samples are contaminated because of insufficient instruction in proper collection technique. This test is used for women and for men if a bladder infection is suspected. If a prostate problem is suspected in men, a more complicated test, called a segmented urine culture (see below), may be used.

For women, how to provide a clean-catch urine sample: First, using cotton, alcohol swabs, gauze, or tissues, cleanse the vaginal opening with plain water or with antibacterial soap, whatever is provided. Start and stop the flow of urine a couple of times to help wash contaminants out of the urethra. Then begin to urinate into a sterile cup, being careful not to let it touch any part of your body or pubic hair. It is important not to let the urine flow, as it normally does, down across the vaginal opening and back across the perineum. This can be avoided by spreading your knees far apart as you sit on the toilet. If you sit backward on the toilet, your knees will be forced far apart and the urine will shoot out so it can easily be caught in the cup. The laboratory actually requires only a small amount of urine, so focus on quality rather than quantity. If you think you have inadvertently contaminated the sample, it's very important that you say so. You may have to wait a half hour or so to get another sample, but it will be worth it. If your report comes back "negative" or "sterile" and you are still having symptoms, a second sample should be taken to look for a low bacterial count.

It is important to remember that even one antibiotic tablet, a dose of Pyridium, or even vitamin C might cause enough change to invalidate a sample, so be sure to tell your doctor what medications, if any, you have taken in the last several days.

Normally, a clean-catch midstream urine sample is sufficient for a diagnosis of uncomplicated cystitis. At times, however, when there may be complicating factors such as multiple recurrences or vaginitis, or a catheter or other instruments have been inserted into the bladder, your doctor may decide to take a catheterized specimen, and in special cases a suprapubic aspiration, to get a specimen that is not contaminated.

For women and men, how to get a catheterized specimen: A very small tube, or catheter, is gently inserted into the urethra and pushed up until its tip is inside the bladder. Any urine that is in the bladder will come out. In women, the procedure takes just ten or fifteen seconds, and is only mildly uncomfortable. In men, since there is less chance of contamination in collecting a midstream urine specimen, this test is performed less frequently. Rarely, a suprapubic aspiration may be indicated. If so, a small needle is inserted through the skin above the pubic bone and pushed into the bladder.

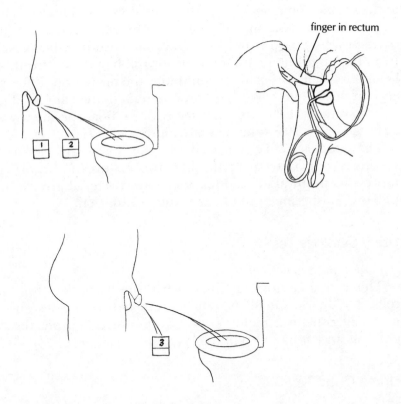

18. **Segmented urine culture for prostatitis.** Step 1: urinate about 2 ounces into cup 1, then, without stopping, urinate several ounces into cup 2. Step 2: Urinate into the toilet until your bladder is almost empty. Step 3: Your doctor will do a prostatic massage. Step 4: Now finish urinating into cup 3. This will empty the bladder and wash out the prostatic secretions released by the massage.

For men, how to provide a segmented urine sample: Your doctor may ask you not to ejaculate for two or three days before your appointment, since a slight inflammatory response normally occurs in the prostate after an ejaculation. This is very important if you want to get a quick and correct diagnosis. Then, on the day you are to give your urine sample, you should drink a lot of water before your appointment. A nurse will give you pre-labeled sterile containers with indications for how much urine should go into each one. The containers will be labeled in order VB^1, VB^2, VB^3, and EPS ("VB" standing for "voided bladder"). He or she will instruct you to release enough urine to cover the bottom of the first container (VB^1). Then a midstream specimen will be collected in the second container (VB^2). Next, the doctor will insert a gloved finger into your rectum and stroke your prostate six or seven times (*prostatic massage*) on either side, and if any prostate fluid emerges from the tip of the penis, a few drops will be placed directly on a laboratory slide for examination under the microscope. The presence of pus (white blood cells) and bacteria in the expressed prostatic secretions (EPS) can be detected. The final specimen will be collected in the VB^3 container (see illustration 17).

The samples will be sent to the lab for a standard culture and sensitivity test. Growth in the first two cultures (VB^1 and VB^2) represents urethral or bladder infections. Bacterial growth in the EPS or VB^3 specimens indicates prostatic infection.

Urine Cytology Test

Used in the diagnosis of cancer

This is a laboratory test in which urine is checked for cancer cells. The first urine of the day is preferred for this test, because it should contain a higher concentration of cells from the bladder wall since it has been in the bladder overnight.

Home Urine Tests

If you are doing intermittent self-start antibiotic therapy, it is important to check your urine for signs of infection before you begin taking antibiotics. This can easily be done with chemically treated dip sticks, which do not test for bacteria but confirm the presence of white blood cells (indicating that the body is fighting infection) and nitrites, by-products of bacterial invasion. To find out if you have an infection, urinate into a cup and immerse the dip stick in the urine for a few seconds. The chemically treated sticks will turn certain colors and can be compared to a color scale on the container. Dip sticks are manufactured by, among others, Boehringer Mannheim Diagnostics (9115 Hague Rd., Indianapolis, IN 46250) and the Ames Co. (P.O. Box 3100, Elkhart, IN 46515) and can be purchased at most pharmacies.

URODYNAMIC TESTS

Urodynamic tests attempt to reproduce the symptoms of voiding dysfunction as closely as possible, to pinpoint whether dysfunction is caused by the failure to store urine properly or to empty it completely. These tests are designed to evaluate changes in volume, flow, and pressure inside the bladder and urethra, as well as the strength of the pelvic muscles.

Cystometrogram

Used in the diagnosis of incontinence and prostate enlargement

In this test, also referred to as *cystometry,* two very small catheters are inserted through the urethra into the bladder. One fills the bladder with either water or carbon dioxide gas, and the other, attached to an electronic monitor, records changes in pressure inside the bladder as it fills and empties.

Uroflow

Used in the diagnosis of incontinence and prostate enlargement

The uroflow exam, also called uroflowmetry, measures your urine flow rate over a period of time and shows the efficiency of bladder emptying. For this test, you will be asked to come to your appointment with a full bladder. When the test begins, you will urinate into a special toilet. The rate at which the urine is excreted will be measured (in milliliters per second) on a graph. This test is useful in identifying urethral obstruction or an unusual pattern in voiding, and in evaluating the success or failure of drug therapy and surgery.

Residual Urine Test

Used in the diagnosis of prostate enlargement and other conditions in which urine may be retained in the bladder

This test will show if the bladder is emptying normally. After the uroflow exam (see page 291) is completed, a catheter will be inserted into the bladder and any remaining urine will be drained and measured.

Urethral Pressure Profile

Used in the diagnosis of stress incontinence and prostate enlargement

The urethral pressure profile (UPP) measures the changes in urethral pressure under a variety of conditions. This test is useful in assessing how well the urethra stays closed during bladder filling and during certain maneuvers such as coughing, straining, etc. (Continence is maintained when the pressure in the bladder is less than or equal to the pressure of the urethral sphincter muscle. Incontinence, as well as voluntary urination, results when the pressure in the bladder *exceeds* the pressure in the urethra.) In this test, two balloon-tipped catheters are inserted into the bladder, with a sensor on each tip. Each catheter is then withdrawn at a constant speed along the entire length of the urethra. As the sensor passes through the urethra, it senses changes of pressure in the urethral wall, and the result, the urethral pressure profile, is printed on a graph.

Electromyography

Used in the diagnosis of stress, reflex, and overflow incontinence

An electromyogram (EMG) is a recording, on a graph or a screen, of the contraction of the muscles surrounding the urethra (the pelvic muscles). In this test, electrical sensors are placed on the perineum, and the activity in the muscles is measured while the bladder is being filled with water, and then while it is emptying. This test determines whether the bladder and sphincter are working in sync, or if they are contracting and relaxing out of sync, causing bladder-sphincter dyssynergia (dis-coordination).

Videourodynamics

Used in the diagnosis of stress, urge, reflex, and overflow incontinence, and prostate enlargement

In addition to VCRs, video games, and video matchmaking, we also have videourodynamics. If you have complicated incontinence, your doctor may request these highly specialized studies, usually available only at incontinence centers or major universities. This technique combines the visual capabilities of video technology with the urodynamic procedures described above to provide instantaneous visualization of the urinary tract—kind of like a moving X-ray.

Voiding Cystourethrogram (VCUG)

Used in the diagnosis of cystitis and incontinence

In this test, a catheter is inserted into your bladder and the bladder is then filled with an opaque liquid that shows up on X-ray. When you have a strong desire to urinate, the catheter is removed and you urinate into a special toilet. While you are voiding, an X-ray or a videotape will be made. This test reveals the shape and capacity of the bladder, whether urine backs up into the ureters, the efficiency of storage and emptying, and if there is urine left in the bladder after voiding.

DRUG GLOSSARY

There are two types of drugs: generic and brand name. Generic drugs contain the same active ingredients as their brand-name counterparts and must also be identical in terms of strength, dosage, and form—i.e., pill, liquid, or injection—but the base in which they are prepared may be somewhat different. For example, the generic may contain sugar or artificial colors and may dissolve faster or slower than a brand name. Generic drugs are generally cheaper than brand-name drugs. *The Pill Book* (see Resources at the end of this section) recommends that you know the following before you take any medication:

- how long it will be before you should see results;
- how long you should take the drug;
- if you can drink alcohol while taking the drug;
- if the drug can safely be combined with other drugs you are taking (including over-the-counter medications);
- what time of day the drug should be taken for maximum benefit;
- which side effects to report; and
- if there is a less expensive, but equally effective, form of the drug that you could take.

If you are taking any drug for a long time, be sure that you are aware of the dangers of overuse and abuse of the drug. Ask your doctor or pharmacist for a list of long-term side effects and more serious problems that can develop or consult the *Physicians' Desk Reference*. Knowing the answers to these questions can help your medication be more effective and safer.

The list below includes only drugs that are commonly used in treating bladder disorders and their common side effects. Other effects can occur. If you need more detailed information on these drugs, ask your doctor or pharmacist, or consult one of the books listed under Resources at the end of the section.

The drugs in this index are listed in families, in alphabetical order under the family name. Within each family (in boldface type), the generic name is given first and the brand names follow in parentheses. Only drugs that are commonly used to treat bladder disorders are included here. If you are looking for a specific drug and don't know which family it is in, you will have to look at the ones listed at the beginning of each family or subgroup within a family. If the drug you are looking for is not here, that does not mean it is not prescribed but probably that it is less frequently prescribed.

ADRENERGIC DRUGS

Adrenergic drugs mimic the action of epinephrine, a hormone made in the adrenal gland and other tissues that affects the activity of muscles. There are two types of adrenergic drugs: *alpha blockers*, which relax smooth muscles, especially the smooth muscles of the bladder neck and urethra; and *alpha agonists*, which stimulate smooth muscles to work more efficiently.

Alpha agonists

ephedrine sulfate (Sudafed), phenylpropanolamine hydrochloride (Ornade, Dexatrim)
Prescribed for: incontinence. These drugs stimulate smooth-muscle activity of the bladder neck and urethra. Although many are potent prescription drugs, alpha agonists are the main ingredient of some over-the-counter nose drops, allergy and cold medications, hemorrhoid preparations, and diet pills as well.

Common side effects: may cause urinary retention, especially in cases of prostate enlargement; may increase prostate enlargement (especially Ornade and Dexatrim) or may cause rapid heartbeat, jumpiness, insomnia, or high blood pressure.

Adverse drug interactions: These drugs should not be taken in conjunction with antidepressants, high blood pressure medications, or drugs used to treat depression such as Marplan, Nardil, or Parnate.

Alpha blockers

phentolamine (Regitine), prazosin hydrochloride (Minipress), terazosin (Hytrin), phenoxybenzamine (Dibenzyline)
Prescribed for: urinary retention caused by an enlarged prostate. These drugs are also used for other conditions that affect the function of the sphincter muscles of the urethra such as interstitial cystitis, urethral syndrome, and prostatodynia when other treatments have failed.

Common side effects: fatigue, diarrhea, dizziness, or dramatic drop in blood pressure on standing (sometimes described as "you stand up, your blood doesn't"), drowsiness, depression, fluid retention, nasal stuffiness, heart palpitations, inhibition of ejaculation. For many people, the initial effects of these drugs can be severe. You can minimize them by taking the first dose at bedtime after a substantial meal. These effects usually diminish to more tolerable levels after a few days or a few weeks.

More serious effects: phenoxybenzamine is known to cause cancer in laboratory animals and thus should not be taken over the long term.

ANALGESICS

Analgesics are drugs that relieve pain by interfering with the transmission of nerve impulses. Non-narcotic bladder analgesics and antispasmodics act directly on the bladder lining, while narcotic analgesics act on the central nervous system. Neither of these two types of analgesics reduces bacterial growth or inflammation; they just make you more comfortable.

Narcotic analgesics

acetaminophen (Tylenol, Percocet, Percodan, Dilaudid) with aspirin or Codeine, meperidine (Demerol)

Narcotic analgesics are drugs that relieve pain by depressing nerve activity in the central nervous system. Formerly most narcotics were derived from opium, but today there are a number of synthetic narcotic drugs as well, which are also habit-forming when taken over the long term.

Occasionally prescribed for: interstitial cystitis, prostate, and bladder cancer.

Side effects: headache, dry mouth, dizziness, drowsiness, sleep, loss of appetite, nausea, constipation.

More serious effects: decreased coordination, shallow breathing, urinary retention, hallucinations, disorientation, flushing of face and neck, rash, increased heart rate, lower libido, anemia, jaundice, decrease in blood sugar.

Adverse drug interactions: these drugs should *not* be taken with alcohol, other tranquilizers, sleeping pills, or antidepressants. Narcotics can enhance the effects of these drugs and lead to stupor, coma, and even death.

Symptoms of overdose: difficulty in breathing, pupils narrowed to a "pinpoint," irregular breathing including cessation of breathing (apnea) for up to a minute, lowered blood pressure and weakening, irregular heart rate, stupor, convulsions, coma.

Use in pregnancy: should not be used.

Non-narcotic analgesics

phenazopyridine hydrochloride (Azodine, Azo-Standard, Baridium, Di-Azo, Phenazodine, Pyridiate, Pyridium)

This drug soothes the irritated bladder lining, reducing both pain and frequency.

Prescribed for: cystitis, interstitial cystitis, prostatitis, prostatodynia.

Side effects: will turn urine orange.

More serious effects: jaundice, anemia, nausea.

These drugs should not be used by people with kidney disease.

ANTIBIOTICS

There are numerous families of antibiotics which can be grouped together because of similar chemical structure and mode of action. Some of them will kill bacteria, while others, classified as antiseptics, merely disturb the bacteria's growth cycle and suppress growth.

The common side effects of antibiotics include loss of appetite, nausea, vomiting, stomach cramps, diarrhea, colitis, drowsiness, dizziness, headache, chills, fever, dry mouth, rash, hives, joint pain, temporary hair loss, and yeast infections. Not all of these physical side effects appear with all antibiotics, but most of them can occur with any of the drugs listed in this section.

More serious effects: shortness of breath, anaphylaxis (strong allergic reaction).

aminoglycosides (Gentamicin, Tobramycin, Amikacin)

These drugs are used for serious infections and are effective against most bacteria affecting the urinary tract. They are poorly absorbed when taken by mouth and are usually given intravenously.

Prescribed for: serious urinary tract infections and acute bacterial prostatitis (ABP).

Serious side effects: temporary or permanent damage to hearing and to the kidneys.

These drugs should be used with caution by people with kidney problems.

Use during pregnancy: possible loss of hearing in the fetus.

erythromycin (E-Mycin, E.E.S., Eramycin, Erythrocin, Robimycin, Wyamycin)

Erythromycin is an antibiotic that is effective against streptococcus and staphylococcus gonococcus bacteria. Since erythromycin is processed by the liver, people with decreased liver function should be carefully monitored while using it.

Prescribed for: chronic bacterial prostatitis (CBP) and urethritis caused by sexually transmitted diseases.

Adverse drug interactions: If you are taking high doses of **theophylline,** an asthma medication, erythromycin can increase its effects. This can cause theophylline toxicity, which can be serious and even fatal in elderly people.

The E-Mycin brand of this drug is specially coated to lessen stomach irritation.

Erythromycin is known to be more effective when the pH of the bloodstream and bladder are more alkaline (pH of 7 or higher), therefore alkalizing the urine by taking a little baking soda could be helpful. If you have high blood pressure, consult your doctor before taking baking soda.

Side effects: general antibiotic side effects.

Use in pregnancy: should not be used.

nitrofurantoin (Furadantin, Macrodantin, Nitrex, Furalan, Furan)

This drug is best taken with food or milk to prevent stomach pain, intestinal irritation, nausea, or diarrhea.

Prescribed for: cystitis.

Side effects: general antibiotic side effects.

More serious effects: difficulty in breathing, asthma, jaundice.

Nitrofurantoin should not be taken by people who have kidney disease or over a long-term period by people who have lung disease.

The effectiveness of this drug is enhanced when the blood and urine are acidic (pH of 6 or lower), so acidifying the urine by drinking *moderate* amounts of acidic juices such as cranberry and citrus might be useful.

Use during pregnancy: may cause fetal blood problems.

penicillin (Penicillin VK), ampicillin (Omnipen), amoxicillin (Amoxil), carbenicillin (Geocillin)

These drugs are best taken on an empty stomach.

Prescribed for: cystitis, gonorrhea, chronic bacterial prostatitis.

Side effects: general antibiotic side effects, especially digestive problems, yeast infections, allergic reactions.

More serious effects: anemia, allergic reactions.

Use during pregnancy: thought to be safe.

probenecid (Benemid)

A derivative of benzoic acid often used in conjunction with penicillin to boost its effectiveness when prescribed for gonorrhea.

cephalosporin: cephalexin (Keflex), cefadroxil (Duricef), cephradine (Anspor, Velosef), cefaclor (Ceclor), cefataxime (Rocefin)

Prescribed for: cystitis and prostatitis.

Side effects: general antibiotic side effects.

More serious effects: colitis (inflammation of the lining of the colon) and other digestive problems.

Cephalosporins are related to penicillin, so if you are allergic to penicillin, you may also have a sensitivity to these drugs. These drugs should not be taken by people who have serious kidney problems. Cephalosporins are most effective when taken between meals, but can be taken with food if serious stomach distress is experienced. Cefataxime is given in an injection or intravenously.

Use during pregnancy: thought to be safe.

quinolones: nalidixic acid (NegGram), cinoxacin (cinobac); fluoroquinolones: Norfloxacin (Noroxin), ciprofloxacin (Cipro)

Prescribed for: cystitis, prostatitis, and kidney infections.

Side effects: general antibiotic side effects.

Use during pregnancy: safety not established.

ANTICHOLINERGIC DRUGS

The drugs in this group relax the bladder muscle and decrease the intensity of bladder contractions, diminishing frequency by delaying the desire to urinate.

oxybutynin chloride (Ditropan), propantheline bromide (Norpanth, Probanthene), dicyclomide (Bentyl)

Prescribed for: reflex incontinence, incontinence caused by uninhibited bladder contractions.

Side effects: blurred vision, headache, dizziness, drowsiness, fatigue, decreased sweating, nausea, nasal congestion, constipation, fever, loss of taste, heart palpitations, bloating, rash, weakness.

More serious effects: difficulty in urination or urinary retention, insomnia, erectile dysfunction.

These drugs should not be taken by people with urinary obstruction from prostate enlargement or other conditions, glaucoma, severe colitis, intestinal obstruction, or asthma. When administered in high temperatures, the effects can be intensified, so caution should be used in such situations.

Elderly people with kidney or liver disease should only use anticholinergic drugs under close supervision. If diarrhea develops, call your physician because this could be a symptom of intestinal obstruction.

Adverse drug interactions: these drugs may intensify the effects of antihistamines, antidepressants, tranquilizers, and narcotics.

These drugs are best absorbed in an acid environment, so avoid taking them at the same time as antacids, calcium, or baking soda—wait at least two hours after taking one before taking the other.

ANTIDEPRESSANTS

These antidepressants have a sedative effect and may work by interfering with the activity of norepinephrine and serotonin, two substances that promote nerve activity, in the nervous system.

imipramine (Tofranil), nortriptyline (Pamelor, Aventyl), desipramine (Norpramin), protriptyline (Vivactil), amitriptyline (Amitrip, Elavil, Emitrip, Endep, SK-Amitriptyline), doxepin hydrochloride (Sinequan), trazadone (Desyrel)

Prescribed for: interstitial cystitis, incontinence.

Side effects: dry mouth, blurred vision, constipation, rash, fatigue, loss of appetite, nausea, changes in blood pressure (high and low), edema, skin sensitivity to sunlight, and others.

More serious effects: urinary retention, disorientation, hallucinations, anxiety, restlessness, insomnia, tingling and numbness in extremities, seizures, loss of libido, depression of bone marrow function, depressed liver function, and others.

People with seizures, urinary retention, glaucoma, heart problems, thyroid overactivity, schizophrenia, diabetes, and other conditions should use these drugs with caution.

Monoamine oxidase (MAO) inhibitors

Commonly referred to as MAO inhibitors, these drugs prevent the breakdown of monoamines, thus increasing the amount of amines, substances that stimulate the central nervous system. It is not clear how these drugs mediate depression, or how they work in reducing bladder pain.

isocarboxazid (Marplan), phenelzine (Nardil), tranylcypromine (Parnate)

Prescribed for: depression.

Side effects: low blood pressure, headache, dizziness, constipation, restlessness, edema, fatigue, dry mouth, blurred vision, loss of appetite, rash.

More serious effects: memory impairment, insomnia, tremors, digestive disruption, and, occasionally, urinary retention.

Adverse drug reactions: the following drugs should *not* be taken while taking MAO inhibitors: central nervous system depressants, amphetamines, methyldopa, levodopa, dopamine, epinephrine, norepinephrine, tryptophane. In addition, avoid foods high in tryptophane and those high in tyramine, especially some cheeses (Cheddar, Camembert, Stilton, Brie, Emmentaler, and Gruyère), beer, wine, pickled herring, chicken livers. These drugs should be discontinued for about ten days before having general anesthesia. People with kidney or liver disorders and congestive heart failure should not take MAO inhibitors.

ANTIHISTAMINES

Histamines are potent substances that are released in the blood-stream in response to the ingestion or internal formation of certain substances, and cause an inflammatory response where they settle. Antihistamine drugs are not able to stop the formation of histamines, but they can counteract their effect by interfering with the ability of histamines to attach themselves to their target sites—a mechanism known as *competitive binding*.

Prescription antihistamines

azatadine maleate (Optimine), brompheniramine maleate (Brombay), terfenadine (Seldane), tripelennamine hydrochloride (PBZ)

Prescribed for: interstitial cystitis, urethral syndrome, prostatodynia.

Side effects: drowsiness, dry mouth, dizziness, disturbed coordination, fatigue, restlessness, headache, nasal stuffiness, sensitivity to sunlight, and others.

More serious effects: urinary frequency, difficult urination, urinary retention, convulsions, anemia, heart palpitations, tightness in the chest.

People who should not use antihistamines are those who have prostate enlargement or other obstruction of the bladder neck, asthma, glaucoma, or ulcers.

Adverse drug interactions: if you are taking MAO inhibitors, you should not take antihistamines.

Non-prescription antihistamine

benadryl (Sudafed, Actifed)
This drug is the most frequently used over-the-counter antihistamine.

ANTI-INFLAMMATORY DRUGS

Non-steroidal anti-inflammatory drugs are commonly used in arthritis, gout, and other inflammatory diseases. These drugs reduce inflammation and have a soothing analgesic effect.

Anti-inflammatories

naproxen (Anaprox, Naprosyn), piroxicam (Feldene), ibuprofen (Advil, Nuprin, Motrin)
Prescribed for: interstitial cystitis, urethral syndrome, prostatitis, prostatodynia.
Side effects: dry mouth, constipation, heartburn, stomach pain, nausea and diarrhea, headache, dizziness, lightheadedness, rash, hearing or visual disturbances, edema, heart palpitations (rarely), drowsiness.
People taking sulfa drugs or probenecid should exercise caution, since these drugs can prolong the effects of naproxen. Everyone who takes the drug for an extended period should have periodic blood tests.

ANTISPASMODICS

hyoscyamine (Cystospaz), hyoscyamine sulfate (Cystospaz-M, Anaspaz)
Hyoscyamine relaxes smooth muscles and inhibits spasms of the smooth muscle of the bladder and urethra. These drugs should not be taken by people with sensitivity to atropine-like drugs or those who have heart problems or glaucoma.

Prescribed for: interstitial cystitis, urethral syndrome, prostato-dynia, cystitis.

Side effects: drowsiness, dry mouth, skin sensitivity to sunlight, constipation, urinary retention.

More serious effects: increased heart rate, dizziness, blurred vision. *If these effects occur, the drug should be discontinued immediately.*

(Urised)

Urised is a combination of urinary antiseptics, atropine sulfate (an extract of belladonna), and hyoscyamine. It also contains methylene blue, which will turn the urine blue or green, depending on how acid (blue) or alkaline (green) it is. Both atropine and hyoscyamine can be toxic in high doses.

Prescribed for: cystitis, interstitial cystitis, urethral syndrome, prostatodynia.

Side effects: the same as for Cystospaz.

More serious effects: severe dry mouth, rapid pulse, dizziness, blurred vision, and urinary retention. *If any of these effects occur, the drug should be discontinued immediately.*

flavoxate hydrochloride (Urispas)

This synthetic antispasmodic drug calms spasms of the bladder muscle and urethra. It is similar in activity and indications to the other drugs in this group. Urispas should not be used by people with obstruction of the urethra from prostate enlargement or other conditions, intestinal obstruction, or glaucoma.

(Pyridium Plus)

This drug is **Pyridium** with the addition of the barbiturate **butabarbital,** a sedative.

Prescribed for: cystitis, interstitial cystitis, prostatitis, prostatodynia.

Side effects: drowsiness, dizziness, nausea, vomiting, diarrhea, difficulties in breathing, rash, orange urine.

More serious effects: anemia, jaundice.

Adverse drug reactions: may increase the effect of **valproic acid (Depakene),** an anticonvulsant medication; alcohol may intensify the effect of this drug. Butabarbital is mildly hypnotic and can be habit-forming.

ANTIVIRAL DRUGS

acyclovir (Zovirax)

Acyclovir is an antiviral drug that can help control or prevent new eruptions of the herpes simplex virus. The drug works by intervening with the DNA synthesis of the virus. It can be used as an ointment (on skin but not in eyes, mouth, or vagina) or taken orally or intravenously.

Prescribed for: urethritis caused by herpes simplex.

Side effects: rash, headache, nausea, dizziness, loss of appetite.

More serious effects: insomnia, heart palpitations, menstrual irregularities, depression, hair loss, muscle cramps, acne, blood clots.

HEPARIN-LIKE DRUGS

sodium pentosanpolysulfate (Elmiron)

Heparin, a sugar-based substance manufactured in the liver, helps to prevent blood clots and is also found in significant quantities in the thin mucous layer of the bladder lining. Elmiron is a synthetic drug, with many properties similar to those of heparin, that has been employed in helping to restore or reinforce the bladder lining.

Prescribed for: interstitial cystitis.

Side effects: diarrhea, transient hair loss, bleeding disorders.

People who have bleeding ulcers or other bleeding disorders should not take Elmiron.

HORMONES

estrogen

Estrogen is a key factor in the development and healthy functioning of the female urinary and reproductive systems. As women enter menopause, the availability of estrogen to these organs decreases, and in some women, lowered estrogen levels affect the tissues of the vagina, causing thinning and dryness of the vaginal walls, while urethral tissues may become brittle and less elastic. Although the dosage of hormone-like drugs is considerably lower in hormone replacement therapy (HRT) than it is in birth control pills, the same drugs are used for both and have similar risks.

Occasionally prescribed for: incontinence, interstitial cystitis, urethral syndrome. Most urologists don't feel the need to prescribe systemic hormones (estrogen or an estrogen-progestagin combination) for bladder or urethral problems and only prescribe a low-dose vaginal cream containing only estrogen or an estrogen patch. The cream can be rubbed on the urethral opening and vaginal walls. This method of administration provides lower exposure, with some of the cream being absorbed through the vaginal walls into the bloodstream. Some women find that the estrogen seems to help, and some get no relief at all.

In general, women taking the Pill have lower risks of ovarian and endometrial (uterine) cancer, but increased risks of high blood pressure and strokes. The controversy over the risks of breast cancer in women taking HRT is far from settled. Some studies show increased risks of breast cancer for women taking HRT and other studies don't.

Side effects: weight gain, edema, breast growth or tenderness, nausea, stomach cramps, jaundice, permanent colasma (skin discoloration), loss of hair, increase in body hair, eye changes that can affect the fit of contact lenses, headache, dizziness.

More serious effects: migraine headaches, depression, loss of interest in sex (libido), varicose veins, increased risk of cancer of the cervix, vagina, and liver, gallbladder disease, heart disease, lung disease, high blood pressure, stroke, accelerated growth of fibroids.

If you are taking estrogens and develop any of the following conditions, *call your doctor:*

- severe abdominal pain
- severe chest pain, cough, shortness of breath
- severe headache, dizziness, weakness, numbness
- eye problems (vision loss or blurring), speech problems
- severe leg pain (in calf or thigh)
- unusual uterine bleeding

MUSCLE RELAXANTS

diazepam (Valium)

Valium acts directly on the brain, suppressing certain activity of the hypothalamus, relaxing muscles, and producing a sedative effect.

Prescribed for: certain types of incontinence, interstitial cystitis, urethral obstruction from prostate enlargement, muscle spasm, or other causes.

Side effects: drowsiness, fatigue, diminished muscle coordination, headache, rash, slurred speech, constipation, low blood pressure.

More serious effects: blurred vision, confusion, depression, incontinence, urinary retention, jaundice, lowered libido, tremor.

Adverse drug reactions: Valium should *not* be mixed with alcohol and other central nervous system drugs.

People who have epilepsy should be monitored carefully while taking this drug. Discontinuing the drug abruptly can cause severe withdrawal symptoms. Valium may be habit-forming.

Use during pregnancy: Valium may cause fetal malformations during early pregnancy.

SULFA DRUGS

Sulfa drugs have long been relied upon in the treatment of urinary tract infections. Today, they are still used alone, or in combination with trimethoprim. People who take sulfa drugs for prolonged periods should have periodic liver function tests. Those who have kidney disease should *not* take sulfa drugs, and those who have liver problems should have periodic liver-function tests.

sulfamethoxazole (Gamazole, Gantanol, Gantanol DS, Urobak)

Prescribed for: cystitis, chronic bacterial prostatitis, and acute bacterial prostatitis.

Side effects: general antibiotic side effects.

Drug interactions: symptoms of overdose are produced when taken with blood thinners, drugs to treat diabetes, methotrexate (chemotherapy drug), aspirin-like drugs, phenytoin, or probenecid. Becomes less effective when taken with large doses of vitamin C, and with para-aminobenzoic acid (PABA), a constituent of folic acid.

Adverse drug interaction: sulfamethoxazole may increase the effects of aspirin, phenytoin, probenecid, phenylbutazone, and certain anticoagulants (blood thinners).

trimethoprim (Cotrim, Proloprim, Trimpex)

Trimethoprim binds to the folic acid in bacterial cells and inhibits their ability to function normally. It quickly achieves high levels in the urine.

Prescribed for: cystitis, chronic bacterial prostatitis, and acute bacterial prostatitis.

Side effects: general antibiotic side effects.

Adverse drug interaction: may increase the effects of phenytoin and other anticonvulsant medications, as well as Valium.

trimethoprim/sulfamethoxazole (Bactrim, Cotrim, Septra)

Side effects: general antibiotic side effects.

More serious effects: sensitivity to strong sunlight, swelling around eyes and soles of feet, jaundice, arthritis-like pain, changes in blood components, general feelings of ill health, unusual bruising, kidney damage.

sulfisoxazole (Azo-Gantrisin, Grantrisin)

In addition to sulfa, Azo-Gantrisin also contains phenazopyridine hydrochloride, most commonly known by the brand name **Pyridium** (see Non-narcotic analgesics).

This drug combines sulfamethoxazole and Pyridium.

Side effects: general antibiotic side effects.

tetracycline hydrochloride: oxytetracycline (Terramycin), tetracycline (Achromycin), doxycycline (Vibramycin), minocycline (Minocin)

Tetracycline, one of the most commonly used antibiotics, works by interfering with protein synthesis in bacterial cells. Because of its wide usage, many strains of bacteria have developed a resistance to it. This drug should not be taken by people with kidney or liver problems. With the exception of doxycycline, milk and other dairy products interfere with absorption, so they should be avoided when taking this drug.

Prescribed for: urethritis or prostatitis (caused by Chlamydia and mycoplasma), cystitis (rarely).

Side effects: general antibiotic side effects, but they can often be quite severe.

More serious effects: tetracycline can interfere with skeletal development in the fetus and in the development of tooth enamel in the fetus and children up to eight years old, and can result in discolored teeth in adulthood and retardation of skeletal development. The drug can also cause skin sensitivity to sunlight.

Adverse drug reactions: Aureomycin, Terramycin, Rondomycin, doxycycline, demeclocycline, and minocycline.

Use during pregnancy: should not be used because it may cause tooth discoloration and could stunt bone growth.

RESOURCES

Handbook of Nonprescription Drugs. 6th ed. Washington, D.C.: American Pharmaceutical Association, 1981.

Physicians' Desk Reference (PDR). Barbara B. Huff, ed. Oradell, NJ: Medical Economics Company. This book, said to be the most often stolen from libraries, contains the official description of more than 2,000 generic and brand name drugs from manufacturers (the information is in a form approved by the Food and Drug Administration). Rather than steal the book, you can probably buy last year's edition at medical bookstores for about $40.

The Pill Book. Lawrence D. Chilnick, ed. New York: Bantam Books, 1986. This excellent guide, in encyclopedia form, covers 1,600 of the most frequently prescribed drugs, including many that are used for bladder disorders. It is both cheaper and easier to read than the *PDR*, and from the layperson's perspective, is just about as informative. In addition to descriptions of drugs, *The Pill Book* contains information on how different types of drugs work in the body and on adverse drug interactions between different drugs and between drugs and food.

Taking Hormones and Women's Health: Choices, Risks and Benefits. The National Women's Health Network, 1325 G Street, N.W., Washington, DC, 20005. This readable, detailed booklet summarizes all of the latest studies on estrogen replacement therapy (ERT) and hormone replacement therapy (HRT). Send $5 for a copy.

GLOSSARY OF
UROLOGICAL TERMS

This glossary is designed to help you become familiar with the highly specialized vocabulary of urology. We have attempted wherever possible to define a term within the text where it first appears. If you do not find a term here, look in the index and check the first reference for a word. Some of these words are quite a mouthful. Therefore, we have provided an approximate phonetic pronunciation in parentheses for all but the most obvious words.

acetylcholine (a-set'-ul-co-leen) A substance that plays an important part in the transmission of nerve impulses in the parasympathetic nervous system, which controls, among other things, the operation of smooth muscles, including those of the bladder and urethra.

acid phosphatase (a'-cid fos'-fa-taze) An enzyme made in the prostate by both normal and cancerous cells. If prostate cancer has spread to other parts of the body, the cancerous cells will continue to manufacture acid phosphatase, and elevated levels of the substance can usually be detected by a blood test.

acute Sudden, severe, and intense, but brief, often used to describe the onset of symptoms.

Alzheimer's (Altz'-heim-erz) **disease** A degenerative brain disorder in which certain memory, speech, intellectual, and muscular functions, including those of the bladder, deteriorate.

androgen (an'-dro-gen) A class of hormones, including testosterone, produced mainly in the testicles, that promote the development and

311

growth of a man's sexual organs, including the prostate, and other characteristics of sexual maturation such as body hair, deepening voice, and sweat glands.

antibodies (an-tea-bod-ees) Protein substances produced in the body that have the unique capacity to bind to foreign substances, thereby incapacitating them.

anticholinergic (an'ti-co'-lin-urg-ic) A drug that interferes with the effects of acetylcholine.

antimicrobial (an'-ti-mi'-cro-bi-al) Interfering with or preventing the growth of bacteria.

antispasmodic (an'-ti-spaz'-mod-ic) **drug** A drug that lessens or eliminates spasms.

asymptomatic (a'-symp-to-mat'-ic) Not having any noticeable symptoms.

autoimmune (aw'-to-im-mune') A condition in which the body produces antibodies to its own tissues.

benign prostatic hyperplasia (hi-per-plas'-i-a) **(BPH)** Non-malignant growth of cells in the prostate gland. This excessive overgrowth of cells results in **benign prostatic hypertrophy (BPH),** the enlargement of the gland itself.

biofeedback A technique in which a person learns to consciously control involuntary responses such as heart rate, brain waves, and muscle contractions, by having these responses electronically monitored and noted through beeps, graphs, or on a computer screen. In terms of muscle development, the readout monitors and records progress.

bladder neck The place where the bladder muscle and the urethra meet.

bladder neck suspension operations Surgery to cure or reduce urinary incontinence. In this procedure, a needle passes surgical thread or sutures around the urethra and returns it, as much as possible, to its original position. The procedure was pioneered by Dr. Armand Peyrera, and modifications have been made by Drs. Burch, Stamey, Raz, and Marshall/Marchetti/Krantz.

bladder-sphincter dyssynergia (dis'-sin-ur'gee-a) Lack of coordination between the bladder muscle and the sphincter muscle of the urethra. In order for continence to be maintained, the bladder muscle must be relaxed while the sphincter remains tightly closed. In order for evacuation of urine to occur, the bladder muscle must contract while the sphincter muscle relaxes.

bladder training Exercises that focus on changing urinary habits and patterns. A person is encouraged to hold urine for increasingly longer periods of time, until the comfortable voiding interval is increased. This technique is used in the treatment of urge incontinence, interstitial cystitis, and urethral syndrome.

blood-prostate barrier The portion of the prostate that prevents substances of a certain pH from entering the prostate. This barrier effectively prevents most antibiotics from entering the prostate, making treatment of infections difficult.

bulbocavernosus (bul'-bo-cav'-er-no'-sus) **muscle** The muscle that surrounds the erectile tissue of the penis and clitoris (including the vagina). During sexual response, these muscles help produce erection by compressing the erectile tissue at the point of contact and preventing drainage of the greatly increased blood supply.

carcinoma (car'-ci-no'-ma) A malignant tumor arising in the epithelial, or top, layers of cells of the skin or mucous membranes.

carcinoma-in-situ (CIS) A cancerous tumor that is contained in one place (localized) and is generally curable.

catheter (cath'-e-ter) A small rubber or plastic tube used to drain urine from the bladder. Catheters for women are about 5 inches long and the ones used for men are about 15 inches long. Catheters used in urological procedures may have two or three channels through which evacuation of the bladder's contents can be monitored, and water, gas, or solutions containing drugs can be instilled into the bladder. An **indwelling catheter** is intended to be left in place for an extended period of time, perhaps permanently. The type most commonly used in the United States is the Foley catheter.

cholinergic (co'-lin-urg-ic) Fibers in the parasympathetic nervous system that release acetylcholine.

chronic In terms of disease, the opposite of acute. Continuing over a long time, without much change. Can also indicate a slow progression from one state to another.

congenital (con-gen'-i-tal) **abnormalities** An anatomical or functional problem that is present at birth. Often such problems remain for life, but sometimes they are outgrown or will disappear spontaneously.

continence (con'-ti-nence) The ability to hold urine until an appropriate time and place can be found to empty the bladder. In the past, continence also referred to the willful abstention from sexual activity.

contraindication (con'-tra-in'-di-ca'-shun) A condition that would make a certain form of treatment inappropriate or dangerous.

cystectomy (sis-tek'-to-mee) Removal of the bladder.

cystocele (sis'-to-seal) A hernia, or intrusion of the bladder into the vagina, usually caused when the vaginal muscles that support the bladder and urethra are stretched or damaged. Urine can pool in the sac that protrudes, becoming stagnant and serving as a convenient place for bacteria to grow. Women with cystoceles may have repeated bladder infections.

cystometry (sis-tom'-e-tree) (See Index of Diagnostic Tests.)

cystoplasty (sis'-to-plas'-tee) Partial removal, replacement, or recon-

313

struction of the bladder. In this procedure, most of the bladder is removed and a piece of bowel is *augmented* or *substituted* for the bladder. Urination takes place through the urethra.

cystoscope (sis-to-scope)   A long, thin, telescope-like instrument fitted with lenses and a fiber-optic light source that is small enough to be inserted through the urethra into the bladder. (See Index of Diagnostic Tests for information on the different procedures done with a cystoscope.)

cystourethrocele (sis-to-u-reeth-ro-seal)   A hernia or protrusion of the urethra and part of the bladder into the vagina (see **cystocele**).

dehydration (dee'-hi-dra'-shun).   A state that occurs when not enough fluid is present to fulfill the body's fluid needs. This state can occur through heavy sweating, excessive urination, or diarrhea, without proper fluid replacement. Severe dehydration is a dangerous condition that may damage the bladder, kidneys, and other organs, and can result in coma and even death.

detrusor (de-tru'-sor) **muscle**   The outer muscular layer of the bladder. Often referred to as the "bladder muscle."

detrusor hyperreflexia (de-tru'-sor hi-per-re-flex'-ee-a)   Hyperactivity or overactivity of the bladder muscle, caused by nerve impulses, often resulting in urge incontinence. Also called **detrusor instability.**

diabetes mellitus (dia'-be'-tes mel-lite'-us)   In this form of diabetes, the body does not produce enough insulin, a hormone produced in the pancreas that regulates the level of sugar (glucose) in the bloodstream and cells. The symptoms are extreme thirst, excessive urination, and an unusually strong appetite. The symptoms may often be brought under control by diet and exercise. Otherwise, daily medications or injections of insulin may be necessary.

dysuria (dis-ur'-ee-a)   Painful urination, most frequently caused by infection or inflammation, but it can also be caused by certain drugs. **Acute dysuria** refers to the sudden onset of painful urination.

endoscopic (en-do-scop'-ic) **procedure**   A procedure done through a tubelike instrument, such as a cystoscope, using a natural body opening such as the urethra, or an incision.

enuresis (in'-ur-ee'-sis)   Involuntary urination. This term is most often applied to bedwetting in children.

epidemiology (ep'-i-de-mee-ol'-o-gee)   The study of the sources, causes, prevalence, and distribution of diseases in the general population or within a certain population. An epidemiologist is someone who studies the interrelationships between these factors.

epinephrine (e-pi-nef-reen)   A hormone that causes blood vessels to contract.

fibrosis   The abnormal development of fibrous, or scar, tissue in an organ or tissue.

gerontologist (ge-ron-tol'-o-gist) An internist who specializes in the problems and diseases of the elderly.

glycosaminoglycans (GAG) (gly-co-sam-een-o-gly'-cans) This thin, filmy, sugar-based coating of the bladder, called GAG for short, is thought to protect the underlying layers from bacteria, toxic substances, and the acidic properties of urine. Some researchers also call this layer **mucin.**

heparin (hep'-a-rin) A sugar-based substance found in mast cells that plays a major role in preventing blood clotting under normal conditions. Sodium pentosanpolysulfate (Elmiron), a drug used in the treatment of interstitial cystitis, is chemically similar to heparin.

histamine (his'-ta-meen) A substance that is released from injured cells and plays a part in the inflammatory process.

Hunner's ulcer A large sore or ulcer that is occasionally seen in the bladders of people with interstitial cystitis. For a long time, the existence of these ulcers was considered the hallmark of interstitial cystitis, but since they are rarely seen, their presence is not considered necessary for a diagnosis of IC.

hysterectomy (his-ter-ek'-to-me) Removal of the uterus. If the entire uterus and cervix are removed, it is a **total hysterectomy.** If the cervix is left, it is a **subtotal hysterectomy.** If the entire uterus plus the tubes and ovaries are removed, it is a **total hysterectomy with salpingo-ovariectomy.** The ovaries should not be removed unless they are diseased or there is another compelling reason.

ileal conduit (ill'-e-al con'-du-it) The surgical diversion of the urine, using a bowel segment to conduct the urine to a stoma constructed in the lower abdomen. The urine then drains into a leg bag.

inflammation From the Latin word meaning "to flame within," inflammation is the response of tissue to damage or injury. Changes in the tissue during inflammation include dilation of blood vessels, increased blood flow, and swelling, resulting in pain, redness, heat, and if the injury is severe, a general feeling of illness.

intravesical (in-tra-ves'-i-cal) **pressure within** In urology, the term is often used to refer to the pressure inside the bladder (which is a sum of the pressure of its contents plus any additional pressure applied to it from outside, such as squeezing with abdominal muscles, coughing, sneezing, laughing, or any sudden movement).

introitus (in-troy'-tus) The entrance to the vagina or other canal in the body, such as the ear canal. Also called the vestibule, the introitus runs from the glans of the clitoris to the **fourchette** (foor-shet'), a membranous fold of tissue where the bases of the inner lips meet at the perineum. The **meatus,** or entrance to the urethra, is located in the introitus slightly above the vaginal opening.

lactobacillus acidophilus (lac'-to-ba-cil'-lus a-ci-do'-fil-us) A bacterium normally found in the intestines and vagina, that produces lactic acid during the fermentation of milk. The presence of normal quantities of this bacterium keeps yeast growth under control.

lamina propria The membranous tissue that separates the inner lining of the bladder from the bladder muscle.

laser surgery The word *laser* is an acronym for *l*ightwave *a*mplification by *s*timulated *e*mission of *r*adiation. A laser "gun" produces a highly concentrated, intense beam of radiation of only one wavelength. The neodymium-YAG laser is a "non-contact" laser that does not touch tissue and is potentially less damaging.

mast cells Cells in the connective tissue that contain both heparin and histamines. When mast cells degranulate, or break up, these substances are released into the surrounding tissue.

meatus (mee-a'-tus) An opening; in urology, the urethral opening located at the vagina in women and at the tip of the penis in men.

micturition (mick-tu-rish-un) A medical term for urination.

mucin (mu'-cin) (See **glycosaminoglycans.**)

mucopolysaccharide (mu-co-pol'-lee-sac'-ca-ride) A carbohydrate molecule found in the bladder lining, joints, and other parts of the body. Forming a gelatinous substance, these molecules help bind cells together.

neurology The study of the nervous system.

neurotransmitter (nu'-ro-trans'-mit-ter) A body chemical that facilitates the transmission of nerve impulses.

nocturia (nock-tur'-ee-a) Waking up at night to urinate.

norepinephrine (nor-e-pi-nef-reen) A hormone similar to epinephrine, which causes blood vessels to contract.

Parkinson's disease A degenerative disease of the nervous system characterized by tremor, weakness, and, eventually, rigidity. Many people with Parkinson's disease also develop reflex incontinence.

pelvic muscles The hammock, or sling, of muscles that support the pelvic organs. The pelvic muscles include the urogenital diaphragm and the pelvic diaphragm (levator ani muscle) in both women and men.

perineal route Cutting through the perineum in order to perform a surgical procedure.

perineometer (per-i-ne'-om-i-ter) The device originally invented by Dr. Arnold Kegel to measure the strength of pelvic muscle contractions.

perineum (pe-ri-ne'-um) The short bridge of flesh between the anus and the vagina in women and the anus and the base of the penis in men.

petechial (pe-te'-kee-al) **hemorrhages** Small broken blood vessels, or hemorrhages in the skin or mucous membranes.

pH (potential for Hydrogen) In chemistry, the pH value describes how acid or alkaline (basic) a substance is. The scale runs from 0 to 14, with 0 being very acid, 14 being very alkaline, and 7 being the neutral value. The values are expressed in logarithm, each number away from neutral being ten times more acidic or alkaline, i.e., pH 5 is ten times as acid as pH 6.

physiology (fiz'-ee-ol'-o-gee)   The study of the chemical and physical (or physiological) processes of an organism.

polyp (pa'-lip)   A tumor growing on a stalk. Sometimes found in the bladder neck, they are almost always benign.

prognosis (prog-no'-sis)   The prediction of the outcome of a condition or disease.

prostatic (pro-stat'-ic) **urethra**   The part of the male urethra that passes through the prostate gland.

prostatitis (pros'-ta-ti'-tis)   Infection, inflammation, pain, or discomfort in the prostate. Prostatic conditions include **acute bacterial prostatitis (ABP), chronic bacterial prostatitis (CBP), non-bacterial prostatitis (NBP),** and **prostatodynia.**

prostatodynia (pros'-tate-o-din'-i-a)   Pain or discomfort in the prostate, perineum, rectum, or bladder of unknown cause. This condition may actually be a mild version of interstitial cystitis.

psychosomatic (si'-co-so-mat'-ic)   The interrelationship of the body and the mind. This term pertains to illnesses said to be caused or greatly influenced by psychological or emotional factors. The concept of psychosomatic illnesses has been generally discredited in medicine, although it is possible for some disorders to have a psycho-emotional component.

pubococcygeus (pew-bo-cox-e-gee-us) **muscle**   Another name for the levator ani muscle, one of the pelvic muscles that hold the pelvic organs in place.

pyuria (pie-ur'-ee-a)   Pus in the urine, sometimes causing the urine to be cloudy.

renal (ree-nal) **pelvis**   The part of the kidney in which urine collects.

salpingo-ovariectomy (sal-pin'-go o-ver-ec'-to-me)   Surgical removal of the egg (Fallopian) tubes and the ovaries, often done in conjunction with a hysterectomy. There should be a compelling reason for the removal of the uterus, tubes, and ovaries.

self-intermittent catheterization   People who cannot urinate on their own use this procedure to drain the bladder every few hours. Even young children can be taught to catheterize themselves effectively.

serotonin (se-ro-tone'-in)   A substance found in the bloodstream, mucous membranes, and in **mast cells** that helps constrict blood vessels and has a major role in sleep and sensory perception. Serotonin cannot be made without the amino acid **tryptophane.**

spina bifida (spi'-na bif'-i-da)   A birth defect in which the spinal column does not close entirely, usually in the lower back. The spinal cord often protrudes through the hole, forming a spina bifida tumor.

stoma An artificially constructed outlet for urine or feces in the wall of the lower abdomen.

suprapubic (sou'-pra-pub'-ic) Above the pubic bone.

suprapubic aspiration (sou'-pra-pub'-ic as-pir-a'-shun) The removal of urine using a syringe and needle inserted into the bladder just above the pubic bone.

trabeculation (tra-bec'-u-la'-shun) As the prostate enlarges and begins to obstruct the urethra, the bladder muscle has to work harder to get the urine out, and irregular bands of thickened muscle tissue (trabeculations) develop in the bladder wall. In between these bands, the thinner areas of the bladder wall may pop out, forming little pouches or "cellules."

transitional epithelium (tranz-i'-shun-al ep'-i-the'-lee-um) The inner lining of the bladder, which is composed of three layers of cells: umbrella cells, so called because they are large and somewhat flattened, intermediate cells, and basal (or base) cells.

transurethral (trans'-u-ree'-thral) **resection (TUR)** An operation on the prostate done by passing a resectoscope through the urethra. Common procedures are **transurethral resection of the prostate (TURP) and transurethral resection of bladder tumor(s) (TURBT).**

trigone (try'-gone) An area of the bladder wall shaped like an upside-down triangle, with its base encompassing both ureters and the apex, or tip, lying near the bladder neck. The bladder nerves are more highly concentrated in this area.

trigonitis (try'-gone-i'-tis) A term that is sometimes used to describe bladder pain. Many urologists feel that this term is too vague to be meaningful.

tryptophane (trip'-to-fane') This essential (meaning that it is not manufactured in the body and therefore must be obtained from food) amino acid is the main building block of serotonin, a substance that helps transmit nerve impulses in the sympathetic nervous system, which controls the activity of smooth muscles. Some people think that foods high in tryptophane may irritate a sensitive bladder.

ureters Two very thin muscular tubes about 8 or 9 inches long that transport urine from the kidneys to the bladder.

urethral pressure profile (UPP) (See Index of Diagnostic Tests.)

urethral syndrome An uncertain and insubstantial diagnosis for a number of bladder conditions, including painful urination, urgency, and frequency.

urethrocele (u-reeth-ro-seal) A hernia in which part of the urethra presses on the vaginal wall.

urinary diversion Surgery in which the urine is diverted from the bladder, either to an internal reservoir constructed of a piece of bowel, or directly through a conduit to a stoma on the skin of the lower abdomen. Two different versions of urinary diversion are the **ileal conduit,** in which the urine passes through an artificially constructed tube of bowel, and the **Koch or Indiana pouch,** in which the urine is collected in an internal reservoir constructed from a piece of bowel.

urodynamic studies   Tests done in a urologist's office, designed to duplicate as nearly as possible the symptoms of incontinence in the way that you actually experience them. This set of tests includes cystometry, uroflowmetry, and urethral profilometry. (See Index of Diagnostic Tests for information on these tests.)

uroflowmetry   (u-ro-flo-me-tree)   (See Index of Diagnostic Tests.)

urogynecology   (u'-ro-gyn-e-col'-o-gee)   Urologists and gynecologists who have a special interest in the urinary disorders of women.

uterine prolapse   The uterus has slipped from its normal position and the cervix is closer to, or may protrude from, the vaginal opening.

vesicoureteral reflux   A condition in which urine backs up from the bladder through the ureters to the kidneys. If untreated, it can cause kidney damage.

vulvovaginal   (vul-vo-vag'-i-nal) **glands**   These tiny mucous-producing glands, also called Bartholin's glands, can be seen where the inner lips meet just below the vaginal opening by the perineum.

REFERENCES

Chapter 1: A New Day for Bladder Disorders

1. Whiting, J. W. M., and Child, I. L.: *Child Training and Personality: A Cross-cultural Study*. New Haven: Yale University Press, 1953, pp. 74–77.
2. Herman, J. R.: *Urology: A View Through the Rectospectroscope*. New York: Harper & Row, 1973, pp. 1–9.
3. Bryan, C., trans.: *Ancient Egyptian Medicine: The Papyrus Ebers*. Chicago: Ares Publishers, 1974.

Chapter 4: Incontinence

1. Walsh, P. C., Gittes, R. F., Perlmutter, A. D., and Stamey, T. A., eds.: "Urinary Incontinence in the Female," *Campbell's Urology*. Philadelphia: W. B. Saunders, 1987, p. 2681.
2. Jeter, K. F.: "Incontinence in the American home: A survey of 36,500 incontinent people," *J. Am. Geriatric Soc.* (in press).
3. Gartley, C. B., ed.: *Managing Incontinence*. Ottawa, IL: Jameson Books, 1985, p. 11.
4. International Continence Society Committee on Standardisation of Terminology: "The standardisation of terminology of lower urinary tract function," *Scand. J. Urol. Nephrol., Supplementum 114*, 1988, pp. 1–7.
5. *The Oxford English Dictionary*. Glasgow: Oxford University Press, 1971, compact edition, p. 1407.
6. Wein, A. J.: "Classification of neurogenic voiding dysfunction," *J. Urol.*, 125:605–609, 1981.
7. Blaivas, J. G., and Olsson, C. A.: "Stress incontinence: Classification and surgical approach," *J. Urol.*, 139:727, 1988.

8. Resnick, N. M., Yalla, S. V., and Laurino, E.: "The pathophysiology of urinary incontinence among institutionalized elderly persons," *N. Engl. J. Med.*, 320(1): 1–7, 1989.

9. Jeter, K. J., ed., *The HIP Report:* 5(4), 1987.

10. Perry, J., and Hullett, L. T.: "The bastardization of Dr. Kegel's exercises," Northeast Gerontological Society Meeting, New Brunswick, NJ, May 20, 1988.

11. Kegel, A. J.: "Early genital relaxation," *Obstet. & Gyn.*, 8(5):547, 1956.

12. Peattie, A. B., and Plevnik, S.: "Cones versus physiotherapy as conservative management of genuine stress incontinence," *J. Neurourol. Urodyn.*, 7(3):265, 1988.

13. Burgio, K. L., Whitehead, W. E., and Engel, B. T.: "Urinary incontinence in the elderly: Bladder/sphincter biofeedback and toileting skills training," *Ann. of Internal Med.*, 103: 507, 1988.

14. Wein, A. J.: "Lower urinary tract function and pharmacologic management of lower urinary tract dysfunction," *Urol. Clin. N. Am.*, 14(2):273–296, 1987.

15. Rud, T.: "The effects of oestrogens and gestagens on the urethral pressure profile in urinary continent and stress incontinent women," *Acta. Obstet. Gynecol. Scand.*, 59:265, 1980.

16. Stanton, S. L.: "Suprapubic approaches for stress and urge incontinence in women," Urinary Incontinence in Adults, NIH Consensus Development Conference, October 3–5, 1988, pp. 57–64.

17. Kelly, M. J., Knielsen, K., Bruskewitz, R., Boskamp, D., and Leach, G. E.: "A pre- and postoperative symptom analysis of patients undergoing the modified pereyra bladder neck suspension for stress urinary incontinence," (in press).

18. Scharf, M., *Waking Up Dry: How to End Bedwetting Forever.* Cincinnati: Writer's Digest Books, 1986.

19. Weider, D. J., and Hauri, P. J.: "Nocturnal enuresis in children with upper airway obstructions," *Int. J. Pediatr. Otorhinolaryngol.*, 9:173–182, 1985.

Chapter 5: Cystitis and Urethritis

1. Parsons, L. C.: "Protocol for the treatment of typical UTI: Criteria for antimicrobial selection," *Urol. (Suppl).*, 32(2):22–25, 1988.

2. Neu, H. C.: "Urinary tract infection in the 1980's," *Seminars in Urology*, 1(2):130–137, 1983.

3. C. M. Kunin, ed., *Detection, Prevention and Management of Urinary Tract Infections.* 4th ed., Philadelphia: Lea & Febiger, 1987, p. 98.

4. Gillenwater, J. Y., et al.: *Gillenwater's Adult and Pediatric Urology.* Chicago: Yearbook Medical Publishers, 1987, p. 247.

5. Kunin, C. M.: "The natural history of recurrent bacteria in schoolgirls," *N. Engl. J. Med.*, 282:1443–1448, 1970.

6. Elster, A. B., Lach, P. A., Roghmann, K. J., and McAnarney, E. R.: "Relationship between frequency of sexual intercourse and urinary tract infections in young women," *S. Med. J.*, 74(6):704–708, 1981.

7. Nicole, L. E., Harding, G. K. M., Preiksaitis, J., and Ronald, A. R.: "The

association of urinary tract infection with sexual intercourse," *J. Infect. Dis.*, 146(5):582, 1982.

8. Fihn, S. D., Latham, R. H., Roberts, P., Running, K., and Stamm, W. E.: "Association between diaphragm use and urinary tract infection," *JAMA*, 254:240–245, 1985.

9. Elster, et al., op. cit.

10. Fihn, et al., op. cit., p. 245.

11. Stamey, T. A., and Timothy, M. M.: "Studies of introital colonization in women with recurrent urinary infections. I: The role of vaginal pH," *J. Urol.*, 114:261, 1975.

12. Ofek, I., and Beachey, E. H.: "General Concepts and Principles of Bacterial Adherence in Animals and Man," in Beachey, ed., *Bacterial Adherence.* London: Chapman and Hall, 1980, pp. 1–29.

13. Corriere, J. N.: "Avoiding 'overkill' in diagnosis and treatment of lower urinary tract infections," *Urol. (Suppl.)*, 32(2):17–21, 1988.

14. Ibid.: 17–18.

15. Stamm, W. E., Counts, G. W., Running, K. R., et al.: "Diagnosis of coliform infection in acutely dysuric women," *N. Engl. J. Med.*, 304:956–958, 1986.

16. Fowler, J. E., Jr.: "Urinary tract infections in women," *Urol. Clin. N. Am.*, 13(4):263, 1986.

17. Kraft, J. K., and Stamey, T. A.: "The natural history of symptomatic recurrent bacteriuria in women," *Medicine*, 56:55–60, 1977.

18. Parsons, C. L.: "Protocol for treatment of typical urinary tract infection: Criteria for antimicrobial selection," *Urol. (Suppl.)*, 32(2), 1988.

19. Corriere, op. cit., p. 18.

20. Hatcher, R. A., et al.: *Contraceptive Technology*, New York: Irvington Publishers, 1986, p. 218.

21. Elster, et al., op. cit.

22. Foxman, B., and Frerichs, R. R.: "Epidemiology of urinary tract infections. II: Diet, clothing and urination habits," *Am. J. Pub. Health*, 75:1314–1328, 1985.

23. Fihn, et al., op. cit., p. 16.

24. Chan, R. C. Y., Reid, G., and Irvin, R. T.: "Competitive exclusion of uropathogens from human uroepithelial cells by lactobacillus whole cells and cell wall fragments," *Infect. Immun.*, 47(84), 1985.

25. Murry, M. T.: "Hydrastis canadensis (goldenseal)," *Phyto-Pharmica*, 1(2), 1987.

26. Andriole, V. T.: "Urinary tract infections in pregnancy," *Urol. Clin. N. Am.*, 2:485–598, 1975.

Chapter 6: The Painful Bladder Syndrome

1. Fall, M., Johansson, S. L., and Aldenborg, F.: "Chronic interstitial cystitis: A heterogenous syndrome," *J. Urol.*, 137:35, 1987.

2. Hunner, G. L.: "A rare type of bladder ulcer in women: Report of cases," *Trans. South. Surg. Gynecol.*, 27:247, 1914.

3. Held, P., Pauley, M., Hanno, P. M., and Wein, A. J., Urban Institute Survey

on Interstitial Cystitis, Workshop on Interstitial Cystitis, National Institutes of Health, Bethesda, MD, August 1987.

4. McDonald, H. P., Upchurch, W. E., and Artime, M.: "Bladder dysfunction in children caused by interstitial cystitis," *J. Urol.*, 80:354, 1958.

5. Held, et al., op cit.

6. Ruggieri, M. R., Hanno, P. M., and Levin, R. M.: "Nitrofurantoin is not a surface active agent in the rabbit urinary bladder," *Urol.*, 29(5):534, 1987.

7. Jokinen, E. J., Alfthan, O. S., and Oravisto, K. J.: "Antitissue antibodies in interstitial cystitis," *Clin. Exp. Immunol.*, 11:333, 1972.

8. Parsons, C. L., Schmidt, J. D., and Pollen, J. J.: "Successful treatment of interstitial cystitis with sodium pentosanpolysulfate," *J. Urol.*, 130:51, 1983.

9. Dixon, J. S., Holm-Bentzen, M., Gilpin, C. J., et al., "Electron microscopic investigation of the bladder urothelium and glycocalyx in patients with interstitial cystitis," *J. Urol.*, 135:621, 1986.

10. Messing, E. M., "Interstitial Cystitis and Related Syndromes," in Walsh, P. C., Gittes, R. F., Perlmutter, A. D., and Stamey, T. A., eds., *Campbell's Urology.* Philadelphia: W. B. Saunders, 1986, pp. 1070–1092.

11. Dixon, J. S., and Hald, T., "Morphological Studies of the Bladder Wall in Interstitial Cystitis," in George, N. J. R., and Gosling, J. A., eds., *Sensory Disorders of the Bladder and Urethra.* Berlin: Springer-Verlag, 1986, pp. 63–70.

12. Hanno, P. M., Levin, R. M., Moson, F. C., Teuscher, C., Zhou, Z. Z., Ruggieri, M., Whitmore, K. E., and Wein, A. J., "Diagnosis of Interstitial Cystitis," *J. Urol.*, 143:278, 1990.

13. Hanno, P. M., Workshop on Interstitial Cystitis, National Institute of Kidney and Digestive Diseases, National Institutes of Health, Bethesda, MD, August 28–29, 1987.

14. Fall, M., Workshop on Interstitial Cystitis, National Institute of Kidney and Digestive Diseases, National Institutes of Health, Bethesda, MD, August 28–29, 1987.

15. Hanno, P. M., and Wein, A. J., "Interstitial cystitis, I & II," *Am. Urol. Ass. Update Series*, 6(9–10), 1987.

16. Sant, G. R., "Interstitial cystitis: Pathophysiology, clinical evaluation, and treatment," *Urol. Annual*, 3, 1989. p. 171.

17. Dunn, M., Ramsden, P. D., Roberts, J. B. M., et al., "Interstitial cystitis, treated by prolonged bladder distention," *Br. J. Urol.*, 49:641, 1977.

18. Fall, M., "Conservative management of chronic interstitial cystitis: Transcutaneous electrical nerve stimulation and transurethral resection," *J. Urol.*, 133:774, 1985.

19. Shanberg, A. M., Baghdassarian, R., and Tansey, L. A., "Treatment of interstitial cystitis with the neodymium-YAG laser," *J. Urol.*, 134:885, 1985.

20. Sant, G. R., "Intravesical 50% dimethyl sulfoxide (RIMSO-50) in treatment of interstitial cystitis," *Urol. (Suppl.)* 29(4):6, 1987.

21. Ibid., p. 19.

22. Messing, E. M., and Stamey, T. A., "Interstitial cystitis: Early diagnosis, pathology and treatment," *Urol.*, 12:381, 1978.

23. Hanno, P. M., Buehler, J., and Wein, A. J., "Use of amitriptyline in the treatment of interstitial cystitis," *J. Urol.*, 141:846, 1989.

24. Wein, A. J., "Pharmacologic treatment of lower urinary tract dysfunction in the female patient," *Urol. Clin. N. Am.,* 12(2), 1985.
25. Fall, M.: "Conservative management of chronic interstitial cystitis: Transcutaneous electrical nerve stimulation and transurethral resection," *J. Urol.,* 133:774–778, 1985.
26. Gillespie, L.: *You Don't Have to Live with Cystitis!* New York: Rawson Associates, 1986, p. 244.
27. Catalona, W. J.: "Bladder Cancer," in J. Y. Gillenwater, et al., eds., *Gillenwater's Adult and Pediatric Urology.* Chicago: Yearbook Medical Publishers, 1987, p. 1024.
28. Mindell, E.: *Earl Mindell's New and Revised Vitamin Bible.* New York: Bantam Books, 1985, p. 80.
29. McGuire, E. J., Lytton, B., and Cornog, J. L., "Interstitial cystitis following colocystoplasty," *Urol.,* 2:28, 1973.
30. Edward Messing, personal communication, September 1989.

Chapter 7: Prostate Problems

1. Stamey, T. A.: *Pathogenesis and Treatment of Urinary Tract Infections.* Baltimore: Williams & Wilkins, 1980.
2. Drach, G. W., Meares, E. M., Jr., Fair, W. R., Stamey, T. A., et al.: "Classification of benign disease associated with prostatic pain: Prostatitis or prostatodynia?" *J. Urol.,* 120:26, 1981.
3. Fair, W. R., Couch, J., and Wehner, N.: "Prostatic antibacterial factor: Identity and significance," *Urol.,* 7:169–177, 1976.
4. Shortliffe, L. M. D.: "Evaluation and Management of Prostatitis," in W. R. Fair, ed., *Mediguide to Urology.* New York: Lawrence Delacorte Pub., 1989.
5. Baert, L., and Leonard, A.: "Chronic bacterial prostatitis: 10 years of experience with local antibiotics," *J. Urol.,* 140:755, 1988.
6. Schaeffer, A. J., Schmiel, J. S., and Grayhack, J. S.: "Natural history of prostatic inflammation," *J. Urol.,* 133(4,2):207A, 1984.
7. *Benign Prostatic Hyperplasia,* National Institute of Diabetes and Digestive and Kidney Diseases, NIH Publication No. 89-3012, December 1988.
8. Blaivas, J. G.: "Pathophysiology and differential diagnosis of benign prostatic hypertrophy," *Urol. (Suppl.),* 33(6):5, 1988.
9. Schafer, W., Rubben, H., Noppeney, R., and Deutz, F. -J.: "Obstructed and unobstructed prostatic obstruction: A plea for urodynamic objectification of bladder overflow incontinence in benign prostatic hypertrophy," *World J. Urol.,* 6:198, 1989.
10. National Kidney and Urological Diseases Advisory Board, 1988, Annual Report.
11. Mebust, W. K., "Surgical management of benign prostatic obstruction," *Urol. (Suppl.),* 32(6):14, 1988.
12. Woolf, C. M., "An investigation of the familial aspects of carcinoma of the prostate," *Cancer,* 13:739, 1960.
13. Winklestein, W., Jr., and Ernster, V. L., "Epidemiology and Etiology," in

G. P. Murphy, ed., *Prostatic Cancer.* Littleton, Mass.: PSG Publishing Co., 1979, pp. 1–17.

14. Winklestein, W., Jr., and Kantor, S., "Prostatic cancer: Relationship to suspend particulate air pollution," *Am. J. Public Health,* 59:1134, 1969.
15. Gleason, D. F., "Veterans Administration Cooperative Urological Research Group, Histologic Grading in Clinical Staging of Prostatic Carcinoma," in M. Tannenbaum, ed., *Urologic Pathology: The Prostate.* Philadelphia: Lea & Febiger, 1977, p. 171.

Chapter 8: Confronting Bladder Cancer

1. *Cancer of the Bladder: Research Report,* National Institutes of Health Publication No. 87-722, May 1987.
2. L. Pickle, *Atlas of U. S. Cancer Mortality, 1950–1980.*
3. Seebode, J. J., and Najem, G. R.: "The role of environmental factors in bladder carcinoma," *Am. Urol. Ass. Update Series,* 3(21), 1984.
4. Soloway, M. S., Morrison, D. A., Shelton, T. B.: "Modalities used in the diagnosis, staging, and evaluation of bladder cancer," *Am. Urol. Ass. Update Series,* 4(5), 1985.
5. Wijkstrom, H., Gustafson, H., and Tribukait, B.: "Deoxyribonucleic acid analysis of the evaluation of transitional cell carcinoma before cystectomy," *J. Urol.,* 132:894, 1984.
6. Lantz, E. J., and Hattery, R. R., "Diagnostic imaging of urothelial cancer," *Urol. Clin. N. Am.,* 11:576, 1984.
7. DeKernion, J. B., Huang, M., Lindner, A., et al.: "Management of superficial bladder tumors and carcinoma-in-situ, with intravesical bacille calmette-Guérin (BCG)," *J. Urol.,* 133:598, 1985.
8. Lamm, D. L., Stogdill, V. D., and Stogdill, B. J.: "Complications of BCH immunotherapy in patients with bladder cancer," *Proc. Am. Urol. Assoc.,* 1984, p. 140A.
9. Koontz, W. W., Prout, G. R., Jr., Smith, W., et al.: "The use of intravesical Thiotepa in the management of non-invasive carcinoma of the bladder," *J. Urol.,* 125:307, 1981.
10. Soloway, M. S.: "Intravesical and systemic chemotherapy in the management of superficial bladder cancer," *Urol. Clin, N. Am.,* 11:623, 1984.
11. Lundbeck, F., Mogensen, P., and Jeppersen, N.: "Intravesical therapy of non-invasive bladder tumors with doxorubicin and urokinase," *J. Urol.,* 130:1087, 1983.
12. Prout, G. R., Jr.: "The surgical management of bladder carcinoma," *Urol. Clin. N. Am.,* 3:149, 1976.
13. Goffinet, D. R., Schneider, M. J., Glatstein, E. P., et al.: "Bladder cancer: Results of radiation therapy in 384 patients," *Radiology,* 117:149, 1975.
14. Studer, U. E., Biedermann, C., Chollet, D., et al.: "Prevention of recurrent superficial bladder tumors by oral Etretinate: Preliminary results of a randomized double-blind, multicenter trial in Switzerland," *J. Urol.,* 131:47, 1984.

Chapter 9: Staying Sexual

1. McCormick, N. B., and Vinson, R. K.: "Interstitial cystitis: How women cope," *Urol. Nursing,* 9(4):14, 1989.
2. Register, C.: *Living with Chronic Illness: Days of Patience and Passion.* New York: The Free Press/Macmillan, 1987.
3. King, R.: "Sexuality and Incontinence," in C. Gartley, ed., *Managing Incontinence.* Ottawa, IL: Jameson Books, 1985, pp. 100–107.
4. Masters, W. H., and Johnson, V. E.: *Human Sexual Response.* Boston: Little, Brown, 1966, p. 228.
5. Ladas, A. K., Whipple, B., and Perry, J. D.: *The G-Spot and Other Recent Discoveries in Female Sexuality.* New York: Holt, Rinehart & Winston, 1983, p. 56.

Chapter 10: Coping Strategies for Everyday Survival

1. Verhovek, S. H., "Albany goal: Giving women restroom 'parity' with men," *The New York Times,* June 13, 1989, p. B-4.
2. John Bouda, *The Non-Wovens Industry Magazine,* March 1989, pp. 46–54.
3. Jeter, K. J.: *The HIP Report,* 5(1), Winter 1987.

INDEX

329